METHODS IN
VITAMIN B-6 NUTRITION
Analysis and Status Assessment

METHODS IN VITAMIN B-6 NUTRITION

Analysis and Status Assessment

Edited by

James E. Leklem

Oregon State University
Corvallis, Oregon

and

Robert D. Reynolds

Beltsville Human Nutrition Research Center
U.S. Department of Agriculture
Beltsville, Maryland

PLENUM PRESS • NEW YORK AND LONDON

Library of Congress Cataloging in Publication Data

Workshop on Vitamin B-6 Analytical Methodology and Criteria for Assessing Nutritional Status, Timberline Lodge, Mount Hood, Or., 1980.
Methods in vitamin B-6 nutrition.

Proceedings of the workshop held June 29-July 2, 1980.
Includes index.
1. Vitamin B6 in human nutrition—Congresses. 2. Vitamin B6—Analysis—Congresses. I. Leklem, James E., 1941-   . II. Reynolds, Robert D., 1943-   . III. Title.
[DNLM: 1. Pyridoxine—Analysis—Congresses. W1 AD559 v. 136/QU 195 M592 1980]
QP772.P9W65 1980   612'.399   80-29553
ISBN 978-1-4684-9903-2   ISBN 978-1-4684-9901-8 (eBook)
DOI 10.1007/978-1-4684-9901-8

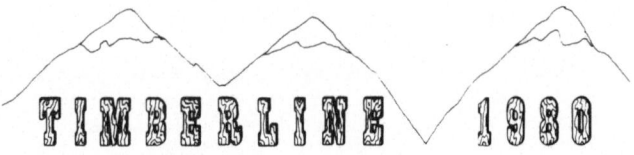

Proceedings of a workshop on Vitamin B-6 Analytical Methodology
and Criteria for Assessing Nutritional Status, held June 29–July 2, 1980,
at Timberline Lodge, Mt. Hood, Oregon

INTRODUCTION

During the period 29 June to 2 July 1980, a Workshop was held at Timberline Lodge, Mt. Hood, Oregon, entitled "Vitamin B-6 Analytical Methodology and Criteria for Assessing Nutritional Status". The papers which follow are the proceedings of that Workshop and represent the combined works of 36 scientists from across the United States and Canada. In addition to the 19 papers, there were seven short presentations which we consider to be at the very frontiers of analytical methods and status assessment for vitamin B-6. These reports discussed such areas as production of specific antibodies to the various vitamers, the synthesis of deuterated vitamers, comparisons of ultraviolet, fluorescence and elctrochemical determinations of the vitamers and the identification of polyamine-pyridoxal Schiff bases in urine. Those reports are not included in this book solely due to their highly tentative and preliminary findings, not because we considered them of any less importance than the papers presented herein. In fact, these reports may well provide the foundations upon which subsequent workshops are developed.

The feeling for the need of such a Workshop in part grew out of a previous workshop held at the Letterman Army Institute of Research, San Francisco, California, 11-12 June 1976. At that time, extensive discussions were held on the requirements of various populations for vitamin B-6, and an underlying feeling was present on how best to determine the nutritional status of individuals and populations in order to properly determine their requirements for vitamin B-6. In the intervening years, many advances were made in the analysis of the various vitamers. Without accurate and appropriate analysis of the desired compounds, it is impossible to determine nutritional status. Thus, we felt that the time was appropriate for these two areas to be brought together and addressed at a common workshop.

Based on discussions with leading scientists in the field of vitamin B-6 research, it was agreed that such a workshop would contribute a needed dimension in terms of nutrition research. The specific goals of the workshop were 1) to discuss and evaluate current and developing methods used to study vitamin B-6 nutrition, 2) similarly, to discuss and evaluate the criteria used for assessment, and 3) to arrive at a consensus in each of these two areas. As an added step in the evaluation process, two scientists working outside the area of vitamin B-6 provided critical analyses and evaluation of the papers and discussion. Bert Tolbert and Robert Stokstad blended their unique backgrounds and talents to provide a penetrating and stimulating discussion of both methodology and status assessment. To them we are deeply indebted and most thankful. The papers contained herein attest to the success of the workshop and the sharing of scientific knowledge.

For the convenience of workers in vitamin B-6 nutrition, the papers in the first section give extensive details on procedures used for the analysis of the various metabolites of interest. The completeness of detail of the nine different analytical procedures should allow this book to be used as a laboratory handbook as well as a source book for comparisons between different methodologies. The second section is an evaluation of how the various methods have been applied in order to determine vitamin B-6 status in different populations. The advantages and shortcomings of each assessment method are presented as a guide to subsequent workers in this field. Finally, the third section gives an evaluation and recommendations on the suggested methods for analysis and status assessment. The ideas presented in this section were derived from the numerous discussion sessions held during the Workshop in which all participants contributed. Thus, the authorship of these two papers could be considered to be the same as the list of participants at the Workshop. Although no point was agreed upon unaminously, each recommendation presented, in our opinion, is a fair representation of the consensus of the majority of the participants. We hope these recommendations are, in fact, accurate representations of the majority and that they will be of value to others in this field.

The Editors

ACKNOWLEDGMENTS

As with any conference, the success of the Timberline 1980 Workshop was the result of the efforts of many persons. Without the generous financial support of the following organizations, this Workshop could not have been held: the Fogarty International Center, the National Cancer Institute, and the National Institute of Arthritis, Metabolism and Digestive Diseases, National Institutes of Health; Human Nutrition, United States Department of Agriculture; the Nutrition Research Institute, Oregon State University; and Hoffman-LaRoche, Inc. The Program Advisory Committee, composed of Myron Brin, Avanelle Kirksey, Ting-Kai Li, and Howerde Sauberlich, provided invaluable advice in the selection of topics and speakers and in the format of the program. Barbara Foos generously donated her artistic talents in designing the artwork which provided the theme that was carried throughout the entire Workshop. Prior to and during the Workshop, the devoted staff of Shirley Cress, Lori Stolsig, and Sherril Knower provided the secretarial services so vital to any successful program. The entire staff at Timberline Lodge was gracious and helpful in every aspect both during the planning stages and during the actual Workshop. Hilda MacMichael deserves special gratitude for her expertise and patience during the editing and numerous typings of the manuscripts for the publication of this book. All the above receive our public appreciation.

One final word of appreciation must go to whatever forces controlled the rumblings and eruptions of Mt. Hood and Mt. St. Helens during the week of the Workshop. Although relatively quiet during that period, the uncertainty contributed to the air of excitement at the Workshop.

CONTENTS

METHODOLOGY OF VITAMIN B-6 ANALYSES

EVALUATION AND RECOMMENDATIONS

VITAMIN B-6 ANALYSIS: SOME HISTORICAL ASPECTS

Esmond E. Snell

Departments of Microbiology and Chemistry
The University of Texas
Austin, TX 78712

The discovery and purification of almost every vitamin or
other physiologically active substance has been achieved only as
methods which permit its detection have been devised. Even crude
methods may suffice to permit isolation of the active compound;
once the purified compound is available and its chemical nature is
known, it becomes possible to modify old methods or devise new ones
that provide enhanced convenience, specificity, and sensitivity.

The history of vitamin B-6 and methodology for its determination illustrates well this sequence of events.

DISCOVERY OF PYRIDOXINE BY ANIMAL ASSAY

As soon as thiamine (B-1) and riboflavin (B-2)--the first two
B-vitamins to be isolated--became available as pure compounds or
as reasonably pure concentrates, it rapidly became obvious to those
attempting to grow rats or chicks on purified diets that additional
trace compounds supplied by crude supplements were essential for
growth. Paul György in 1934 first used the term "vitamin B_6" (1)
to designate one such substance in crude feed supplements that cured
a florid dermatitis that developed in rats fed a purified diet
supplemented with vitamins B-1 and B-2. Such diets lacked many of
the B-vitamins now known to be required for rat growth; indeed,
crude fractions that supplied certain unidentified growth requirements (e.g. pantothenic acid) were quickly added to them. Rat
growth assays based on these incomplete diets nevertheless permitted
isolation of a crystalline vitamin in five different laboratories
during 1938 (Table 1), and this permitted, in turn, the characterization and synthesis of pyridoxine in 1939. As additional
substances required for animal growth were defined, these early

Table 1. Isolation of Pyridoxine (Rat Assay)

Authors	Date	Source	Reference
Lepkovsky	1938(Feb)	Rice bran	(2)
Keresztesy & Stevens	1938(Feb, May)	Rice bran	(3)
György	1938(April)	Yeast (Peter's eluate)	(4)
Kuhn & Wendt	1938(May)	Yeast	(5)
Ichiba & Michi	1938	Rice bran	(6)

diets were greatly improved and the stage was set for the accurate determination of vitamin B-6 by animal assay.

DISCOVERY OF PYRIDOXAL AND PYRIDOXAMINE BY MICROBIOLOGICAL ASSAY

We turn now to the origins of microbiological assays for this vitamin. Moeller (7) first recognized, very shortly after its isolation in 1938, that pyridoxine was required for growth of Bacterium acetylcholini, Lactobacillus plantarum, and several other lactic acid bacteria. During 1938-1941, Moeller (7), Schultz, et al. (8), and Eakin and Williams (9) identified pyridoxine as a growth factor for various yeasts, and Beadle and Tatum (10) pre-pared mutants of Neurospora that required this vitamin. The time seemed ripe for the use of certain of these organisms for the microbiological assay of pyridoxine by methods analogous to that introduced so successfully for riboflavin in 1939 by Snell and Strong (11).

Vitamin B-6, however, proved to be more complex. When the quantitative response of Lactobacillus casei or Streptococcus faecalis to pyridoxine was tested, we found (12) that the amount of the vitamin apparently required for growth was extraordinarily large when filter-sterilized pyridoxine was added to the medium, but was substantially decreased when pyridoxine was heat sterilized with the medium (Fig. 1). The growth effect for the yeast, Saccharomyces carlsbergensis, was unaffected by this treatment. Furthermore, natural materials were far more active in supporting growth of S. faecalis or of L. casei than their "pyridoxine" content, as indicated by assay with yeast, would predict (13) (Table 2). Substances possessing such enhanced activity were formed from pyridoxine by feeding this vitamin to deficient animals, and were excreted in the urine (13). Highly active substances also were formed from pyridoxine or its esters by ammonia treatment (14)

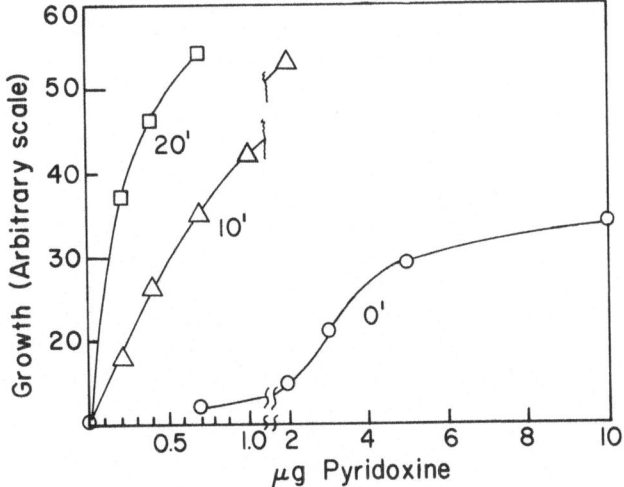

Fig. 1.   Effect of sterilizing (120°) pyridoxine with the growth
medium for 0, 10, or 20 minutes on its growth-promoting
activity for Streptococcus faecalis. Modified from (12).

Table 2.   The "Pyridoxine" Content of Natural Products
Assayed With Two Organisms Against a Pyridoxine
Standard. Modified from Reference (13).

Material	S. cerevisiae GM	S. faecalis
	"Pyridoxine equivalents", µg/g	
Yeast extract	16	16,800
Rat tissues		
Brain (PN-def)[a]	0.33	900
Brain (" + PN)[b]	3.1	8,800
Liver (PN-def)	0.27	540
Liver (" + PN)	0.84	5,600
Rat urine (24 hr.)		
PN-deficient	0.07	96
" + PN	4.2	2,480

[a]21-day old animals were fed a vitamin B-6-free diet
for 35 days.
[b]Diet supplemented with 3 µg of pyridoxine/g.

or by mild oxidation (14,15). These findings pointed unmistakably
to an aldehyde and an amine derived chemically from pyridoxine
(Fig. 2) as the active compounds and led directly in a collaborative project to the synthesis of pyridoxal and pyridoxamine (16,17).

These three forms of vitamin B-6 showed approximately equal
activities in promoting growth of yeast, Neurospora, and higher
animals (Table 3). However, for lactic acid bacteria and
Tetrahymena, pyridoxal, pyridoxamine or both were far more effective than pyridoxine in promoting growth. Indeed, we concluded
that pyridoxine per se has no growth-promoting activity for lactic
acid bacteria; its slight apparent activity at high concentrations
results from non-enzymatic formation of traces of pyridoxal or
pyridoxamine in the growth media.

To determine whether pyridoxal and pyridoxamine occurred
naturally, we chose S. carlsbergensis to measure total vitamin B-6
(PN + PM + PL), S. faecalis to determine pyridoxal plus pyridoxamine, and L. casei to measure pyridoxal only. When the most
active form of vitamin B-6 was used as the standard for each
organism, values were obtained (Table 4) consistent with the view
that natural materials contain all three forms of vitamin B-6.
In addition, the active material for L. casei was destroyed by
agents that destroy pyridoxal, a fraction of the total activity
(i.e., pyridoxamine, but not pyridoxal or pyridoxine) was destroyed
by nitrous acid, etc. Pyridoxal and pyridoxamine were shown in
this way to occur naturally, and vitamin B-6 to be a complex of the

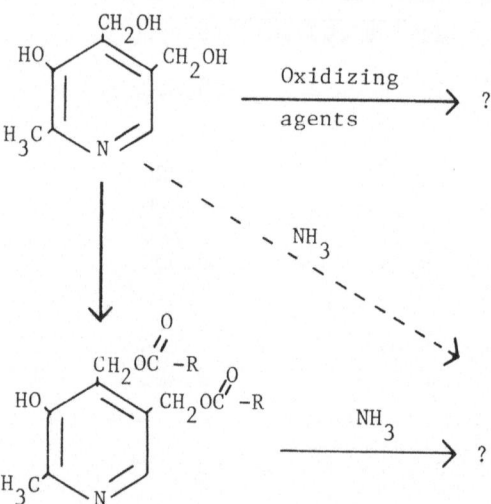

Oxidizing
agents

→ ?

Destroyed by carbonyl reagents
(HCN, Acetone + NaOH)

Forms phenylhydrazone

Undamaged by HONO

i.e. an aldehyde (pyridoxal)

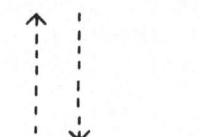

NH_3

→ ?

NH_3 specific for formation

Destroyed by HNO_2

Undamaged by carbonyl reagents

i.e. an amine (pyridoxamine)

Fig. 2. Production of compounds with high activity for lactic
         acid bacteria by various chemical treatments of
         pyridoxine. Abstracted from (14).

Table 3. Comparative Growth-Promoting Activities of Pyridoxine (PN),
          Pyridoxal (PL) and Pyridoxamine (PM) for Various Organisms

Organism	Activity % of Most Active Form			
	PN	PL	PM	Reference
Bacteria				
Lactobacillus casei	(0.085)[a]	100	(0.70)	18
Streptococcus faecalis R	(0.015)	69	100	18
Clostridium welchii	(0.08)	35	100	19
Yeasts				
Saccharomyces carlsbergensis	86	100	94	18
Saccharomyces cerevisiae GM	100	33-98	13-52	18
Fungi				
Neurospora sitophila 299	88	100	100	18
Protozoa				
Tetrahymena geleii	(0.16)	100	100	20
Higher animals				
Chicks (inject)	100	100	100	21[b]
" (diet)	100	50	80	21,22[c]
Dogs (inject)	100	100	100	23
Rats (inject)	100	100	100	18,21[b]
" (diet)	100	50	65	21,22[c]
Mice (inject)	100	100	100	22

[a]Parentheses indicate uncertainty whether pyridoxine per se has any
activity: see text.
[b]In these comparisons, the vitamin supplements were given intraperitoneally or by dropper.
[c]In these comparisons the supplements were mixed into the diet.

Table 4. Pyridoxal, Pyridoxamine and Pyridoxine Content of Yeast Extract Before and After Various Treatments. Adapted from (24).

Sample	L. casei (pyridoxal std)	S. faecalis (pyridoxamine std)	S. carlsbergensis (pyridoxine std)
		μg per g	
Yeast extract	1.0	11.7	13.0
" + HNO$_2$	1.3	0.4	5.5
Pyridoxamine	7.0 x 10^3	1000 x 10^3	1100 x 10^3
" + HNO$_2$	3.0 x 10^3	1.1 x 10^3	470 x 10^3
Yeast extract	1.0	11.7	13.0
" + NaCN + NH$_4$Cl	0.01	11.0	11.6
Pyridoxal	1000 x 10^3	1000 x 10^3	1000 x 10^3
" + NaCN + NH$_4$Cl	2 x 10^3	1 x 10^3	2 x 10^3

three compounds. The amounts of each of these compounds present was increased by acid hydrolysis, indicating that each occurred partly in "bound" forms.

This differential assay for vitamin B-6 revealed that pyridoxamine and pyridoxal are the predominant forms of vitamin B-6 in metabolically active tissues (Table 5), while pyridoxine was most abundant in cereal grains and extracts of higher plants (25).

An interesting discrepancy exists between data in Tables 4 and 5, which show that yeast contains essentially no pyridoxine, and Table 1, which indicates that both Gyorgy and Kuhn isolated pyridoxine from yeast. Documentation requirements were apparently rather lax in 1938: Gyorgy's report specifies doses of the purified material required to cure acrodynia in rats, but contains no analysis, melting point, or other data to establish the identity of the isolated product. Kuhn's report, on the other hand, gives analyses that correspond exactly to pyridoxine. I was brash enough some 30 years ago to ask Professor Kuhn how he managed to isolate pyridoxine from a source material that contained none. He smilingly attributed this to the use of nitric acid at various points in the isolation procedure--a point not made in his described procedure. Nitric acid contains some nitrous acid, and in the presence of reducing materials, more would be formed. Kuhn thought that sufficient nitrous acid was present to convert pyridoxamine to pyridoxine. Isolations from rice bran do not present this anomaly; pyridoxine is by far the most common form of vitamin B-6 in this material (Table 5).

Table 5. Distribution of Various Forms of Vitamin B-6 as Determined by Differential Microbiological Assay. Adapted from (25).

Sample	Pyridoxal	Pyridoxamine	Pyridoxine
		µg per g	
Rat liver	29	9	9 (+5)
Rat heart	16	9	1 ($\overline{+}$3)
Rat brain	9.2	4	4 ($\overline{+}$2)
Rat kidney	33	13	10 ($\overline{+}$6)
Beef liver	7	31	-3 ($\overline{+}$4)
Yeast, brewers	4.9	36	-1 ($\overline{+}$4)
Egg, whole	5.6	1.2	0 ($\overline{+}$0.9)
Carrot	2.1	0.3	7 ($\overline{1}$1)
Whole wheat	1.9	3.7	9 ($\overline{+}$2)
Rice bran extract	1.9	10	79 ($\underline{\overline{+}}$11)

DISCOVERY OF PYRIDOXAL PHOSPHATE BY ENZYMATIC ASSAY

We turn now to identification of combined forms of vitamin B-6. Both Gyorgy (26) and Kuhn and Wendt (5) recognized that vitamin B-6 occurred naturally in combined form; indeed, the first step in purification of the vitamin by the latter workers was a prolonged dialysis of yeast juice, during which the vitamin remained in the non-dialyzable fraction. They postulated that the vitamin was part of some unidentified enzyme present in yeast. Uzawa in 1942 (27) described an unidentified coenzyme required for the action of tryptophananse from E. coli while Gale and his coworkers (28), beginning about 1940, described a series of bacterial amino acid decarboxylases, some of which also required an uniden- tified, heat stable coenzyme. Gunsalus and coworkers then showed that S. faecalis grown in media low in vitamin B-6 contained almost no tyrosine decarboxylase activity, but that this activity appeared when washed cells were incubated with pyridoxal or when dried cells were incubated with pyridoxal plus ATP (29). These findings indicated that the coenzyme was a phosphorylated pyridoxal, and by phosphorylation of pyridoxal with $SOCl_2$ and silver phosphate a phosphorylated derivative was prepared with coenzymatic activity (29). Shortly thereafter, Wood et al. (30) showed that pyridoxal phosphate also was the coenzyme for tryptophanase. Initially, it was uncertain in which position the pyridoxal was phosphorylated, but the phosphate moiety was eventually shown to be present at the 5' position; i.e. the coenzyme was pyridoxal 5'-phosphate (31).

Comparative microbiological assays with S. faecalis and S. carlsbergensis led Rabinowitz and Snell (32) to the discovery of pyridoxamine 5'-phosphate and the conclusion that it comprises much of the combined vitamin in yeast extract. Today we know, of course, that both PLP and PMP are essential coenzymatic forms in transamination reactions, and the fact that both are generally distributed in tissues is no longer surprising. Certain lactic acid bacteria lack pyridoxal kinase and are auxotrophic for PMP or PLP (33). Finally, as first shown by Wada et al., pyridoxine 5'-phosphate also occurs naturally (34); it accumulates in a mutant of E. coli auxotrophic for pyridoxal, indicating that it lies before pyridoxal in the biosynthetic sequence leading to these compounds (35).

From this rather extended historical account of the discovery of the six major forms of vitamin B-6, it should be apparent that many of the currently used methods for vitamin B-6 analysis, i.e., assay with higher animals, with microorganisms, or with enzymes, are direct outgrowths of methods used for discovery of the vitamin itself and its coenzyme forms. Now that all of the vitamins and other requirements for animal and microbial growth are known and available in pure form, it is a simple matter to construct basal diets or basal media that specifically lack vitamin B-6, but are

complete in other respects. Since they supply growth essentials
other than vitamin B-6 which might otherwise be supplied in part by
samples to be assayed, such diets or media should yield assay
results of improved precision, and it seems unnecessary to dwell
on such modified procedures here. An account of the development
of vitamin assay methods through about 1950, including those for
vitamin B-6, has been published (36). Rather, I shall consider
some of the advantages of the various methodologies, and some of
the problems they have in common.

ANIMAL ASSAYS--ADVANTAGES AND DISADVANTAGES

Assay with rats or chicks has one major advantage over all
other methods of vitamin B-6 assay: the sample can be fed directly
and the problems associated with other methods--complete extraction
without destruction, conversion to a form or forms showing equal
response in the assay procedure, etc.--can be left to the enzymatic
machinery of the animal. It is not that the animal necessarily
solves these problems completely (we have seen, for example, that
pyridoxamine and pyridoxal may be less active than pyridoxine when
fed in some diets), but rather that experimental animals are likely
to solve it in approximately the same way as farm animals and man.
If the ultimate use for analytical figures is for guidance in the
construction of adequate animal diets, then animal assay seems a
preferable procedure.

Why then are such assays so little used? The answers are
obvious. Accurate assay requires large numbers of animals and a
time period measured usually in weeks. The methods are therefore
very slow and very expensive. Furthermore, analytical results are
useful in a far wider context than construction of diets, and for
some of these uses rapid procedures are needed that are applicable
to much smaller samples than those required for animal assay, or
that determine one or another single form of the vitamin. Microbiological, enzymatic and chemical or physical methods provide
these advantages; they share, however, the problem of extracting
the vitamin quantitatively from the sample.

EXTRACTION OF VITAMIN B-6 AND ITS COMPLICATIONS

It is useful to review the chemical nature of the various
forms of vitamin B-6 that occur in tissue samples, and to consider
what may happen to them during processing, storage and extraction.
The six forms usually encountered are shown in Fig. 3. In addition,
conjugates of vitamin B-6 of unknown structure were reported to
occur in rice bran extract (37), urine (38), and perhaps other
materials. These reports have not been reevaluated since the
discovery of multiple forms of vitamin B-6, hence the current
status of such conjugates is not clear. The three phosphorylated
compounds, PLP, PMP, and PNP, comprise most of the vitamin B-6 in

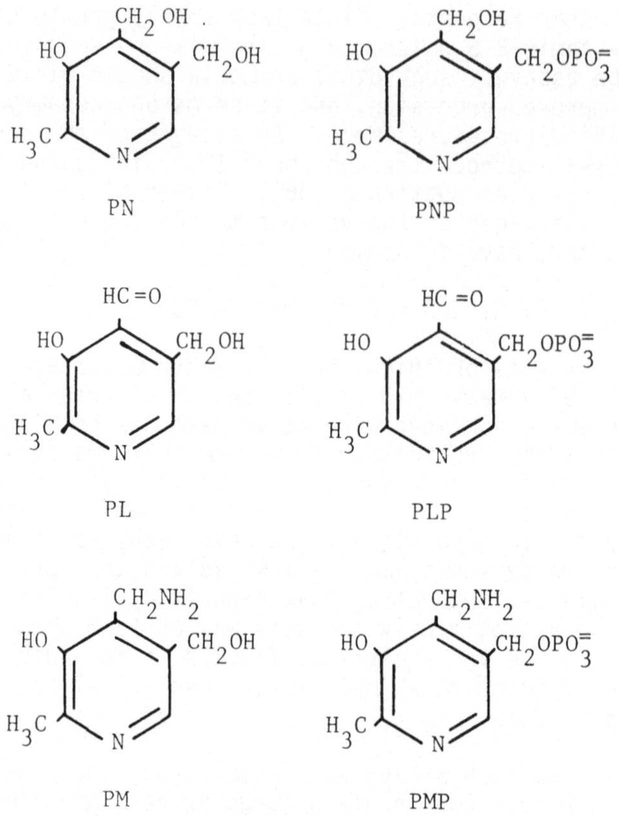

Fig. 3. Structures of the major naturally-occurring compounds
with vitamin B-6 activity.

tissues. PL, PM, and PN arise from them by phosphatase action--
intestinal alkaline phosphatase in an effective catalyst—or by
acid hydrolysis, but not by alkaline hydrolysis. Rubin and
Scheiner first showed that the pH optimum for hydrolysis of PLP
and PMP lies between 1.5 and 2.0 (39); as a consequence, low
concentrations of acid (e.g. 0.055N H_2SO_4) bring about more rapid
hydrolysis of these compounds, and more rapid liberation of
vitamin B-6 from some tissues than do higher acid concentrations,
provided always that the acid is added in amounts that exceed the
buffer capacity of the sample (39,40). However, extraction with
0.055N acid is not as effective for some materials as higher acid
concentrations (39), a fact that may reflect the occurrence of
still unidentified conjugates of the vitamin in such samples.

Dilute solutions of PM and PN are stable in hot dilute mineral acids or alkalis; pyridoxal also is stable in acid, but is slowly destroyed in hot alkali, where its aldehydic nature indicates that air oxidation to 4-pyridoxic acid, anaerobic dismutation to a mixture of 4-pyridoxic acid and pyridoxine, and self-condensation reactions are to be expected. All three compounds (and presumably their 5'-phosphates) are destroyed by light (41); extractions should therefore be conducted in subdued or red light.

Although the pure compounds are stable, one should not assume stability in the presence of an excess of other materials supplied by tissues and tissue extracts. We have seen that traces of pyridoxal and pyridoxamine are readily formed by heating pyridoxine in bacteriological media. PM and PL (and also their phosphates) are readily interconverted by nonenzymatic transamination (Equation 1 (42)), a reaction that may explain the high pyridoxamine

1. α-Amino acid + PL $\rightleftharpoons$ α-Ketoacid + PM

content of dried yeast and yeast extract.

The reaction in equation 1 results in a transformation in the form of vitamin B-6, but no loss in amount. Several reactions are known, however, that can lead to destruction of pyridoxal (or pyridoxal phosphate). These include reaction with histidine to form compound I (43) (Fig. 4), an analogous reaction with tryptophan (42) to form compound II (presumed structure, Rabinowitz and Snell, unpublished), reaction with glycine to form compound III (44) and reaction with cysteine to form compound IV (45). The latter compound is formed under some conditions during heat processing of milk products (44); although active in place of vitamin B-6 for Neurospora sitophila, it is essentially inactive in experimental animals and man.

All of these reactions proceed as a consequence of the pre-liminary interaction between PL or PLP and an amino acid to form the Schiff's base, V, as depicted in Fig. 5. With most α-amino acids, V equilibrates with VI and leads by partial reaction a through e to reversible, nonenzymatic transamination reactions (Equation 1). Under appropriate conditions with amino acids of suitable structure, e.g. histidine (→I), tryptophan (→II), cysteine (→thiazolidine →IV), glycine (→III), other elements of the same or another amino acid residue can add to V to yield the products indicated. But under mild conditions in aqueous solutions at physiological pH values, the Schiff's base V (or VI in solutions of PM and α-ketoacids) itself may be stable. Thus, if pyridoxal is mixed with a hydrolyzed casein solution and chromatographed, pyridoxal will be found in many different locations as a result of V formation; only under acid conditions, where Schiff's bases are largely hydrolyzed, is a single zone due to pyridoxal found. PN

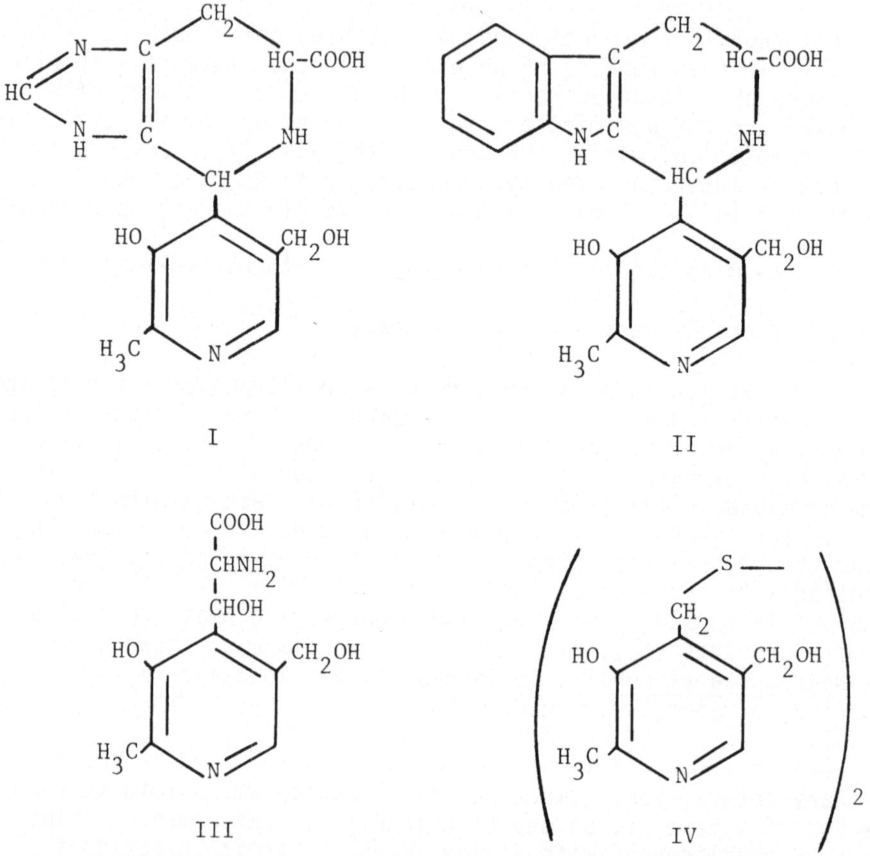

Fig. 4. Structures of reaction products between pyridoxal and
(I) histidine, (II) tryptophan, (III) glycine, and
(IV) cysteine.

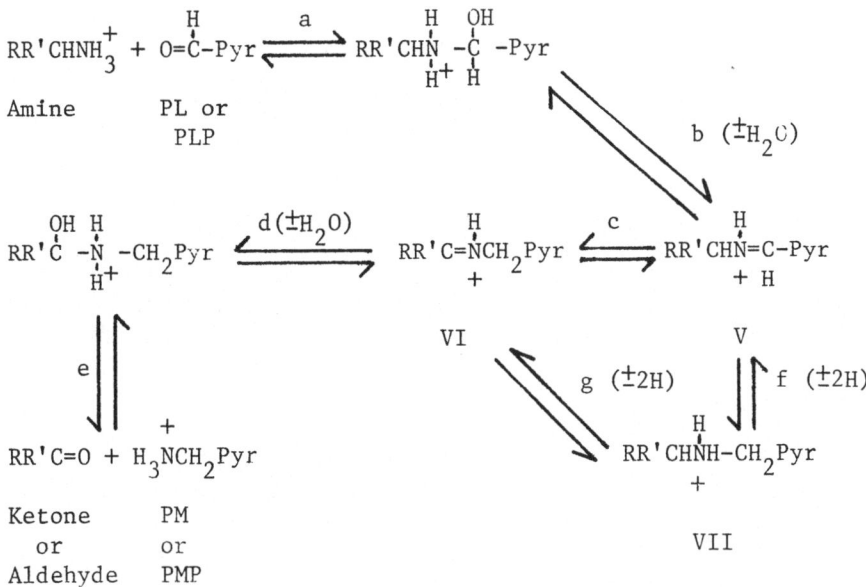

Fig. 5. Formation of Schiff's bases between pyridoxal and amino
         acids (V) or pyridoxamine and keto acids (VI) and their
         interconversion.

and PM, under these conditions, migrate as single, discrete zones.
One of the non-standard forms of vitamin B-6 in urine appears to
be a similar adduct formed from pyridoxal and urea with loss of
water (46).

    PLP in enzyme proteins so far studied is invariably combined
with the protein through formation of a Schiff's base (V, Fig. 5)
with an ε-amino group of a specific lysine residue, as first
recognized by Fischer (47) in phosphorylase. This is the only
covalent link so far established between vitamin B-6 and protein
in any native protein (additional non-covalent forces--ionic links
and hydrophobic attractions--also operate), and it is labile to
acid. Several authors have recently described difficulties in
recovering PLP from tissue samples and ascribe this difficulty to
its "combination" in an undefined manner with protein. Although
I can readily believe in the difficulties experienced, I think the
explanation needs further documentation. Gregory (48), however,
has provided evidence that peptide-linked ε-pyridoxyllysine (VII,
Fig. 5, where R' = H and R = -CH₂CH₂CH₂CHNH₂COOH) is formed as a
"degradation" product of vitamin B-6 during storage of certain
foods. This product is readily formed by reduction of PLP-
containing proteins (reaction f, Fig. 5). Many pyridoxylamines
and pyridoxylamino acids of the same chemical nature have been

synthesized (49) and their properties studied. If air oxidation,
which leads to PM or PL via reactions f and g of Fig. 5, is
avoided, they are generally inactive for bacteria auxotrophic for
vitamin B-6 (50), but are partially or completely active in
supporting growth of Neurospora (50) or rats (49,51), in which
amine oxidases permit regeneration of PM or PL.

There is little doubt that some of the difficulties in vitamin
B-6 analysis stem from formation of one or several of the adducts
of the vitamin with amino acids discussed here. A systematic
study of the conditions that lead to their formation would provide
the basic information necessary for avoiding this source of assay
errors.

THE ASSAY METHODS

I have emphasized the need for detailed investigation of
extraction procedures because these seem to me to be the weakest
point in current methodology. If quantitative extraction of
vitamin B-6 from tissues could be achieved without appreciable
change in the distribution of vitamin forms, then any of several
assay procedures could be selected without difficulty to meet the
investigators' research objectives. With purified diets now available any experimental animal will provide reliable assays marred
only by differences in relative activities of PN, PM, and PL when
mixed in the diet. Even this factor can be minimized or eliminated
in rats by adding suitable antibiotics to the ration (52).

Similarly, a great many microorganisms with fully defined
nutritional requirements are now known that are auxotrophic for
vitamin B-6, and differences in their growth response to individual
vitamin forms permit a choice of an appropriate assay organism,
again depending upon the research objectives.

A few enzymatic methods that permit the specific estimation of
pyridoxal phosphate or of PLP plus PMP (53) are listed in Table 6.
However, over 50 enzymes that require PLP as coenzyme are now known;
any one of them could be employed for PLP (or, with the transaminases,
PLP plus PMP) estimation. One hopes that in the future, we will not
have to deal with the special peculiarities of such large numbers
of similar methods! The choice between such methods will ultimately
depend on the availability, cost, and stability of the apoenzyme
required, and upon the ease and sensitivity of the end measurements.
Future developments, through use of coupled systems (e.g. pyridoxal
kinase plus PNP (PMP) oxidase) could permit the estimation of all
forms of vitamin B-6 as PLP.

Table 6.   Some Enzymatic Methods for Estimation of Coenzymatic
Forms of Vitamin B-6[a]

Methods that Determine Only PLP
    Tryptophanase

$$\text{Trp} + H_2O \xrightarrow{\text{ApoE (+PLP)}} \underline{\text{Indole}} + \underline{\text{Pyruvate}} + NH_3$$

$$\text{S-}\underline{o}\text{-Nitrophenylcysteine} \xrightarrow{\text{ApoE (+PLP)}}$$

$$\underline{\text{o-Nitrothiophenol}} + \text{Pyruvate} + NH_3$$

Tyrosine Decarboxylase

$$\text{Tyr} \xrightarrow{\text{ApoE (+PLP)}} \text{Tyramine} + \underline{CO_2}$$

D-Serine Dehydratase

$$\text{D-Ser} \xrightarrow{\text{ApoE (+PLP)}} \text{Pyruvate} + NH_3$$

γ-Cyanoaminobutyric Acid Synthase

$$NC\text{-}S\text{-}CH_2CH_2CHNH_2COOH + CN^- \xrightarrow{\text{ApoE (+PLP)}}$$

$$\underline{CNS^-} + N\equiv CCH_2CH_2CHNH_2COOH$$

Methods that Determine PLP + PMP
    Glutamate-oxaloacetate transaminase

$$\text{Asp} + \alpha\text{-K.G.} \xrightleftharpoons{\text{ApoE (+PLP or PMP)}} \underline{\text{Glu}} + \underline{\text{Oxaloacetate}}$$

---

[a]The product most commonly determined is underlined.

I have not yet considered chemical methods for vitamin B-6.
Chemical methods depending upon the phenolic nature of pyridoxine
and utilizing the color developed when either 2,6-dichloroquinone
chlorimide (54) or diazo reagents (55) couple at the unsubstituted
p-position of pyridoxine achieved early prominence. They appear
not to have survived the complexity introduced by recognition of
multiple forms of the vitamin, but are still of value for control
purposes in certain areas.

I have reserved mention of one of the most promising procedures, based upon separation of individual forms of vitamin B-6 by absorption methods, for the last. Toepfer and his colleagues (57) first used chromatographic separation on Dowex columns for the quantitative separation on PN, PL and PM prior to their estimation by other procedures. A number of investigators have developed these methods more fully, and used them together with isotopically labelled pyridoxine for investigating the time course of metabolism of vitamin B-6 in animals (e.g. 57,58). Current advances in high performance liquid chromatography now permit separation of all six major forms of the vitamin on a single column (e.g. 59). Used in conjunction with a suitable system for detection and quantification of the individual vitamin forms, such systems are of great analytical promise. Provided the extraction problem can be satisfactorily solved, these procedures should give us analytical tools of unprecedented precision and sensitivity for future investigations of vitamin B-6 distribution and metabolism.

LITERATURE CITED

1. György, P. (1934) Vitamin B-2 and the pellagra-like dermatitis of rats. Nature 133, 448-449.
2. Lepkovsky, S. (1938) Crystalline factor I. Science 87, 169-170.
3. Keresztesy, J. C. & Stevens, J. R. (1938) Vitamin B-6. Proc. Soc. Exp. Biol. Med. 38, 64-65; J. Am. Chem. Soc. 60, 1267-1268.
4. György, P. (1938) Crystalline vitamin B-6. J. Am. Chem. Soc. 60, 983-984.
5. Kuhn, R. & Wendt, G. (1938) Über das antidermatitische Vitamin der Hefe. Ber. Deut. Chem. Ges. 71B, 780-782.
6. Ichiba, A. & Michi, K. (1938) Isolation of vitamin B-6. Sci. Papers Inst. Phys. Chem. Res. (Tokyo) 34, 623-626.
7. Moeller, E. F. (1938) Vitamin B-6 (Adermin) als Wuchsstoff für Milchsäurebakterien. Z. Physiol. Chem. 254, 285-286.
8. Schulz, A., Atkin, L. & Frey, C. N. (1939) Vitamin B-6, a growth promoting factor for yeast. J. Am. Chem. Soc. 61, 1931.
9. Eakin, R. E. & Williams, R. J. (1939) Vitamin B-6 as a yeast nutrilite. J. Am. Chem. Soc. 61, 1932.
10. Beadle, G. W. & Tatum, E. L. (1941) Genetic control of biochemical reactions in Neurospora. Proc. Natl. Acad. Sci. U.S. 27, 499-506.
11. Snell, E. E. & Strong, F. M. (1939) A microbiological assay for riboflavin. Ind. Eng. Chem., Anal. Ed. 11, 346-351.
12. Snell, E. E. (1942) Effect of heat sterilization on growth-promoting activity of pyridoxine for Streptococcus faecalis R. Proc. Soc. Exp. Biol. Med. 51, 356-358.

13. Snell, E. E., Guirard, B. M. & Williams, R. J. (1942)
     Occurrence in natural products of a physiologically active
     metabolite of pyridoxine. J. Biol. Chem. 143, 519-530.
14. Snell, E. E. (1944) The vitamin B-6 group. I. Formation
     of additional members from pyridoxine and evidence concerning
     their structure. J. Am. Chem. Soc. 66, 2082-2088.
15. Carpenter, L. E. & Strong, F. M. (1944) Determination of
     pyridoxine and pseudopyridoxine. Arch. Biochem. 3, 375-388.
16. Snell, E. E. (1944) The vitamin activities of pyridoxal and
     pyridoxamine. J. Biol. Chem. 154, 313-314.
17. Harris, S. A., Heyl, D. & Folkers, D. (1944) The structure
     and synthesis of pyridoxamine and pyridoxal. J. Biol. Chem.
     154, 315-316; J. Am. Chem. Soc. 66, 2089-2092.
18. Snell, E. E. & Rannefeld, A. N. (1945) The vitamin B-6
     group. III. The vitamin activity of pyridoxal and pyri-
     doxamine for various organisms. J. Biol. Chem. 157, 475-489.
19. Boyd, M. J., Logan, M. A. & Tytell, A. A. (1948) The growth
     requirements of Clostridium perfringens (welchii) BP6K. J.
     Biol. Chem. 174, 1013-1025.
20. Kidder, G. W. & Dewey, V. C. (1949) Studies on the bio-
     chemistry of Tetrahymena. XII. Pyridoxine, pyridoxal and
     pyridoxamine. Arch. Biochem. 21, 58-65.
21. Sarma, P. S., Snell, E. E. & Elvehjem, C. A. (1946) The
     vitamin B-6 group. VIII. Biological assay of pyridoxal,
     pyridoxamine, and pyridoxine. J. Biol. Chem. 165, 55-63.
22. Luckey, T. D., Briggs, G. M., Elvehjem, C. A. & Hart, E. B.
     (1945) Activity of pyridoxine derivatives in chick nutrition.
     Proc. Soc. Exptl. Biol. Med. 58, 340-344.
23. Sarma, P. S., Snell, E. E. & Elvehjem, C. A. (1946) The
     vitamin B-6 group. IX. Comparative growth and antianemic
     potencies of pyridoxal, pyridoxamine and pyridoxine for dogs.
     Proc. Soc. Exptl. Biol. Med. 63, 284-286.
24. Snell, E. E. (1945) The vitamin B-6 group. IV. Evidence
     for the occurrence of pyridoxamine and pyridoxal in natural
     products. J. Biol. Chem. 157, 491-505.
25. Rabinowitz, J. C. & Snell, E. E. (1948) The vitamin B-6
     group. XIV. Distribution of pyridoxal, pyridoxamine, and
     pyridoxine in some natural products. J. Biol. Chem. 176,
     1157-1167.
26. Gyorgy, P. (1964) The history of vitamin B-6. Introductory
     remarks. Vitam. Horm. 22, 361-365.
27. Uzawa, S. (1943) Formation of indole from L-tryptophan (VII).
     Separation of apo- and co-tryptophanase. J. Osaka Med. Assoc.
     42, 1637.
28. Gale, E. F. (1946) The bacterial amino acid decarboxylases.
     Advan. Enzymol. 6, 1-32.

29. Gunsalus, I. C., Bellamy, W. D. & Umbreit, W. W. (1944) A
     phosphorylated derivative of pyridoxal as coenzyme of tyrosine
     decarboxylase   J. Biol. Chem. 155, 685-686.
30. Wood, W. A., Gunsalus, I. C. & Umbreit, W. W. (1947) Function
     of pyridoxal phosphate. Resolution and purification of the
     tryptophanase enzyme of Escherichia coli. J. Biol. Chem.
     170, 313-321.
31. Heyl, D., Luz, E., Harris, S. A. & Folkers, K. (1951)
     Phosphates of the vitamin B-6 group. I. The structure of
     codecarboxylase. J. Am. Chem. Soc. 73, 3430-3433.
32. Rabinowitz, J. C. & Snell, E. E. (1947) The vitamin B-6
     group. XII. Microbiological activity and natural occurrence
     of pyridoxamine phosphate. J. Biol. Chem. 169, 643-650.
33. McNutt, W. S. & Snell, E. E. (1948) Phosphates of pyridoxal
     and pyridoxamine as growth factors for lactic acid bacteria.
     J. Biol. Chem. 173, 801-802.
34. Wada, H., Morisue, T., Nishimura, Y., Morino, W., Sakamota, Y.
     & Ichihara, K. (1959) Enzymatic studies on pyridoxine
     metabolism. Proc. Japan Acad. 35, 299-304.
35. Dempsey, W. B. (1966) Synthesis of pyridoxine by a pyridoxal
     auxotroph of Escherichia coli. J. Bacteriol. 92, 333-337.
36. György, P., ed. (1950) Vitamin Methods, vol. I (571 pp.)
     and vol. II (740 pp.). Academic press, N.Y.
37. Scudi, J. V. (1942) Conjugated pyridoxine in rice bran
     concentrates. J. Biol. Chem. 145, 637-639.
38. Scudi, J. V., Buhs, R. P. & Hood, D. B. (1942) The metab-
     olism of vitamin B-6. J. Biol. Chem. 142, 323-328.
39. Rubin, S. H. & Scheiner, J. (1946) The availability of
     vitamin B-6 in yeast to Saccharomyces carlsbergensis. J.
     Biol. Chem. 162, 389-390.
40. Rabinowitz, J. C. & Snell, E. E. (1947) The vitamin B-6
     group. Extraction procedures for the microbiological
     determination of vitamin B-6. Ind. Eng. Chem., Anal. Ed.
     19, 277-280.
41. Cunningham, E. & Snell, E. E. (1945) The vitamin B-6 group.
     VI. The comparative stability of pyridoxine, pyridoxamine,
     and pyridoxal. J. Biol. Chem. 158, 491-495.
42. Snell, E. E. (1945) The vitamin B-6 group. V. The
     reversible interconversion of pyridoxal and pyridoxamine by
     transamination reactions. J. Am. Chem. Soc. 67, 194-197.
43. Heyl, D., Harris, S. A. & Folkers, K. (1948) The chemistry
     of vitamin B-6. VI. Pyridoxylamino acids. J. Am. Chem.
     Soc. 70, 3429-3431.
44. Metzler, D. E., Longenecker, J. B. & Snell, E. E. (1954)
     The reversible catalytic cleavage of hydroxyamino acids by
     pyridoxal and metal salts. J. Am. Chem. Soc. 76, 639-644.

45. Wendt, G. & Bernhart, F. W. (1960) The structure of a sulfur-containing compound with vitamin B-6 activity. Arch. Biochem. Biophys. 88, 270-272.

46. Barnett, G. E. & Pearson, W. N. (1969) Isolation and identification of a new urinary metabolite of ^{14}C-pyridoxine in the rat. Fed. Proc. 28, 559 (Abst. 1669).

47. Fischer, E. H., Kent, A. B., Snyder, E. R. & Krebs, E. G. (1958) The reaction of sodium borohydride with muscle phosphorylase. J. Am. Chem. Soc. 80, 2906-2907.

48. Gregory, J. F. & Kirk, J. R. (1978) Assessment of storage effects on vitamin B-6 stability and bioavailability in dehydrated food systems. J. Food Science 43, 1801-1808.

49. Heyl, D., Harris, S. A. & Folkers, K. (1952) Chemistry of vitamin B-6. VIII. Additional pyridoxylideneamines and pyridoxylamines. J. Am. Chem. Soc. 74, 414-416.

50. Snell, E. E. & Rabinowitz, J. C. (1948) The microbiological activity of pyridoxylamino acid. J. Am. Chem. Soc. 70, 3432-3434; Rabinowitz, J. C. & Snell, E. E. (1953) The microbiological activity of pyridoxylamines. J. Am. Chem. Soc. 75, 998.

51. Gregory, J. F. & Kirk, J. R. (1978) Vitamin B-6 activity for rats of ε-pyridoxyllysine bound to dietary protein. J. Nutr. 108, 1192-1199.

52. Linkswiler, H., Baumann, C. A. & Snell, E. E. (1951) Effect of aureomycin on the response of rats to various forms of vitamin B-6. J. Nutr. 43, 565-573.

53. Schreiber, G., Eckstein, M., Oeser, A. & Holzer, H. (1964) Zur Bestimmung von Pyridoxal-5-phosphorsaureester mit Apoaspartatamino-transferase aus Bierhefe. Biochem. Zeit. 340, 35-40.

54. Scudi, J. V. (1941) On the colorimetric determination of vitamin B-6. J. Biol. Chem. 139, 707-720.

55. Ormsby, A. A., Fisher, A. & Schlenk, F. (1947) Note on the colorimetric determination of pyridoxine, pyridoxal and pyridoxamine. Arch. Biochem. 12, 79-81.

56. Toepfer, E. W. & Lehmann, J. (1961) Procedure for chromatographic separation and microbiological assay of pyridoxine, pyridoxal, and pyridoxamine in food extracts. J. Assoc. Off. Agric. Chem. 44, 426-430.

57. Contractor, S. F. & Shane, B. (1971) Metabolism of (^{14}C)pyridoxol in the pregnant rat. Biochim. Biophys. Acta 230, 127-136.

58. Dahlquist, G., Lindstedt, S. & Tiselius, H.-G. (1969) Studies on the distribution and elimination of (^{3}H$_8$)pyridoxine in mice. Acta Physiol. Scand. 75, 427-432.

59. Vanderslice, J. T., Stewart, K. K. & Varmas, M. M. (1979) Liquid chromatographic separation and quantitation of B-6 vitamers and their metabolite, pyridoxic acid. J. Chromatogr. 176, 280-285.

MICROBIOLOGICAL ASSAY OF VITAMIN B-6 IN FOODS

Marilyn Polansky

Beltsville Human Nutrition Research Center
United States Department of Agriculture
Beltsville, MD 20705

In 1939, only a year after the isolation of vitamin B-6 and 5 years after its discovery, Schultz et al. (1) and Eakin et al. (2) reported that vitamin B-6 was effective in yeast growth stimulation and that this stimulation might be useful as a method for determination of vitamin B-6. In 1943, Atkin et al. (3) presented a microbiological method for determining pyridoxine (PN), the only known form at that time, using a strain of Saccharomyces carlsbergensis (culture 4228), now renamed Saccharomyces uvarum (ATCC 9080) by American Type Culture Collection. This yeast was especially selected for its specific response to pyridoxine. The initial yeast used in the yeast growth method for assay of vitamin B-6 was not specific. In a pyridoxine-free medium, S. uvarum grows very slightly, but when pyridoxine was added to the medium an extensive growth was observed. With a few exceptions the yeast method gave results that agreed reasonably well with results obtained by the rat growth method. This same year, Stokes, et al. (4) presented a method for determining vitamin B-6 by using a mold, Neurospora sitophila as the test organism. Also in 1943, Siegel et al. (5) reported modifications of the Williams yeast growth method for determination of pyridoxine in acid extracts of natural products. Results they obtained by microbiological procedure also agreed with those obtained by animal biological assay. Snell in 1942 (6) reported that by using certain lactic acid bacteria for assay of vitamin B-6, compounds other than pyridoxine contributed to the vitamin B-6 activity of natural products. In 1944, he reported that these active substances were two new forms of vitamin B-6, an amine, PM, and an aldehyde, PL (7). By using either PL or PM as a standard of comparison with Streptococcus lactis, he found values for vitamin B-6 content of natural materials to be similar to those indicated by the yeast assay, whereas S. lactis failed to respond to PN when used as the standard.

The following year, this same laboratory reported that S. uvarum gave activity for PN, PL, and PM and that the activity of PL and PM closely approached the activity of PN (8). They suggested that three separate microorganisms might be used for the individual detection of PN, PL, and PM; a strain of Lactabacillus casei responds principally to PL and a strain of Streptococcus faecalis R responds to both PL and PM (9). These organisms used in conjunction with S. uvarum comprised the differential assay (10). They found PL and PM to be the predominant forms of vitamin B-6 in hydrolyzed animal tissues and yeasts, with only slight indications or none at all of the presence of PN, and PN to be more evident in plant materials occurring in amounts as large or larger than those of PL or PM.

In the mid 1950's, our laboratory investigated the use of the microbiological assay using S. uvarum for determining the vitamin B-6 content of the edible portion of foods as offered on the retail market. At the beginning of our vitamin B-6 studies, it was assumed that S. uvarum gave approximately equal activity to the three forms of vitamin B-6. However, a critical evaluation of the Atkin yeast method by Parrish (11) and confirmed in this laboratory revealed that the growth response of the test organism to the three forms was not equivalent. Growth rates in basal medium supplemented by PN and PL were similar, but PM produced a slower rate of growth. Parrish made several modifications of the Atkin yeast method to improve the sensitivity of the assay (11,12).

Most of these modifications were verified in our laboratory. The inoculum is grown in a liquid culture medium and the cells washed twice before using as inoculum. The casein hydrolysate for the basal medium was prepared in the laboratory. An inorganic source of nitrogen was included in the medium as well as addition of tryptophan, histidine, methionine, isoleucine, and valine.

The pH of the medium was adjusted to 4.5. The basal medium was steamed for 10 minutes and added aseptically to the previously sterilized assay tubes. Our procedure uses 16 x 150 mm screw capped tubes with two glass beads per tube with a hole drilled in the cap. The tubes are sterilized with the caps on, sterile medium is added through the hole in the cap, and each tube is inoculated through the same hole. Under the conditions in our laboratory, contamination

has not been evident. The assay tubes are incubated on a constant
rotary shaker at 30° for 22 hours. The typical growth response
obtained with S. uvarum for PN, PL, and PM during our early work
when percent transmission was plotted against concentration is
shown in Fig. 1. PN and PL yield quite similar and sometimes
almost superimposable growth responses while the PM gives a lower
response.

EXTRACTION

    Vitamin B-6 occurs naturally as PN, PL, and PM, together with
the phosphorylated derivatives of each form which frequently occur
in association with proteins. Yeast cannot utilize the phosphorylated forms of the vitamin. Therefore, to obtain the total
vitamin B-6 content of natural materials, dephosphorylation must
first be carried out. In 1943, Atkin et al. (3) stated that although
vitamin B-6 is relatively soluble, it is extracted from most plant
and animal tissues with difficulty. They found that acid extraction
increases the vitamin B-6 content of extracts as measured by the
yeast method. The efficiency of the extraction depends upon the

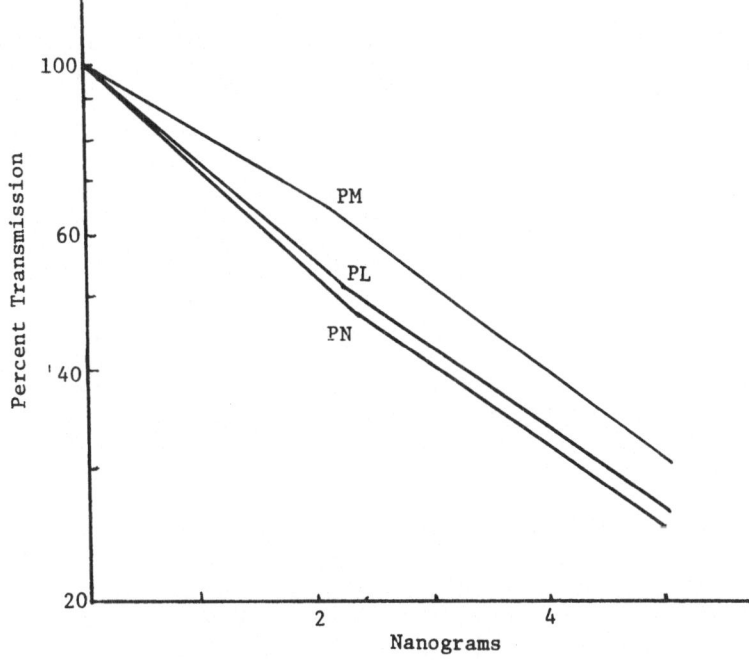

Fig. 1. Typical growth response obtained with S. uvarum during
         early years when percent transmission was plotted against
         concentration.

volume of the extraction medium as well as the concentration of
acid. For most substances extraction of a finely divided sample
containing between 2 and 4 micrograms of PN with 180 ml of 0.055 N
H_2SO_4 at 9 kg (20 lbs) pressure for 1 hour yielded maximal values.
This procedure was not satisfactory for wheat and wheat products,
but was if the acid concentration was increased to 0.44 N.
Rabinowitz and Snell in 1947 (13) found that hydrolysis in 0.055 N
HCl at 20 pounds pressure for 5 hours gave maximal values for all
products tested except a rice bran concentrate. Rice bran concentrate required hydrolysis with 2 N acid for maximal release of
vitamin B-6. This procedure was also adequate for some other plant
products, but inferior to treatment with 0.055 N acid for yeast
and animal products. The extraction procedures used by these two
groups were quite similar and were verified in our laboratory. The
superiority of low concentrations of acid (0.055 N) over high
concentrations for extraction of vitamin B-6 was also observed in
our laboratory for animal products (14). Extraction of meat products with 0.44 N HCl instead of 0.055 N HCl gave approximately
the same pyridoxine and pyridoxal values, but only about half of
the pyridoxamine.

To determine the necessary acid concentration for plant products, comparisons of the amounts of vitamin B-6 in extracts
obtained with increasing concentrations of acid were made on whole
wheat samples (Fig. 2) (15). The extracts were chromatographed on
Dowex 50 columns to determine the effect of the extraction on the
individual vitamin B-6 components. The amounts of the components
and total vitamin B-6 released in the whole wheat extracts were
identical for 0.44 N HCl and 1.0 N HCl when autoclaved 5 hours. The
values for PL were the same for 0.055 N, 0.44 N, and 1.0 N HCl. PN
and PM were incompletely freed by 0.055 N HCl. Autoclaving with
0.44 N HCl for 2 hours was found to be equivalent to a 5-hour autoclaving period, and was the procedure adopted for use in the analyses
of plant products by our laboratory. It was desirable to keep the
acid concentration as low as possible because of the effect of the
salt concentration, after the pH adjustment of the extract, on the
ion exchange resin.

The effectiveness of enzymatic digestion in dephosphorylation
of vitamin B-6 by several enzymes was also checked in our laboratory
Digestion with clarase gave values for most products that were
similar to those obtained with the 5-hour acid hydrolysis as was
observed by Atkin et al. (3). The other enzymes studied were not
satisfactory.

CHROMATOGRAPHIC SEPARATION

Since S. uvarum did not measure the three forms equally, it
was important to develop procedures to separate PN, PL, and PM and

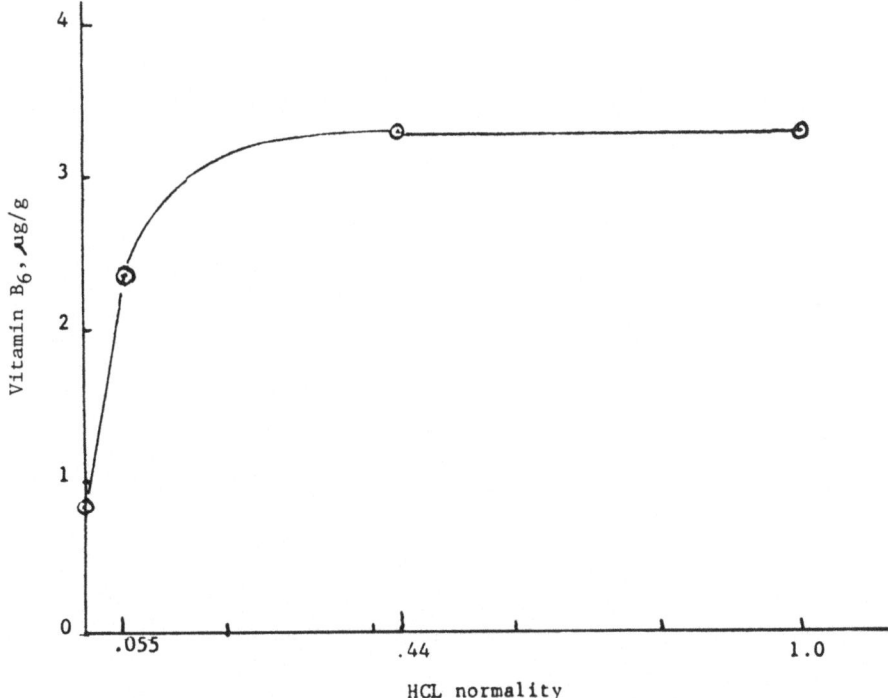

Fig. 2.   Amounts of vitamin B-6 extracted from whole wheat with
increasing concentrations of HCl.

determine them individually to obtain more reliable vitamin B-6
values on a wide variety of foods. After a lengthy investigation
of cation exchange resins, Dowex AG 50W-X8 (100-200 mesh), in the
potassium form was found to give a complete separation of the three
forms (Fig. 3) (16). The desired amount of sample was placed on
the ion exchange column. The column was washed and PL, PN, and PM
were eluted in succession. The completeness of absorption of PN,
PL, and PM by the resin was determined by running a microbiological
assay on the combined forerun and the 100 ml wash prior to elution.
The growth response observed in this fraction measured as PL was
termed "leakage" and was usually only about 1% of the total vitamin
B-6. This may be one of the forms of vitamin B-6, an unknown
factor stimulating yeast growth, or a fortuitous combination of
substances in food extracts stimulating yeast growth in the assay

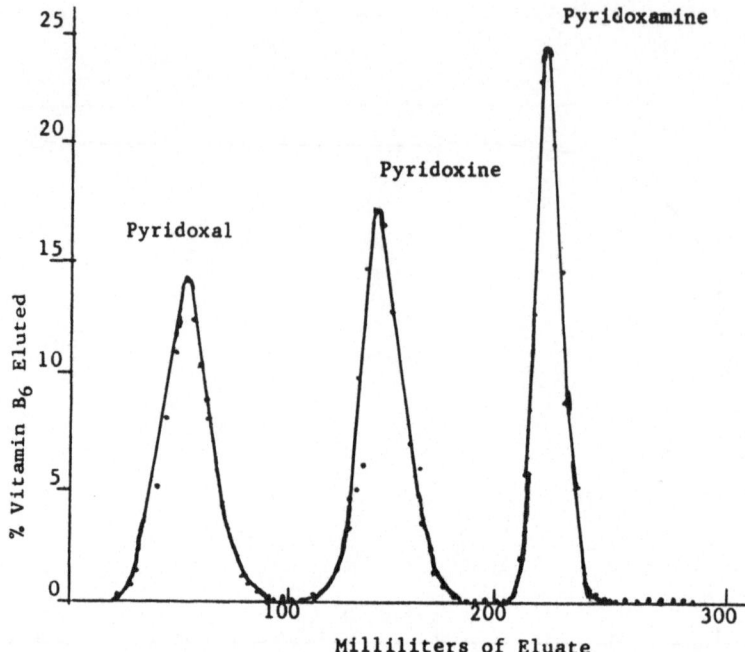

Fig. 3.   Chromatographic fractionation of vitamin B-6 components
          with Dowex AG 50W-X8 (100-200 mesh) resin.

medium.   The percent recovery calculated from 12 experiments for
the three forms eluted from the Dowex resin column are shown in
Table 1.   The three forms were put on the column singularly or as
a mixture of the three forms and the average recoveries were 97%
or greater.   These same recoveries were obtained when from 5 to 50
ng of each form of the vitamin was passed through the column.

The procedure for the microbiological assay of the vitamin B-6
components in food samples (17) as developed in our laboratory is
given in outline form in Table 2.   All work with solutions containing
vitamin B-6 is performed in a darkened laboratory.   The use of red
or gold fluorescent light is suitable.   The ground or finely divided
food sample was extracted by autoclaving in the presence of 0.055
N HCl for 5 hours for animal products or 0.44 N HCl for 2 hours for
plant products at 15 pounds steam pressure.   The extracts were
adjusted to pH 4.5, made to volume, filtered, and an aliquot put
on the column.   The column was washed with 100 ml of hot 0.02 M
KOAc at pH 5.5.   Much of the salts and other materials from the
extract passed through the column with the washing and were calculated against the PL standard as leakage.   PN, PL, and PM remained

Table 1. Percent Recovery of PN, PL, and PM when Separated
with Dowex AG 50W-X8 (100-200 Mesh) Resin

PN		PL		PM	
Eluted with 0.1 M KOAc pH 7		Eluted with 0.04 M KOAc pH 6		Eluted with $KCl-K_2HPO_4$ pH 8	
One[a]	Mix[b]	One[a]	Mix[b]	One[a]	Mix[b]
99 ± 3.2	98 ± 3.5	97 ± 4.6	100 ± 3.6	100 ± 2.5	99 ± 3.3

[a] Only one form of vitamin B-6 was put on the resin column.
[b] A mixture of all three forms was put on the column.

on the column. PL was removed with 100 ml boiling 0.04 M KOAc, pH
6.0, pyridoxine next with 100 ml boiling 0.1 M KOAc at pH 7.0; and
pyridoxamine with 100 ml boiling $KCl-K_2HPO_4$ at pH 8.0. After
adjusting the volume, the chromatographed fractions were placed in
culture tubes with the assay medium, inoculated with a suspension
of yeast cells, and incubated 22 hours at 30° with constant shaking.
Growth of yeast was measured by percent transmission in a spectrophotometer at 550 nm with the inoculated blanks set at 100% transmission. Currently, absorbance is measured and the inoculated
blank is set at zero. Standard solutions were also chromatographed
for preparation of standard curves from which PN, PL, and PM in
extracts can be determined. Microbiological assays of the fractions
were made at five levels in triplicate along with standards for each
component. The absorbance is plotted against ng of eluted standards
PN, PL, or PM per tube. The amount of PN, PL, or PM per sample
tube is interpolated from the standard curve and reported in ng PN,
PL, or PM per g of sample. Our procedure, with few improvements,
is still used today. The detailed procedure is included at the end
of this paper.

Table 3 shows the difference obtained by chromatographing a
sample that contains a high percentage of PM. Only about two-thirds
of the vitamin B-6 content of this sample was obtained when analyzed
directly. The microbiological assay of extracts that are not
separated can lead to low vitamin B-6 values for samples that are
high in PM, because the test organism gives a lower growth response
to this form.

Table 2.   Vitamin B-6 Assay of Foods

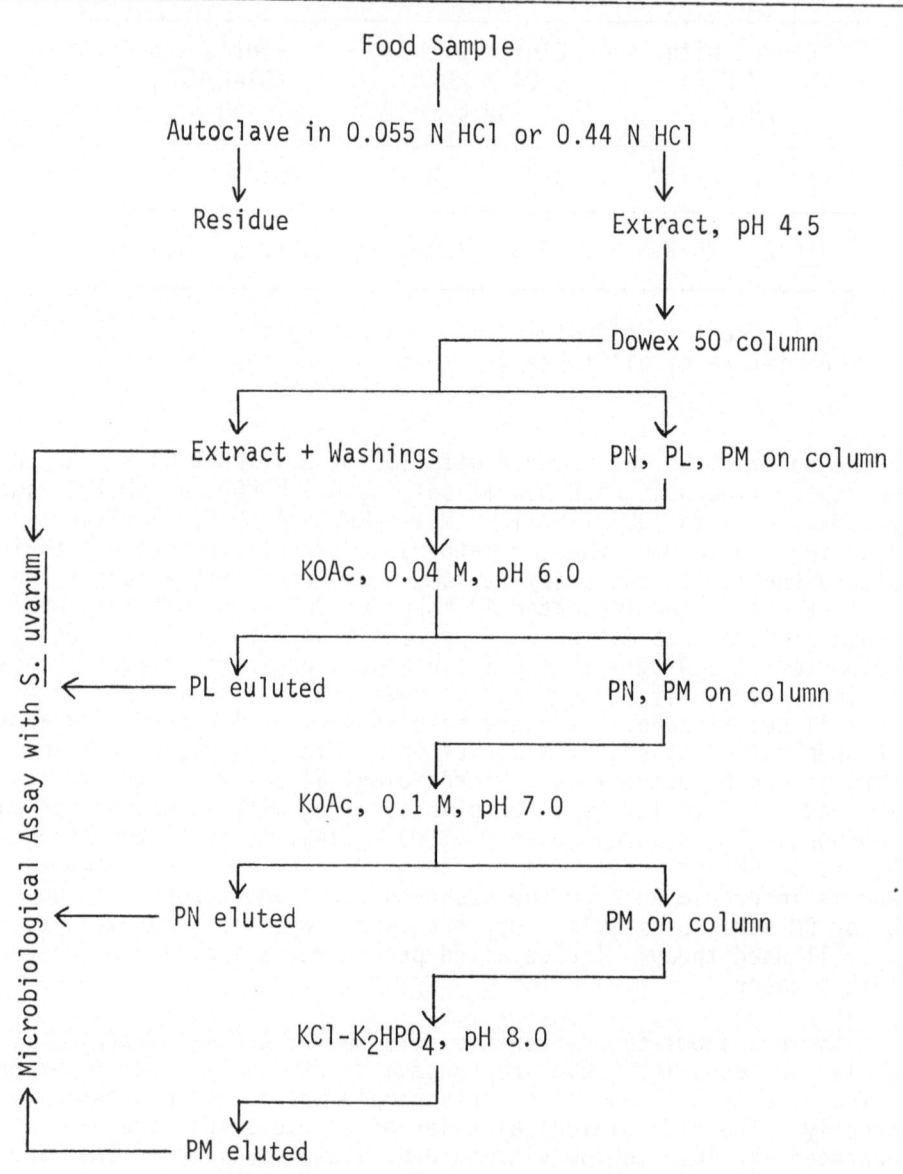

Food Sample

Autoclave in 0.055 N HCl or 0.44 N HCl

Residue   Extract, pH 4.5

Dowex 50 column

Extract + Washings   PN, PL, PM on column

KOAc, 0.04 M, pH 6.0

PL euluted   PN, PM on column

KOAc, 0.1 M, pH 7.0

PN eluted   PM on column

KCl-K$_2$HPO$_4$, pH 8.0

PM eluted

Microbiological Assay with S. uvarum

Table 3.   Vitamin B-6, μg/g

Sample	Chromatographed				Not Chromatographed
	PN	PL	PM	Total	Total
Condensed milk	0.05	0.20	0.35	0.60	0.38

The animal growth test is still considered the true assay for
a nutrient. Vitamin B-6 values obtained by rat bioassay were compared to free and total vitamin B-6 values of a few selected food
samples assayed by our microbiological procedure on nonfractionated
extracts and on the individual fractions of PN, PL, and PM obtained
by chromatographing the extracts (18). Table 4 shows values for
free and total vitamin B-6 on chromatographed samples. The values
for the free vitamin B-6 were approximately one-third of the total
vitamin B-6 with the exception of the dry milk sample in which the
free vitamin B-6 was approximately 90% of the total vitamin B-6.
Table 5 gives vitamin B-6 values for the bioassay, for fractionated
PN, PL, and PM, for their total, and for nonfractionated samples.
The rat bioassay values agreed with the total vitamin B-6 values
obtained microbiologically on chromatographed extracts as the 95%
confidence limits for these values overlap. There appeared to be
differences at the tested level of comparison between bioassay
values and those obtained microbiologically on unfractionated
extracts of nonfat dry milk solids and whole wheat flour. The
microbiological assay value was somewhat greater. There was also
a difference between the microbiological assays on whole wheat flour
between the chromatographed and non-chromatographed extracts. From
these data, it was concluded that the bioassay measures free and
combined forms of vitamin B-6 and that the bioassay values agree
with the values obtained microbiologically on chromatographed,
fractionated extracts of these samples. The Texas group that did
the bioassay also assayed these samples microbiologically using the
procedures, including fractionation, developed in our laboratory.
The chromatographed total vitamin B-6 values for the two laboratories
are shown in Table 6. Agreement between the data obtained by the
two laboratories working independently was strong evidence that the
chromatographic fractionations of extracts and the microbiological
procedures were reproducible and could be used routinely for the
determination of the three forms of vitamin B-6 in foods.

Table 4. Free and Total Vitamin B-6 Values for Selected
         Food Samples[a]

Sample	Total of Vitamin B-6 Components	
	Free	Hydrolyzed
	µg/g	µg/g
Ground beef, dried	5.04	15.93
Lima beans, dried	1.93	6.72
Milk solids, nonfat, dry	3.66	4.06
Whole wheat flour	1.17	3.50

[a]Microbiological assay of chromatographed extracts.

ASSAY MICROORGANISMS

It is now 25 years since we at Beltsville set out to determine
the vitamin B-6 content of foods, and there is a renewed interest
in this vitamin and its content in foods. Haskell in 1978 (19)
stated that "The microbiological assay still is the method of choice
for the determination of the vitamin B-6 content of foods." She
stated that most cultures of S. uvarum grow with approximately equal
efficiency in response to PL, PN, and PM. She further states that
since these three forms of the vitamin also have equal activity for
animals and humans, S. uvarum is well suited to the estimation of
total vitamin B-6 in foods. She did give one objection to S. uvarum
as an assay organism. Some cultures apparently grow only about 80%
as well on PM as they do on PL or PN. Under conditions used in our
laboratory, S. uvarum does give a lower growth response for PM than
for PN or PL.

Fig. 4 shows the growth response of PN, PL, PM, and of a mixture
of equal amounts of each form over a concentration range of 1-10 ng/
tube using a newly purchased S. uvarum culture. The absorbance
instead of percent transmission is read and plotted against vitamin
B-6 concentration. S. uvarum gives similar growth response for PN
and PL, but still gives a lower response to pyridoxamine. An equal
molar mixture of the three forms gives a growth response that is
less than PN and PL and greater than PM as expected. The growth
response of the yeast to the three forms is similar to that observed
in our laboratory in the earlier years. To verify that the proper
amounts of vitamins were being assayed, the extinction coefficients
for PN, PL, and PM were measured and found to be very close to those
reported; therefore, our standard solutions are assumed to be correct.

Table 5. Vitamin B-6 Values of Selected Food Samples by Bioassay and Microbiological Assay Procedures

| Sample | Bioassay | Vitamin B-6 in µg/g | | | | |
| | | Microbiological Assay Fractionated | | | | Not Fractionated |
		PN	PL	PM	Total	Total
Ground beef, dried	13.2 (10.4-16.9)[a]	0.8 (0.6-1.0)	6.4 (5.7-7.1)	8.7 (8.2-9.3)	15.9 (14.6-17.3)	14.3 (12.7-16.0)
Lima beans, dried	7.1 (5.8-8.8)	5.0 (4.7-5.4)	1.0 (0.8-1.2)	0.7 (0.7-0.7)	6.7 (6.1-7.3)	7.4 (6.8-8.1)
Milk solids, nonfat, dry	3.2 (2.6-3.8)	0.1 (0.1-0.1)	2.5 (2.3-2.7)	1.4 (1.3-1.5)	4.0 (3.7-4.4)	4.5 (4.2-4.8)
Whole wheat flour	2.9 (2.4-3.6)	2.5 (2.3-2.6)	0.6 (0.5-0.6)	0.4 (0.4-0.5)	3.5 (3.3-3.7)	4.3 (4.0-4.6)

[a]95% confidence limits, low and high, respectively.

Table 6. Comparison of Vitamin B-6 Values by
Microbiological Assay Procedure from
Two Laboratories

Sample	Total Vitamin B-6 from Chromatographed Extracts	
	Texas	Beltsville
	µg/g	µg/g
Ground beef, dried	14.91	15.93 (14.55-17.31)[a]
Lima beans, dried	6.99	6.72 (6.11- 7.33)
Milk solids, nonfat, dry	3.68	4.06 (3.73- 4.39)
Whole wheat flour	3.51	3.50 (3.27- 3.73)

[a]95% confidence limits, low and high, respectively.

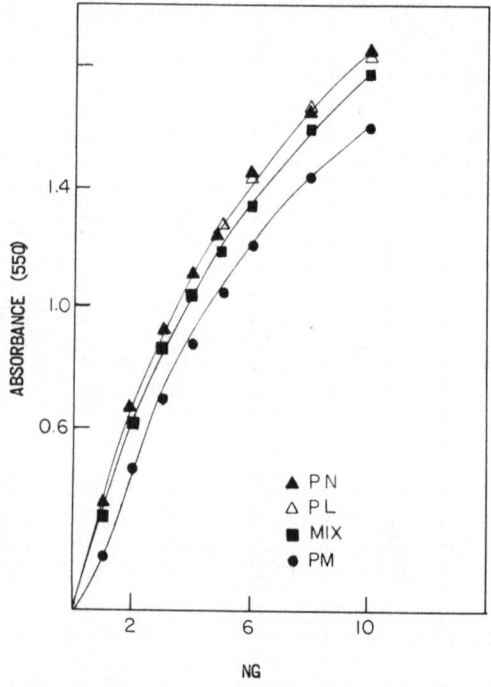

Fig. 4. Representative growth of S. uvarum (newly purchased) to
PN, PL, PM, and of a mixture of equal amounts of each
form over a concentration range of 1-10 ng/tube (30°,
22 hours, HN medium).

Recently, Guilarte and coworkers from Johns Hopkins Medical
Institution (20) reported that Kloeckera brevis (ATCC 9774), renamed
K. apiculata by American Type Culture Collection, should be the ideal
microorganism for the microbiological assay of total vitamin B-6.
They showed that K. apiculata responds equally to all three forms
of vitamin B-6 at a dosage range of 2-10 ng molar equivalent of PN.
On the other hand, S. uvarum did not show an equal growth response
to any of the three forms. They proposed that K. apiculata be used
with a standard solution concentration range of 2-10 ng of vitamin
B-6 as the standard turbidimetric microbiologic assay system for
vitamin B-6 in biologic materials. Fig. 5 shows the growth response
of S. uvarum to PN, PL, and PM grown in our laboratory at Beltsville
under conditions normally used for the microbiological assay, and
Fig. 6 shows the growth response of K. apiculata to the three forms
grown at the same time under the same conditions. Under our normal
microbiologic assay conditions, we observe growth responses for the
two yeasts that are similar but not equal for all three forms of
vitamin B-6. S. uvarum gives a similar response to PN and PL while
the response to PL for K. apiculata was a little less. The response
to PM was considerably less for both test organisms under our
routine laboratory conditions. With our normal conditions, we do
not see equal growth to the three forms for K. apiculata as did the
Johns Hopkins researchers.

Two other groups of researchers used K. apiculata for vitamin
B-6 determinations. Daoud and coworkers (21) used S. uvarum and
K. apiculata to measure the vitamin B-6 retention in canned garbanzo
beans. They found that the use of K. apiculata as the test organism
resulted in slightly but consistently higher values for total vitamin
B-6 content in all samples tested throughout the study than values
obtained using S. uvarum. They stated that this could be due to
the difference in the response of the two organisms toward the
different forms of vitamin B-6. No comparison of growth response
between the two yeasts was given. They stated that growth of
K. apiculata responds nearly equally to PN, PL, and PM while S.
uvarum responds nearly equally to PN and PL but responds to a lesser
degree to PM. Barton-Wright (22) reported that K. apiculata shows
virtually equal activity to all three forms of the vitamin B-6
complex. These differences in growth response to the three forms
may be due to the differences in growth conditions between our
laboratory and the others. In Table 7 growth conditions used by
the various laboratories are compared. The laboratories all used
different agar slants to carry the yeast culture. The Wort agar
used in our laboratory does not appear to be satisfactory for K.
apiculata but the growth curves shown were made while the yeast was
being transferred in liquid medium right after the culture was
received. The way in which the inoculum is prepared probably affects

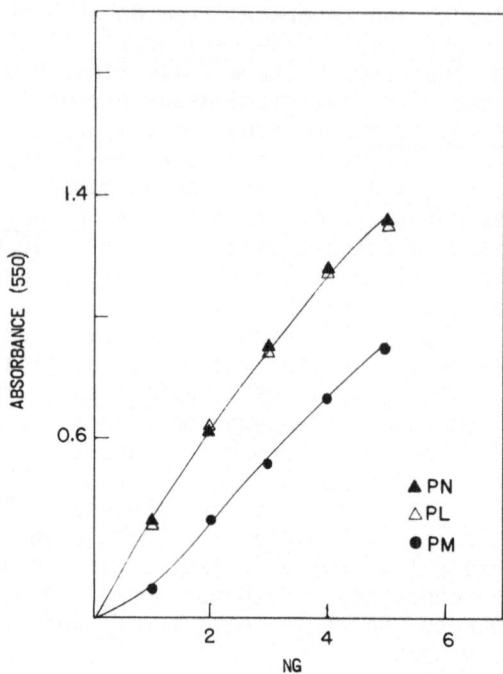

Fig. 5. Growth response of S. uvarum to PN, PL, and PM grown
         under our normal laboratory conditions (30°, 22 hours,
         HN medium).

the sensitivity of the assay. The pH of the basal medium is not the
same for each laboratory and may be critical to the growth response
of K. apiculata to each or all forms of vitamin B-6, as was the pH
of the medium for S. uvarum particularly for its response to PL.

     The time of incubation for three of the laboratories was
essentially the same but Daoud incubated the K. apiculata assay for
48 to 60 hours compared to 15 to 18 hours for S. uvarum. This would
tend to indicate a slower and/or lower growth rate for K. apiculata.
The Johns Hopkins group and our laboratory grew both organisms for
the same length of time. The Johns Hopkins group did show a lower
growth response to K. apiculata than to S. uvarum. The basal medium
was different for each laboratory and is probably the most critical
factor in obtaining equal response to the three forms. Each laboratory used a different medium, but the Johns Hopkins laboratory,
Daoud's group, and our laboratory grew both organisms on the same
medium within their respective laboratories. Therefore, comparisons
within a laboratory should be valid. Time has not allowed us to
further investigate K. apiculata for use in the microbiological
assay, but studies are in progress.

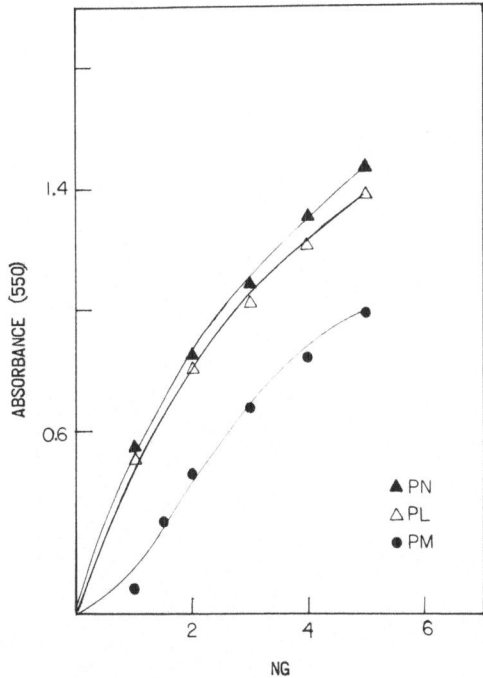

Fig. 6. Growth response of K. apiculata to PN, PL, and PM grown
         under normal growth conditions for S. uvarum and at the
         same time as results for Fig. 5 (30°, 22 hours, HN
         medium).

     Obviously, it is essential that the growth responses to the
three forms of vitamin B-6 of any test organism be checked in the
individual laboratory under the conditions of the laboratory doing
the assay before proceeding to do routine determinations.

SUMMARY

     The microbiological assay has been associated with vitamin B-6
since it was discovered. The microbiological method using S. uvarum,
which was selected for its specific response to vitamin B-6, is
still the most widely used method for the estimation of total vitamin
B-6 in foods. Since the yeast grows only on the free forms of
vitamin B-6, foods must be hydrolyzed to release the vitamin from
phosphate and protein. To obtain the most accurate vitamin B-6
values, especially for foods high in PM, the three forms should be
separated by ion exchange chromatography and each form assayed
against its own standard and the total vitamin B-6 content calculated.
The chromatographic separation corrects for the lower growth response

Table 7. Comparison of Growth Conditions for K. apiculata

Laboratory	Agar	Inoculum	Basal Medium	pH	Time
					hr
Barton-Wright	Malt, yeast, glucose, B-6	Liquid stock Medium + B-6	Complete synthetic with malt extract	4.8-5.0	24
Daoud et al.	--	--	Complete synthetic	-	48-60
Guilarte et al.	Lactobacilli	Agar	Bacto-Pyridoxine-Y	-	21-24
Polansky	Wort	Basal Medium + B-6	Complete synthetic with casamino acids	4.5	22

All laboratories incubated samples at 30°.

of the test organism to PM and also improves the specificity of the assay. Under our routine laboratory conditions following the procedures for S. uvarum, K. apiculata does not give equal growth response to the three forms of vitamin B-6, and it is essential that the growth responses of K. apiculata be investigated further.

Although the microbiological method is slow and tedious, it is highly specific, and thus more reliable then existing methods for use with crude extracts or even partially purified food samples. Presently, newer methods for determining vitamin B-6 utilizing modern technology are being developed. Perhaps some of these may prove to be as reliable as our microbiological procedure.

PROCEDURE FOR CHROMATOGRAPHIC SEPARATION AND MICROBIOLOGICAL ASSAY OF VITAMIN B-6 COMPONENTS IN FOOD EXTRACTS

REAGENTS

(a) 0.01 M potassium acetate pH 4.5; pH adjusted with acetic acid.

(b) 0.02 M potassium acetate pH 5.5; pH adjusted with acetic acid.

(c) 0.04 M potassium acetate pH 6.0; pH adjusted with acetic acid.

(d) 0.1 M potassium acetate pH 7.0; pH adjusted with acetic acid or KOH.

(e) KCl-K_2HPO_4 solution pH 8.0; 74.6 g KCl and 17.4 g K_2HPO_4 dissolved in 800 ml water adjusted to pH 8.0 with acetic acid solution and final volume made to 1 liter.

(f) Ion exchange resin--Dowex AG 50W-X8, 100-200 mesh.

(g) Acid hydrolyzed casein. Mix 100 g of vitamin-free casein with 500 ml of constant-boiling HCl (ca 5 N HCl, 208 ml conc HCl made to 500 ml with water) and reflux 8 hours.

Remove the HCl from the mixture by distillation under vacuum until a very thick syrup remains, keeping the temperature of the water bath below 80°. Dissolve the syrup in water and concentrate again in the same manner. Redissolve the syrup in water.

Adjust to pH 4 with 40% NaOH, add water to bring the volume to 600 ml, add 40 g of activated charcoal of the Darco G-60 type, stir 4 hours, and filter with vacuum through a Buchner funnel with a thin pad of HCl-washed filtercel. If filtrate is not clear, add 20 g of Darco to the filtrate, stir for 1 hour, and refilter.

Repeat with a fresh 10 g portion of Darco and filter. When solution is clear and colorless, make to 1 liter with water. Two to 3 ml of 6 N HCl may be added before making to volume to lengthen the time before microbial growth occurs. Store in refrigerator. (1 ml equals 100 mg hydrolyzed casein.)

(h) Vitamin solution I. Dissolve 10 mg thiamine and 1 g inositol in 200 ml water, and make to 1 liter. Store in refrigerator. (1 ml equals 10 micrograms thiamine, and 1 mg inositol.)

(i) Vitamin solution II. Dissolve 10 mg biotin in 100 ml 50% alcohol-water. Store in refrigerator. (1 ml equals 100 micrograms biotin.)

Dissolve 200 mg calcium pantothenate and 200 mg niacin in 200 ml water; add 8 ml of the biotin solution; make to 1 liter with water. Store in refrigerator. (1 ml equals 200 micrograms each calcium pantothenate and niacin, 0.8 micrograms biotin.)

(j) Salt solution I. Dissolve 17 g KCl, 10.3 g $MgSO_4 \cdot 7H_2O$, 100 mg $FeCl_3 \cdot 6H_2O$, and 100 mg $MnSO_4 \cdot H_2O$ in about 800 ml water. Add 2 ml conc HCl. Dissolve 5 g $CaCl_2 \cdot 2H_2O$ in about 100 ml water; add to the first solution and make to 1 liter with water. Store in refrigerator. (1 ml equals 17 mg KCl, 5.03 mg $MgSO_4$, 50 micrograms $FeCl_3$, 89.3 micrograms $MnSO_4$, and 3.77 mg $CaCl_2$.)

(k) Salt solution II. Dissolve 22 g KH_2PO_4 and 40 g $(NH_4)_2HPO_4$ in water and make to 1 liter. Store in refrigerator. (1 ml equals 22 mg KH_2PO_4 and 40 mg $(NH_4)_2HPO_4$.)

(l) "Tween 80" solution. Weigh 2.5 g of "Tween 80" in a small beaker. Transfer with warm (45°) water and make to 500 ml volume. Store in refrigerator. (1 ml equals 5 mg "Tween 80".)

(m) 1 + 1 citric acid solution. Dissolve 50 g of citric acid in 50 ml of water. Store at room temperature in a bottle with a plastic stopper.

(n) 1 + 2 ammonium phosphate solution. Dissolve 25 g $(NH_4)_2HPO_4$ in 50 ml water. Store at room temperature in a bottle with a plastic stopper.

WORK IN SUBDUED LIGHT WITH ALL SOLUTIONS CONTAINING VITAMIN B-6.

(o) PN standard solutions.

(1) Stock solution, 10 μg/ml. Dissolve and dilute 12.16 mg USP PN·HCl Reference Standard (previously dried 5 days over P_2O_5) to 1 liter with 1 N HCl. Store in a red glass-stoppered bottle in a refrigerator.

(2) Intermediate solution, 1.0 µg/ml. Dilute 10 ml stock solution (o-1) to 100 ml with H_2O.

(3) Working solution, 1.0 ng/ml. Dilute 5 ml intermediate solution (o-2) to 500 ml with H_2O and mix. Dilute 10 ml to 100 ml with H_2O. Prepare fresh for each assay.

(p) PL standard solutions.

(1) Stock solution, 10 µg/ml. Prepare as for PN (o-1), except use 12.18 mg PL·HCl of high purity.

(2) Intermediate solution, 1.0 µg/ml. See (o-2).

(3) Working solution, 1.0 ng/ml. See (o-3).

(q) PM standard solutions.

(1) Stock solution, 10 µg/ml. Prepare as for PN (o-1) except use 14.34 mg PM·2HCl of high purity.

(2) Intermediate solution, 1.0 µg/ml. See (o-2).

(3) Working solution, 1.0 ng/ml. See (o-3).

(r) Mixed PN, PL, PM solutions for liquid broth culture. Pipet 2 ml each of (o-2), (p-2), and (q-2) (1.0 µg/ml) into a liter volumetric flask and make to volume with water.

(s) Citrate buffer solution. Dissolve 100 g potassium citrate and 20 g citric acid and make to 1 liter with water. Store in refrigerator. (1 ml equals 100 mg potassium citrate and 20 mg citric acid.)

(t) Basal medium stock solution (for 200 tubes). To make 1 liter of medium add to about 400 ml water: 100 ml citrate buffer (s), 100 ml hydrolyzed casein solution (g) or 10 g Vitamin Assay Casamino Acids, 50 ml vitamin solution I (h), 25 ml vitamin solution II (i), 50 ml salt solution I (j), and 50 ml salt solution II (k). Dissolve 100 g dextrose in the liquids. Dissolve 22 mg DL-tryptophan, 27 mg L-histidine hydrochloride, 100 mg DL-methionine, 216 mg DL-isoleucine, and 256 mg DL-valine in 10 ml of 10% HCl in a small beaker and add to the above. Add 20 ml "Tween 80" solution (l). Adjust to pH 4.5 with 1+1 citric acid (m) or 1+2 $(NH_4)_2HPO_4$ (n). Make to 1 liter with water; store in Pyrex bottle plugged with cotton in refrigerator. Prepare not longer than 24 hours before use. When ready, steam for 10 minutes and cool.

(u) Test organism. <u>Saccharomyces uvarum</u>, American Type Culture
Collection No. 9080.

(v) Agar culture medium. Suspend 25 g of Bacto-Wort agar in about
400 ml water in a marked 500 ml wide mouth Erlenmeyer flask. Plug
with cotton, steam for about 10 minutes to dissolve the agar, adjust
the volume to 500 ml. Pipet the hot agar in 10 ml amounts into
20 x 150 mm test tubes, plug with absorbent cotton and autoclave
for 15 minutes at 15 pounds pressure. Inasmuch as this medium has
an acid reaction, care should be taken to avoid overheating which
will result in a softer medium. Tilt the hot agar tubes to form
slants and cool in this position.

(w) Liquid culture medium. Pipet 5 ml of mixed solution (r) for
liquid broth culture tubes into 16 x 150 mm test tubes, containing
two glass beads (4 mm), plug with absorbent cotton, autoclave for
10 minutes at 15 pounds pressure. Add 5 ml of steamed vitamin B-6-
free basal medium (t) under aseptic conditions. Store in refrigerator
at 4^0.

(x) Inoculum rinse. Pipet 5 ml of water into test tubes, plug
with absorbent cotton, and autoclave for 10 minutes at 15 pounds
pressure. Add 5 ml of steamed vitamin B-6-free basal medium (t)
under aseptic conditions. Store tubes in refrigerator at 4^0.

CULTURE CARE

    Maintain the <u>S. uvarum</u> culture by weekly transfers on Wort
agar slants (v). Incubate these freshly seeded agar slants at 30^0
for 24 hours and then refrigerate.

ASSAY INOCULUM

    Incubate cells for inoculum on agar at 30^0 for 24 hours just
before use. Transfer cells with loop under aseptic condition to
liquid broth culture tubes (w). Plug with absorbent cotton held
in place with masking tape, and place the tubes on the shaker at
30^0 for 20 hours. Replace the cotton plugs aseptically with
sterile rubber stoppers; centrifuge at 2500 rpm for 1.5 minutes.
Decant the liquid and resuspend in 10 ml of inoculum rinse (x).
Separate by centrifugation at 2500 rpm for 1.5 minutes. Decant the
liquid, resuspend in a second 10 ml of sterile inoculum rinse,
centrifuge for 1.5 minutes and decant. The cells suspended in the
third 10 ml of inoculum rinse are the assay inoculum.

PREPARATION OF EXCHANGE RESIN AND COLUMN

    To 250 g Dowex AG 50W-X8 (100-200 mesh) in the hydrogen form
add excess 6 N KOH until the supernatant liquid is blue to litmus.
Let settle, decant, and rinse the resin with water until the super-

natant liquid is clear. Add about 600 ml of 3 N HCl, stir, and
heat for one-half hour in a boiling water bath. Decant and repeat
this treatment with 3 N HCl two more times. Rinse the resin until
the rinse water is neutral. Add 6 N KOH until pH is strongly basic
and stir for one hour. Rinse with water until rinse water is neutral.
Suspend in 2 M KOAc and store in refrigerator until needed. Just
before use, wash resin with water until the water is pH 7.0. The
resin can be regenerated beginning with the 3 N HCl treatment.

      Pour 30 ml of the prepared resin into 19 x 380 mm column with
water. After the resin settles in the column, place a plug of
glass wool on top of the resin. Rinse the column with 50 ml hot
water followed by two 50 ml portions of hot 0.01 M KOAc, pH 4.5 (a).
The pH of the last buffer rinse from the column should be 4.5;
otherwise, more rinsing with (a) would be required. Do not permit
the level of the liquid on the column to fall below the top glass
wool plug at any time.

EXTRACTION

      Fresh, frozen, or dried samples should be ground or in a finely
divided state. Generally 1 or 2 gram samples are used for dry products and up to 20 grams for fresh products. The weighed sample
is placed in a 500 ml wide-mouth Erlenmeyer flask and suspended in
200 ml of 0.44 N HCl for plant products or in 200 ml of 0.055 N
HCl for animal products. The plant products in the 0.44 N HCl are
autoclaved at 15 pounds steam pressure for 2 hours and the samples
extracted in 0.055 N HCl are autoclaved for 5 hours at 15 pounds
steam pressure. The samples are cooled to room temperature,
adjusted to pH 4.5 with 6 N KOH, brought to 250 ml volume in a
volumetric flask, and filtered through Whatman No. 40 filter paper.
Generally, 40 to 200 ml of filtered aliquot are put through the
resin column.

CHROMATOGRAPHY

      Put desired amount of the filtered extract on the ion exchange
column in approximately 50 ml portions and allow to pass completely
through with no regulation of the flow. Wash the beaker and
column three times with about 5 ml portions of hot 0.02 M potassium
acetate pH 5.5 (b), followed by a similar washing of the sides of
the column. Wash the column with the same solution until a total
of 100 ml of the 0.02 M potassium acetate pH 5.5 solution is used.
PL is eluted with two 50 ml portions of boiling 0.04 M potassium
acetate pH 6.0 (c), collecting the eluate in a 100 ml volumetric
flask. PN is eluted with two 50 ml portions of boiling 0.1 M
potassium acetate pH 7.0 (d) collecting the eluate in a 100 ml
volumetric flask. The PM is eluted with two 50 ml portions of

boiling $KCl-K_2HPO_4$ pH 8.0 solution (e). Collect PM in a 250 ml
beaker. Adjust pH to 4.5. Make eluates of PN and PL to 100 ml
volume and PM to 200 ml unless otherwise desired.

For standard PN, PL, and PM, mix 10 ml each of 1.0 µg/ml
standard solution (o-2), (p-2), (q-2), neutralized with KOH and
make to pH 4.5 with acetic acid. Put this solution on the column,
wash and elute the fractions according to the above procedure. Make
the eluted PN and PL standards to 100 ml, and the eluted PM, after
pH is adjusted to 4.5, to 200 ml. Dilute the eluted standards to
contain 1.0 ng/ml.

MICROBIOLOGICAL ASSAY PROCEDURE

Heat clean tubes and glass beads at 260° for 2 hours. Place
two 4 mm glass beads in each 16 x 150 mm screw-cap glass culture
tube. For the standard curve, pipet in triplicate the appropriate
freshly prepared standard (o-3), (p-3), (q-3) to give 0.0, 0.0, 1.0,
2.0, 3.0, 4.0, 5.0 ng PN, PL, or PM per tube. Similarly prepare
a set of tubes for the eluted standards, omitting the blanks. Dilute
the sample eluates from the chromatographic column to contain about
1 ng vitamin B-6 component per ml. Pipet 1, 2, 3, 4, and 5 ml of
the diluted eluates into triplicate tubes. Pipet water into all
tubes to bring the volume to 5 ml per tube. Cap the tubes with
plastic caps with a 1/8 inch hole through the top. Autoclave the
entire set for 10 minutes at 15 pounds steam pressure. Cool the
tubes to room temperature. Using an automatic pipet with sterilized
delivery attachments, pipet 5 ml of the steamed medium (t) through
the hole in the cap. Cover the tubes with sterile cheesecloth and
place in refrigerator. Remove from refrigerator one hour before
inoculation. Aseptically inoculate through the cap of each tube,
except the first set of 0.0 level for the standard curves, with 1
drop of the assay inoculum of the suspended cells of S. uvarum.
Take care to maintain a uniform suspension of the cells since they
may settle out during the inoculation step. Incubate the tubes on
a rotary shaker at 30° for 22 hours. Steam the tubes in the autoclave for 5 minutes, cool, and remove the caps. Read the absorbance
at 550 nm on a spectrophotometer. To read the uninoculated blank,
set at 0 with water. To read the inoculated blank, set at 0 with
the uninoculated blank. Mix the nine inoculated blank tubes and
with this mixture set 0 on the instrument to read all other tubes.

CALCULATIONS

Average the readings of the triplicate tubes and plot absor-
bence against ng of eluted standard PN, PL, or PM per tube. Determine by interpolation the amount of PN, PL, or PM per sample tube.
Report µg of PN, PL, and PM per g of sample.

LITERATURE CITED

1. Schultz, A. S., Atkin, L. & Frey, C. N.   (1939) Vitamin B-6, a growth promoting factor for yeast. J. Am. Chem. Soc. 61, 1931.
2. Eakin, R. E. & Williams, R. J.   (1939) Vitamin B-6 as a yeast nutrilite. J. Am. Chem. Soc. 61, 1932.
3. Atkin, L., Schultz, A. S., Williams, W. L. & Frey, C. N. (1943) Yeast microbiological methods for determination of vitamins-pyridoxine. Ind. & Eng. Chem., Anal. Ed. 15, 141-144.
4. Stokes, J. L., Larson, A., Woodward, C. R., Jr. & Foster, J. W. (1943) A Neurospora assay for pyridoxine. J. Biol. Chem. 150, 17-24.
5. Siegel, L., Melnick, D. & Oser, B. L. (1943) Bound pyridoxine (vitamin B-6) in biological materials. J. Biol. Chem. 149, 361-367.
6. Snell, E. E., Guirad, B. M. & Williams, R. J. (1942) Occurrence in natural products of a physiologically active metabolite of pyridoxine. J. Biol. Chem. 143, 519-530.
7. Snell, E. E. (1944) The vitamin activities of "pyridoxal" and "pyridoxamine". J. Biol. Chem. 154, 313-314.
8. Snell, E. E. & Rannefeld, A. N. (1945) The vitamin B-6 group. III. The vitamin activity of pyridoxal and pyridoxamine for various organisms. J. Biol. Chem. 157, 475-479.
9. Snell, E. E. (1945) The vitamin B-6 group. IV. Evidence for the occurrence of pyridoxamine and pyridoxal in natural products. J. Biol. Chem. 157, 491-505.
10. Rabinowitz, J. C. & Snell, E. E. (1948) The vitamin B-6 group. XIV. Distribution of pyridoxal, pyridoxamine, and pyridoxine in some natural products. J. Biol. Chem. 176, 1157-1167.
11. Parrish, W. P., Loy, H. W. & Kline, O. L. (1955) A study of the yeast method for vitamin B-6. J. Assoc. Off. Agric. Chem., 38, 506-513.
12. Parrish, W. P., Loy, H. W. & Kline, O. L. (1956) Further studies on the yeast method for vitamin B-6. J. Assoc. Off. Agric. Chem. 39, 157-166.
13. Rabinowitz, J. C. & Snell, E. E. (1947) Vitamin B-6 group. Extraction procedure for the microbiological determination of vitamin B-6. Ind. & Eng. Chem., Anal. Ed. 19, 277-280.
14. Polansky, M. M. & Toepfer, E. W. (1969) Vitamin B-6 components in some meats, fish, dairy products, and commercial infant formulas. Agric. & Food Chem. 17, 1394-1397.
15. Polansky, M. M., Murphy, E. W. & Toepfer, E. W. (1964) Components of vitamin B-6 in grains and cereal products. J. Assoc. Off. Agric. Chem. 47, 750-753.
16. MacArthur, M. J. & Lehmann, J. (1959) Chromatographic separation and fluorometric measurement of vitamin B-6 components in aqueous solutions. J. Assoc. Off. Agric. Chem. 42, 619-622.

17. Toepfer, E. W. & Polansky, M. M. (1970) Microbiological assay of vitamin B-6 and its components. J. Assoc. Off. Agric. Chem. 53, 546-550.

18. Toepfer, E. W., Polansky, M. M., Richardson, L. R. & Wilkes, S. (1963) Comparison of vitamin B-6 values of selected food samples by bioassay and microbiological assay. Agric. & Food Chem. 11, 523-525.

19. Haskell, B. E. (1978) Analysis of vitamin B-6. In: Human Vitamin B-6 Requirements, pp. 61-71, Nat. Acad. Sci., Washington, DC.

20. Guilarte, T. R., McIntyre, P. A. & Tsan, M. (1980) Growth response of the yeasts Saccharomyces uvarum and Kloeckera brevis to the free biologically active forms of vitamin B-6. J. Nutr. 110, 954-958.

21. Daoud, H. N., Luh, B. S. & Miller, M. W. (1977) Effect of blanching, EDTA, and $NaHSO_4$ on color and vitamin B-6 retention in canned garbanzo beans. J. Food Sci. 42, 375-378.

22. Barton-Wright, E. C. (1971) The microbiological assay of the vitamin B-6 complex (pyridoxine, pyridoxal, and pyridoxamine) with Kloeckera brevis. Analyst 96, 314-318.

MICROBIOLOGICAL ASSAY OF VITAMIN B-6 IN BLOOD AND URINE[1]

Lorraine T. Miller and Margaret Edwards

Department of Foods and Nutrition
Oregon State University
Corvallis, OR 97331

Although new, more precise techniques have been developed for the determination of vitamin B-6, the microbiological assay of this vitamin in blood and urine is still an important and valuable method. The assay organism used in our laboratory to measure vitamin B-6 is the yeast, Saccharomyces uvarum (formerly, S. carlsbergensis). Vitamin B-6 determination with this organism is simple, convenient, reproducible, and sensitive. In this paper, we will present the background for our choice of this organism and our procedure for determining plasma and urinary vitamin B-6.

The background for choosing S. uvarum goes back to studies done in the 1960's by Storvick and her associates. They were attempting to apply a differential microbiological method of vitamin B-6 determination to blood and to find an appropriate hydrolysis procedure to extract this vitamin from its bound form. Assaying acid-hydrolyzed whole blood with S. uvarum, Storvick and Peters (1) obtained values that were about one and a half times those obtained on the protein-free filtrate. When this same sample of acid-hydrolyzed blood was assayed with either Streptococcus faecium or Lactobacillus casei, the vitamin B-6 values they obtained were many times greater than those measured with the same organisms on the protein-free filtrate. In addition, these values from the hydrolyzed blood were 20-50 times greater than those obtained with S. uvarum. These results were unexpected because S. uvarum responds

---
[1]Oregon Agricultural Experiment Station Technical Report No. 5574.

to the three forms of vitamin B-6, while S. faecium responds to
pyridoxal (PL) and pyridoxamine (PM), and L. casei to PL only.
Thus these two lactic acid-producing microorganisms were measuring
something in acid-hydrolyzed blood which shows vitamin B-6 activity
for them but not for S. uvarum.

Since more vitamin B-6 activity in blood was obtained with
hydrolysis, Storvick and Peters investigated the effect of varying
the length of hydrolysis time. The results again suggested that
additional vitamin B-6 activity was either released or formed during
hydrolysis for S. faecium and L. casei. These two organisms measured
an increase in apparent vitamin B-6 activity from 30 minutes to a
peak between 10 and 24 hours, and then a decrease and leveling off
by 72 hours. S. uvarum, on the other hand, not only gave much lower
values than the other two organisms, but the peak in vitamin B-6
activity was at 2 hours and then activity decreased sharply to
unmeasurable amounts beyond 10 hours.

Evaluating the responses to these microorganisms to vitamin
B-6 in hydrolyzed blood must take into account the interrelationships
that exist between the nutrients and antagonisms that may occur.
S. uvarum, for example, will synthesize vitamin B-6 if thiamin is
not present in the medium (2). For S. faecium and L. casei, there
is the consideration of the interrelationship between alanine and
vitamin B-6. L. casei can grow in a vitamin B-6-free medium containing relatively large amounts of D-alanine and peptides. In the
absence of vitamin B-6, S. faecium is stimulated by relatively
large amounts of alanine-containing peptides. S. uvarum is
unaffected by the presence of alanine and peptides(3).

Haskell and Wallnofer (4) showed that the increase in apparent
vitamin B-6 activity with length of hydrolysis time, as measured
by S. faecium and L. casei, reflected the increase in D-alanine and
free amino acid content of the blood hydrolysate. D-alanine, which
was not detected in unhydrolyzed blood or in samples hydrolyzed 2
hours or less increased with hydrolysis time between 2 and 20 hours,
suggesting that this isomer was formed from the L-alanine in blood.
The amino groups also increased steadily during hydrolysis. Apparent
vitamin B-6 activity as measured by S. uvarum, did not increase
with length of hydrolysis.

A method using L. casei for the determination of PL in blood
has been developed by Anderson and her associates (5). In this
procedure serum is hydrolyzed with acid for only one hour to
minimize isomerization of L-alanine to D-alanine, and formation of
pyridoxamine from the reaction of PL with amino groups. In addition,
the basal medium was improved with the addition of L-alanine and
L-tryptophan. Assay values are reproducible, in spite of a high
final dilution (1 to 100 or 200). Recovery of pyridoxal added to

the serum was 100%, but conversion of pyridoxal phosphate standards to pyridoxal was not complete, averaging 87%.

The procedure used in our laboratory for determining vitamin B-6 in blood and urine with S. uvarum is presented in detail. Preparation of the reagents and the inoculum are essentially the same as for the AOAC method (6), except that we eliminate the chromotographic step, substitute Difco Vitamin Assay Casamino Acids for acid-hydrolyzed casein in the preparation of the basal medium, use a 6-hour culture instead of a 24-hour one, and read the assay tubes directly in an Evelyn colorimeter.

The standard curves we obtain for the three forms with this procedure are shown in Fig. 1. When the three B-6 vitamers are expressed as free bases, the curves are similar except that there is a lag in the response of the yeast to PM at the lower concentrations.

To extract vitamin B-6 from blood or plasma, the protein is precipitated with 10% trichloroacetic acid (TCA). The precipitate is washed twice with TCA to remove any remaining vitamin B-6. The supernatant and washings are subsequently autoclaved at 121^0 for 30 minutes to remove the TCA and to extract the vitamin B-6. We have designated the values we obtain as "total vitamin B-6" because this treatment is sufficient to cleave the phosphate from pyridoxal phosphate (PLP) almost completely. Recovery of PL, added as PLP to the plasma before precipitation, ranges between 85% and 100%. Recovery of PL added to plasma before the addition of TCA is from 90% to 100%.

In Table 1 typical values for plasma total vitamin B-6 and PLP, as measured with the tyrosine decarboxylase apoenzyme method (7), in ten subjects are compared. Values for plasma total vitamin B-6 are higher than those for pyridoxal phosphate, suggesting that a small portion of the vitamin B-6 in plasma is in the free form.

Plasma total vitamin B-6, which includes both free vitamin B-6 and PLP, is a more sensitive indicator of the absorption of oral loading doses of vitamin B-6 than plasma PLP. This is illustrated in Fig. 2, which shows the changes in plasma total vitamin B-6 and PLP in 5 subjects receiving an oral dose of pyridoxine (PN). Half an hour after the ingestion of 4 mg of PN·HCl the rise in plasma total vitamin B-6 was 3-4 times higher than that of PLP (9).

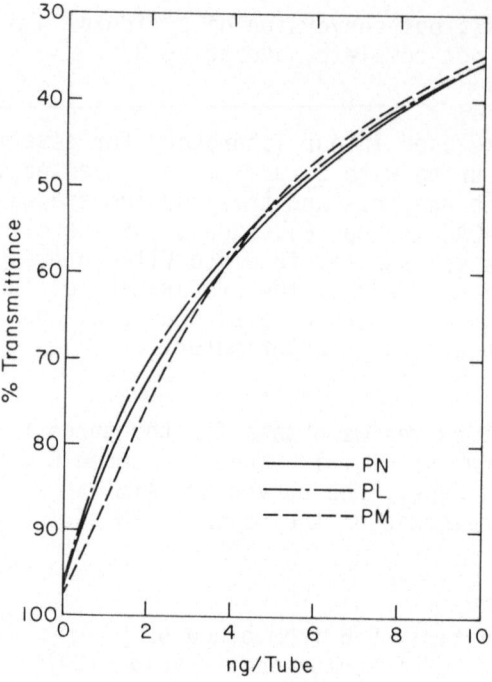

Fig. 1.   The response of S. uvarum to PN, PM, and PL as free bases.
          Instrument was set at 100% transmittance with negative
          blank.

Table 1.   Plasma Total Vitamin B-6 and PLP,
           in nmol/100 ml, in 10 Men (8)

Total B-6[a]	PLP[b]
4.73	3.04
4.97	3.68
4.78	4.41
4.14	3.18
5.73	4.66
4.97	4.04
4.91	4.27
2.60	2.31
3.43	2.54
6.62	4.83

[a]Assayed with S. uvarum.
[b]Determined by tyrosine decarboxylase
apoenzyme method (7).

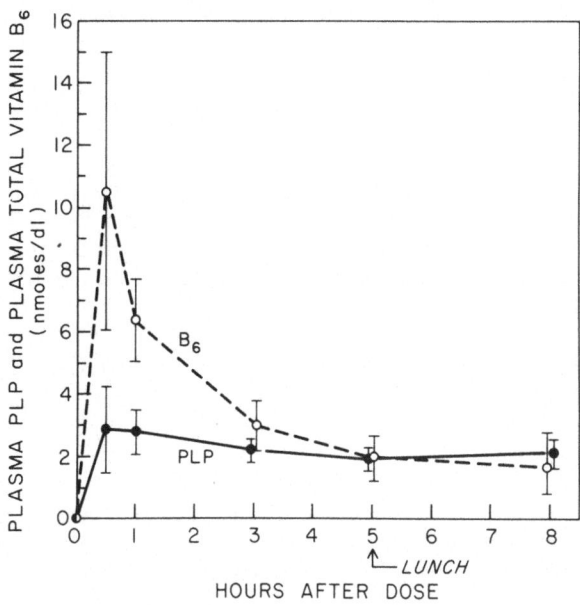

Fig. 2.   Plasma total vitamin B-6 and PLP in 5 subjects to whom
          4 mg of PN·HCl had been administered orally (9).

        S. uvarum is commonly used to measure urinary total and free
vitamin B-6. Total vitamin B-6 is determined in acid-hydrolyzed
urine; free vitamin B-6 is measured in unhydrolyzed urine. The
procedures follow. From Table 2 it can be seen that total vitamin
B-6 content in urine is about 1-1/2 to 2-1/2 times that of free
vitamin B-6. Urinary total and free vitamin B-6 reflect the
dietary intake of the vitamin, which was determined from 3-day
dietary records.

Table 2.   Urinary Free and Total Vitamin B-6
           in 4 Women (10)

| B-6 Intake | Urinary B-6 | | Total/ |
	Free	Total	Free
mg/day	µg/24 hr		ratio
1.9	157	229	1.5
1.6	73	128	1.8
1.8	60	114	1.9
1.0	37	86	2.3

Urine is reported to contain substances that are inhibitory to
S. uvarum (11). We have not experienced this problem. Growth of
the yeast is proportional to the amount of hydrolyzed or unhydrolyzed
urine used and is not depressed by increasing amounts of urine in
the assay tubes. Recovery of PN added to the urine is about 95%.

To summarize, we have given a brief description of the procedures we use to assay plasma and urinary vitamin B-6 with S. uvarum.
Although this method is not specific, it is nevertheless a sensitive
and convenient one for satisfactorily measuring vitamin B-6 status
in population groups.

PROCEDURE FOR ASSAYING VITAMIN B-6 IN BLOOD AND URINE USING S. UVARUM

Reagents

Vitamin solution I. Dissolve 10 mg thiamin and 1 g inositol
in about 200 ml water, and make to 1 liter. Store in refrigerator.
(1 ml = 10 µg thiamin, and 1 mg inositol.)

Vitamin solution II. Dissolve 10 mg biotin in 100 ml 50%
alcohol-water. Store in refrigerator. (1 ml = 100 µg biotin.)

Dissolve 200 mg calcium pantothenate and 200 mg niacin in
about 200 ml water; add 8 ml of the biotin solution, make to 1
liter with water. Store in refrigerator. (1 ml = 200 µg each
calcium pantothenate and niacin, 0.8 µg biotin.)

Salt solution I. Dissolve 17 g KCl, 10.3 g $MgSO_4 \cdot 7H_2O$, 100 mg
$FeCl_3 \cdot 6H_2O$, and 100 mg $MnSO_4 \cdot H_2O$ in about 800 ml water. Add 2 ml
conc HCl. Dissolve 5 g $CaCl_2 \cdot 2H_2O$ in about 100 ml water; add to
the first solution and make to 1 liter with water. Store in
refrigerator. (1 ml = 17 mg KCl, 5.03 mg $MgSO_4$, 50 µg $FeCl_3$,
89.3 µg $MnSO_4$, and 3.77 mg $CaCl_2$).

Salt solution II. Dissolve 22 g KH_2PO_4 and 40 g $(NH_4)_2HPO_4$
in water and make to 1 liter. Store in refrigerator. (1 ml = 22 mg
KH_2PO_4 and 40 mg $(NH_4)_2HPO_4$.)

"Tween 80" solution. Weigh 2.5 g of "Tween 80" in small
beaker. Transfer with warm (45°) water and make to 500 ml volume.
Store in refrigerator. (1 ml = 5 mg "Tween 80".)

1 + 1 citric acid solution. Dissolve 50 g of citric acid in
50 ml of water. Store at room temperature in a bottle with a
plastic stopper.

1 + 2 ammonium phosphate solution. Dissolve 25 g $(NH_4)_2HPO_4$ in 50 ml water. Store at room temperature in a bottle with a plastic stopper.

Citrate buffer solution. Dissolve 100 g potassium citrate and 20 g citric acid and make to 1 liter with water. Store in refrigerator. (1 ml = 100 mg potassium citrate and 20 mg citric acid.)

Basal medium stock solution. To make 1 liter of medium, add the following to about 400 ml water:

        100 ml citrate buffer
         50 ml vitamin solution I
         25 ml vitamin solution II
         50 ml salt solution I
         50 ml salt solution II
         20 ml "Tween 80" solution
         10 g Vitamin Casamino Acids (Difco #0288-02)
        100 g dextrose

Amino acids as listed below dissolved in 10 ml 1N HCl:

         22 mg DL - tryptophan
         27 mg L - histidine hydrochloride
        100 mg DL - methionine
        216 mg DL - isoleucine
        256 mg DL - valine

Adjust to pH 4.5 with 1 + 1 citric acid or 1 + 2 $(NH_4)_2HPO_4$. Make to 1 liter with water. If this is to be used within 24 hours store in refrigerator. Otherwise freeze and thaw when needed. Before using, measure out required amount in a flask, plug with cotton, and steam for 10 minutes.

Preparation of Standard Solutions

1. Stock Standards.
    a. Pyridoxine - 10 µg/ml. Weigh out 12.16 mg PN·HCl and make to 1 liter with 1N HCl.
    b. Pyridoxal - 10 µg/ml. Weigh out 12.77 mg PL·HCl and make to 1 liter with 1N HCl.
    c. Pyridoxamine - 10 µg/ml. Weigh out 14.33 mg PM·2HCl and make to 1 liter with 1N HCl.

These standards are stable for at least one year if stored in brown bottles in the refrigerator.

2. Intermediate Standards - 100 ng/ml. These are prepared on the day of assay. Dilute 1 ml of the desired stock standard to 100 ml with water.

3. Working Standards - 1 or 2 ng/ml. Dilute either 1 or 2 ml of the intermediate standard to 100 ml with water.

Preparation of Inoculum

1. Stock culture. Saccharomyces uvarum (carlsbergensis) 4228 is obtained from American Type Culture Collection as no. 9080 and maintained by transfer on Bacto Lactobacilli Agar AOAC or Bacto-Wort Agar slants at least every three weeks.

Prepare agar according to directions on label, transfer 10 ml of hot agar to culture tubes, plug with cotton, sterilize by auto-claving for 15 minutes at 121^0. Cool in slanted position and then store in refrigerator.

2. Inoculum broth. Pipet 5 ml of basal medium into 18 x 150 mm culture tubes, add 5 ml of a mixture of standards, described below, plug with cotton, autoclave at 121^0 for 10 minutes, cool and store in refrigerator.

The mixture of standards is prepared by adding 0.2 ml of each of the 3 vitamin B-6 stock standards (10 µg/ml) to water and making mixture to 1000 ml.

3. Inoculum rinse. Add 5 ml water and 5 ml basal medium to culture tubes, plug with cotton and sterilize by autoclaving at 121^0 for 15 minutes. Cool. Store in refrigerator.

4. Inoculum. On the day of assay, transfer a loopful of the S. uvarum from an agar slant previously incubated 24 hours at 30^0. Incubate for 6 hours at 30^0. Hold in refrigerator a few hours if necessary. Shortly before it is to be used, centrifuge the culture for 5 minutes and wash twice with 10 ml portions of inoculum rinse. After second washing, centrifuge and resuspend the cells in 10 ml inoculum rinse.

Preparation of Samples

It is imperative to work in subdued light with all solutions containing vitamin B-6.

Blood or plasma. Add slowly with stirring, 2 ml of blood or plasma to 10 ml of 10% trichloroacetic acid (TCA). Allow precipitated sample to stand at room temperature for 30 minutes, stirring it 3-4 times. Centrifuge at top speed for 10 minutes at room temperature. Decant the supernatant into a 50-ml beaker. Resuspend the precipitate in 5 ml of 10% TCA. Centrifuge and add the washing to the supernatant. Repeat this washing step. Autoclave the supernatant and washings at 121° for 30 minutes. When cool, adjust pH of the hydrolysate to 4.5 with dilute KOH. Quantitatively transfer the sample to a 50-ml glass stoppered cylinder, dilute to 40 ml with water and mix.

Urine. Total vitamin B-6 is measured in hydrolyzed urine. Add 10 ml of urine to 50 ml of 0.1 N HCl. Autoclave mixture at 121° for 30 minutes. When cool, adjust the pH of the hydrolysate to 4.5 with KOH, dilute to 100 ml, mix and filter through Whatman no. 1 filter paper.

Hydrolysates can be stored in the refrigerator for assay later. If stored longer than one day, pour a layer of toluene over the sample.

Before assay, dilute hydrolysates to an appropriate volume to obtain a final vitamin B-6 concentration of 1-2 ng/ml.

To determine free vitamin B-6, substitute water for 0.1 N HCl and omit the heating step in the above procedure.

Assay Procedure

The assay is run in Evelyn tubes (21 x 175 mm). Neoprene-coated test tube racks, holding 40 tubes, are used to prevent scratching of tubes. Add 2 glass beads to each tube.

To duplicate tubes, add 0.0, 0.5, 1.0, 2.0, 3.0, 4.0, and 5.0 ml, respectively, of the working standard solution containing either 2 ng/ml of pyridoxine for urine or 1 ng/ml of pyridoxal for blood or plasma. Make volume in each tube up to 5 ml with water. Tubes containing no standard serve as positive blanks.

Add 1.0, 2.0, 3.0, 4.0, and 5.0 ml, respectively, of diluted samples containing approximately 1 or 2 ng of vitamin B-6/ml to duplicate or triplicate tubes and make up to 5 ml with water. Insert two tubes containing 5 ml water for negative blanks. Tubes are covered with a rectangle of cotton about one-half inch thick, cut somewhat larger than the surface of the rack and wrapped in cloth. This cover is secured with rubber bands. Tubes may be plugged with cotton if preferred.

Autoclave the entire assay at 121^0 for 10 minutes. When cool, add aseptically to each tube 5 ml of basal medium which has been previously steamed for 10 minutes and cooled. A syringe mounted in a holder and adjusted to deliver 5 ml is convenient for this addition.

Inoculate each tube except the negative blanks with one drop of freshly prepared inoculum. This can easily be done using a syringe mounted on a ring stand and fitted with a no. 24 hypodermic needle, which delivers about 100 drops/ml inoculum.

Incubate the assay tubes in a rotary shaker at 30^0 for 22 hours. Steam the assy tubes for 5 minutes to stop growth. Cool. Mix each tube well to suspend the cells evenly and read percent transmittance in an Evelyn colorimeter with a 660 nm filter. Adjust instrument to read 100% transmittance with the negative blank. Read positive blanks and then use one to reset the instrument at 100% transmittance for reading the remaining tubes.

Plot percent transmittance values of the standard tubes against ng/tube of standard. Determine ng vitamin B-6 in each sample tube by reference to this curve. Divide ng value of each sample tube by ml of sample. Average ng/ml sample values from the 5 levels and multiply by the dilution factor to obtain ng/ml blood or urine.

ACKNOWLEDGMENTS

We wish to acknowledge the support of Oregon Agricultural Experiment Station funds and USDA Grant No. 616-15-177.

LITERATURE CITED

1. Storvick, C. A. & Peters, J. M. (1964) Methods for the determination of vitamin B-6 in biological materials. Vit. and Hormones 22, 833-854.
2. Rabinowitz, J. C. & Snell, E. E. (1951) The nature of the requirement of Saccharomyces carlsbergensis for vitamin B-6. Arch. Biochem. Biophys. 33, 472-481.
3. Haskell, B. E. & Snell, E. E. (1970) Microbiological determination of the vitamin B-6 group. In: Methods in Enzymology (McCormick, D. B. & Wright, L. D., eds.), vol. 18A, pp. 512-519, Academic Press, New York.
4. Haskell, B. E. & Wallnofer, U. (1967) D-Alanine interference in microbiological assays of vitamin B-6 in human blood. Anal. Biochem. 19, 569-577.
5. Anderson, B. A., Peart, M. B. & Fulford-Jones, C. E. (1970) The measurement of serum pyridoxal by a microbiological assay using Lactobacillus casei. J. Clin. Pathol. 23, 232-242.

6. Horwitz, W., ed. (1980) Official Methods of Analysis of
    the Assoc. Off. Anal. Chem., 13th ed., pp. 768-769,
    Washington, DC.
7. Rose, D. P. (1974) Assessment of tryptophan metabolism and
    vitamin B-6 nutrition in pregnancy and oral contraceptive users.
    In: Biochemistry of Women: Methods for Clinical Investigation
    (Curry, A. S. and Hewitt, J. V., ed.), pp. 317-349, C.R.C.
    Press, Inc., Cleveland, OH.
8. Lindberg, A. S. (1980) The effect of wheat bran on the bio-
    availability of vitamin B-6 in humans. M.S. Thesis, Oregon
    State University.
9. Wozenski, J. R., Leklem, J. E. & Miller, L. T. (1980) The
    metabolism of small doses of vitamin B-6 in men. J. Nutr.
    110, 275-285.
10. Miller, L. T., Dow, M. J. & Kokkeler, S. C. (1978) Methionine
    metabolism and vitamin B-6 status in women using oral contra-
    ceptives. Am. J. Clin. Nutr. 31, 619-625.
11. Rabinowitz, J. C. & Snell, E. E. (1949) Vitamin B-6 group.
    XV. Urinary excretion of pyridoxal, pyridoxamine, pyridoxine,
    and 4-pyridoxic acid in human subjects. Proc. Soc. Exp. Biol.
    Med. 70, 235-240.

MICROASSAY OF PYRIDOXAL PHOSPHATE USING TYROSINE APODECARBOXYLASE

Lawrence Lumeng, Alec Lui and Ting-Kai Li

VA Medical Center and Departments of
Medicine and Biochemistry
Indiana University School of Medicine
Indianapolis, IN 46223

Pyridoxal 5'-phosphate (PLP) assay based on the coenzyme-
dependent decarboxylation of L-tyrosine by tyrosine apodecarboxylase
(EC 4.1.1.25) was the first enzymatic method developed in vitamin
B-6 analysis. Originally isolated from Streptococcus faecalis
and partially purified by Epps (1) in 1944, this apoenzyme was
subsequently used by Umbreit et al. (2) and Baddiley and Gale (3)
to identify the coenzyme role of PLP in decarboxylation reactions.
In these early studies, manometry was employed to follow the
generation of CO_2 as a function of PLP and sensitivity was low.
Although sensitivity was later improved by making certain rearrange-
ments and mechanical changes in the assay system (4,5), it was
still insufficient to detect PLP concentrations below 10 ng/ml of
plasma.

In 1962, Hamfelt (6) introduced a new approach to PLP assay
with tyrosine apodecarboxylase by use of uniformly labeled (^{14}C)-
tyrosine as substrate and isolation of (^{14}C)tyramine on paper
chromatography. This approach greatly improved sensitivity and
allowed determinations of PLP in small samples; however, the isolation of (^{14}C)tyramine by paper chromatography was cumbersome.
In 1968, Maruyama and Coursin (7) modified the procedure by using
(1-^{14}C)tyrosine. Accordingly, the rate of decarboxylation of
(1-^{14}C)tyrosine was measured by determining the residual radioactive counts in the reaction mixture after chasing away the $^{14}CO_2$.
Sundaresan and Coursin (8) subsequently improved their method by
trapping the $^{14}CO_2$ in alkali. In 1970, Chabner and Livingston (9)
further refined the assay procedure by partially purifying the
tyrosine apodecarboxylase approximately 60-fold before use.

The method described in this paper is based on those reported by Sundaresan and Coursin (8) and Chabner and Livingston (9). The major features of the method include: deproteinization of assay samples with trichloroacetic acid (TCA) followed by extraction of TCA with diethyl ether, partial purification of a commercially available apoenzyme isolated from S. faecalis to eliminate con-taminating pyridoxal kinase, the use of citrate as buffer and the use of a higher concentration of L-tyrosine. We have used this method successfully to assay the PLP content of blood plasma, liver, brain, and skeletal muscle (10-12). We have also compared results obtained by this method with those by chromatographic separation and fluorometric assay (13) and investigated in detail the ability of TCA to extract PLP from blood plasma.

REAGENTS

L-(1-^{14}C)tyrosine solution: 10.5 mM in 0.1 M sodium citrate buffer pH 6.0 (specific radioactivity, 23 µCi/mmol). This solution is heated to 80° to solubilize the tyrosine and is kept at 58°-62° until use.

PLP standard solution, 20 ng/ml, in 0.1 M sodium citrate buffer, pH 6.0. The concentration of PLP is determined by its molar absorptivity, ε_{388} = 6600 M^{-1} cm^{-1} in 0.1 M NaOH (14).

Methyl benzethonium hydroxide, 1M in methanol.

Fluoralloy TLA, 32.2 g in 2.5 liters of toluene and 1.25 liters of methoxyethanol. Fluoralloy TLA (Beckman Instrument, Inc.) is a mixture of 30.3 g of 2-(4'-tert-butylphenyl)-5-(4"-biphenyly)-1,3,4-oxadiazole and 1.9 g of 2-(4'-biphenylyl)-6-phenylbenzoxazole.

Tyrosine apodecarboxylase, about 100 U/ml; diluted 1:10 in 0.3 M sodium citrate buffer, pH 6.0, immediately before use.

Sodium citrate buffers, 0.1 M and 0.3 M, pH 6.0.

Hydrochloric acid, 5 M.

TCA, 75%

Peroxide-free diethyl ether, water-saturated.

PROCEDURE

PLP assay is performed in 25 ml Erlenmeyer flasks fitted with stoppers and center wells supplied by Kontes Glass Co. (Cat. no. K882310 and K882320). For the standard curve, the reaction mixture contains 0.1 ml of tyrosine apodecarboxylase (about 1 U), 0-0.2 ml

(0-4 ng) of the PLP standard solution, 1.0 ml of L-(1-^{14}C)tyrosine
solution and 0.1-0.3 ml of the 0.1 M sodium citrate buffer (pH 6.0)
in a final volume of 1.4 ml. For the unknown samples, the reaction
mixture contains 0.1 ml of the apoenzyme, 0.1 ml of an unknown
sample, 1.0 ml of L-(1-^{14}C)tyrosine solution, 0.1 ml of the 0.3 M
sodium citrate buffer (pH 6.0) and 0.1 ml of water. Before the
addition of L-(1-^{14}C)tyrosine, the flasks are preincubated for 30
minutes at room temperature to permit reconstitution of the holoenzyme. The reaction is started by adding L-(1-^{14}C)tyrosine, and
the flasks are immediately capped with rubber stoppers fitted with
center wells. The center wells contain a folded filter paper and
0.2 ml of methyl benzethonium hydroxide in methanol. The flasks
are then incubated at 32^{0} in a Dubnoff shaking water bath for 20
minutes, and the reaction is terminated by injection of 1 ml of 5 M
HCl through the stopper. To ensure complete trapping of ^{14}CO$_2$
after acidification, the flasks are incubated for an additional 60
minutes at 32^{0}. The stopper and center well are then removed and
the well and its contents are put into a counting vial containing
5 ml or 20 ml of the Fluoralloy scintillation fluid. ^{14}CO$_2$ is
counted in a liquid scintillation spectrometer. The efficiency of
this ^{14}CO$_2$ trapping system is close to 100%. All the assays are
performed in duplicate. The reaction flasks and samples are protected from natural light by the use of darkened room and yellow
fluorescent lights in order to avoid photolysis of PLP.

Preparation of the L-(1-^{14}C)Tyrosine Solution

L-tyrosine, 1.2 g, is dissolved in 1.2 liter of 0.1 M sodium
citrate buffer, pH 6.0, by heating to 80^{0}. This solution is
filtered through filter paper under vacuum. To 1 liter of this
warm solution, 1.13 g of L-tyrosine in 125 ml of 0.15 M HCl is
added and the solution refiltered. Then 250 µCi of L-(1-^{14}C)tyrosine,
40-60 mCi/mmol (New England Nuclear Corp., Boston, MA), is added.

Preparation of Tyrosine Apodecarboxylase

All steps are carried out at near 0^{0}. One g of commercially
available, dried S. faecalis cells grown in pyridoxine-deficient
medium (Sigma Chemical Co., St. Louis, MO, or Worthington Biochemical
Corp., Bedford, MA; 1 mg will release 300-400 µl of CO$_2$ in 30 minutes
at pH 5.5 and 37^{0} in the presence of added excess PLP) is suspended
in 10 ml of 10 mM sodium citrate buffer, pH 6.0. This suspension
is then homogenized in a Potter-Elvehjem teflon-glass homogenizer

and centrifuged at 25,000 x g for 10 minutes. The supernatant
fraction is collected and the pellet is resuspended in another 10
ml of 10 mM sodium citrate buffer. The resultant suspension is
then sonicated for 6 minutes (6 pulse of 1 minute) with a Savant
model 500 Insonator (0.5-inch sonohorn) at an output meter setting
of 75. These steps involving centrifugation, resuspension, and
sonication are repeated 5 times and 60 ml of supernatant solution
are collected. The supernatant solution is brought to 60% saturation by adding solid $(NH_4)_2SO_4$ with mechanical stirring (390 g/l).
The suspension is centrifuged at 25,000 x g for 20 minutes and the
precipitate is discarded. The supernatant solution is brought to
85% saturation with $(NH_4)_2SO_4$ (183 g/l), and the precipitate containing most of the tyrosine apodecarboxylase activity is redissolved
in 5 ml of a solution of 0.3 M sodium citrate, pH 6.0, 24% (v/v)
glycerol, and 2 mM mercaptoethanol. The enzyme suspension is then
dialyzed overnight against two changes of 1 liter of the same buffer.
This partially purified apoenzyme, usually 8-12 U/mg protein and
about 100 U/ml (1 unit is defined as the amount of enzyme that
catalyzes the decarboxylation of 1 μmol of tyrosine per minute in
the presence of excess PLP under the conditions of the assay
described above), is stable at -20° for several months.

Standard Curve

Under the conditions of the assay described above, the rate
of $^{14}CO_2$ generation is constant for at least 20 minutes. The rate
of production of $^{14}CO_2$ remains a linear function of PLP concentration up to 4 ng (Fig. 1).

PROPERTIES OF TYROSINE APODECARBOXYLASE

The tyrosine apodecarboxylase prepared by the above method is
free of pyridoxal kinase. Thus, the apoenzyme is specific for PLP
even when ATP is concurrently present (Table 1). Although Chabner
and Livingston (9) had further purified the apoenzyme by means of
Sephadex G-200 chromatography, this added step is not essential
for the purpose of PLP assay.

Allenmark and Servenius (15) have recently characterized this
enzyme by isoelectric focusing and purified it by chromatography
on phenyl-sepharose. They reported that the enzyme from S. faecalis
is heterogeneous, with one form exhibiting a pI of 4.5 and another,
pI of 3.2. Based on Sephadex G-200 chromatography, the molecular
weight is about 200,000 (9).

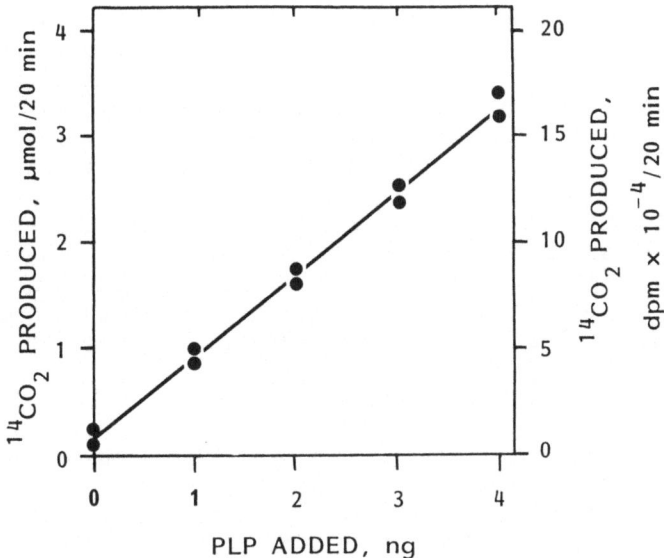

Fig. 1. Standard curve in PLP assay by tyrosine apodecarboxylase.

Table 1. Specificity of PLP Assay by
Tyrosine Apodecarboxylase

B-6 Vitamer (3 ng) Added	ATP-Zn^{2+} Added	$^{14}CO_2$ Produced
	mM	μmol/20 min
-	-	0.08
PLP	-	2.24
PMP	-	0.12
PN	-	0.06
PL	-	0.07
PM	-	0.07
PN	1	0.07
PL	1	0.09
PM	1	0.08

The kinetic properties of tyrosine apodecarboxylase have been determined only with partially purified apoenzyme preparations.   The pH optimum is 5.5; and at pH 6.0, the activity is decreased to half of that at pH 5.5 (1).   The Km for L-tyrosine is in the range of 0.6-1.66 mM (8,9) and for PLP, 0.17 μM (8).   Sulfate (4), trichloro-acetic acid (2), Ag^+, Cu^{2+}, Hg^{2+}, Fe^{2+}, Fe^{3+}, Pb^{2+}, KCN, NH_2OH, and N_2H_4 (1) are known inhibitors of tyrosine decarboxylase.   Acetate and citrate solutions are suitable buffers for assaying this enzyme, although the activity is 14% lower in citrate buffer (1).

In the present method, PLP assay is performed in citrate buffer at pH 6.0 because L-tyrosine is more soluble at this pH than pH 5.5 and citrate buffer has a higher buffer capacity than acetate at pH 6.0.   These modifications allow the use of a high concentration (i.e. 7.5 mM) of L-tyrosine as substrate in the reaction.

PREPARATION OF BIOLOGICAL SAMPLES

Venous blood samples are collected in 2 mM sodium EDTA (pH 7.4) as anticoagulant and plasma is separated by centrifugation.   To 1.8 ml of plasma, 0.2 ml of 75% TCA is added and is mixed thoroughly on a Vortex mixer.   The treated samples are then heated to 37° for 10 minutes and centrifuged for 15 minutes at 18,000 x g and 4°. The clear supernatant is collected and is extracted with 4 volumes of water-saturated diethyl ether 4 times.   Residual ether is then evaporated with a jet of air.   The final pH of the samples should be $\gtrsim 4.5$.

Samples of liver and skeletal muscle, approximately 0.1 g in size, are weighed and put individually into 10 ml of cold sodium phosphate buffer (pH 7.4, 80 mM).   These samples are immediately homogenized by means of a Polytron PT 20 homogenizer at a power setting of 6 for 30 seconds.   Aliquots of the homogenate, 0.5 ml, were added to 1.3 ml of water and 0.2 ml of 75% TCA.   This mixture is then centrifuged at 18,000 x g for 15 minutes and the super-natant is extracted with ether.

The whole brain of each rat is quickly removed after decapi-tation and weighed.   It is then homogenized in 20 ml of water and 1.7 ml of 10% metaphosphoric acid with a Potter-Elvehjem tissue grinder.   The brain homogenate is then heated to 80° for 15 minutes and centrifuged at 18,000 x g for 15 min.

Precision of the Method

For the determination of PLP in blood plasma, the within-run precision expressed as coefficient of variation is 7.0% (23.5 $\pm$ 1.6 ng/ml, mean value $\pm$ SD, n = 12).   The between-run precision is 7.9% (n = 12).

Recovery of PLP Added In Vitro

Table 2 summarizes the ability of TCA to extract PLP from blood plasma, liver, brain, and skeletal muscle. The recovery of added authentic PLP exceeded 90% in all instances. These results are considerably higher than the recovery values of 68-69% for plasma PLP reported by Srivastava and Beutler (16).

Recovery of Plasma (^{14}C)PLP in Experiments In Vivo

It is known that the ingestion of pyridoxine in man raises significantly the plasma content of PLP, PA, and PL (13). Additionally, in isolated rat hepatocytes, the addition of (^{14}C)PN to the incubation suspension results in rapid conversion of this B-6 vitamer to radiolabeled PLP, PA, and PL and leads to release of these radioactive compounds into the medium (13). Accordingly, the completeness of TCA extraction of endogenously synthesized PLP in plasma was evaluated by injecting (^{14}C)PN into rats and determining the ability to recover (^{14}C)PLP from blood plasma after deproteinization.

(4,5-^{14}C)PN (12 μCi/μmol) (Amersham Corp., Arlington Heights, IL), 1 μmol, was injected intraperitoneally into each of 4 rats and 30 minutes later, venous blood was collected in 2 mM EDTA and the plasma separated. The plasma samples were then deproteinized by adding 1.8 ml aliquots to 0.2 ml of 75% TCA. After incubation at 37° for 10 minutes and centrifugation, the TCA in the supernatant fraction was extracted by diethyl ether. The protein precipitate was washed 3 times with 7.5% TCA and the washings were collected.

Table 2. Recovery of PLP Added In Vitro

Tissue or Body Fluid (n)	PLP, ng/sample Endogenous	Added	% Recovery of Added PLP
Liver (8)	212-325[a]	600	104 $\pm$ 6[b]
Brain (15)	286-495	600	90 $\pm$ 14
Muscle (5)	165-427	600	111 $\pm$ 2
Irradiated Blood Plasma (12)[c]	1.8-5.3	40.	96 $\pm$ 8

[a]Range.
[b]Mean value $\pm$ SD.
[c]Irradiated 8 hours at room temperature in an open Petri dish under a long wave-length UV lamp.

Finally, the precipitated protein pellet was redissolved in NaOH.
Based on scintillation counting (Table 3, experiment A), 99% of
the radioactive counts in plasma was in the supernatant fraction
and the washings. The (^{14}C)-labeled B-6 compounds in the supernatant
fraction were then separated by cation-exchange chromatography (13).

Table 3. Extraction of (^{14}C)PLP from Blood Plasma

	Experiment[a]	
	A	B
% of counts[b] in extraction fractions:		
Supernatant fraction	68.5 + 2.4[c]	68.0 + 2.7
Washings	30.5 + 2.3	30.2 + 2.6
Protein precipitate	1.0 + 0	1.8 + 0.2
% of counts in B-6 compounds:		
PLP	48.0 + 2.9	55.5 + 3.9
PA	9.1 + 0.9	6.5 + 0.7
PMP	4.2 + 0.5	4.8 + 3.9
PL	28.2 + 2.1	29.6 + 3.8
PN	9.5 + 2.4	2.6 + 0.8
PM	1.0 + 0.2	1.0 + 0.2
Mean counts as (^{14}C)PLP in supernatant fraction and washings	2.17×10^5	2.02×10^5
Mean counts in protein precipitate	5.88×10^3	6.76×10^3
% (^{14}C)PLP extracted by TCA	97.4	96.8

[a] n = 4 for each experiment.
[b] dpm.
[c] mean value + SD.

The distribution of counts in PLP, PA, PMP, PL, PN, and PM was 48,
9, 4, 28, 10 and 1% respectively. If it is assumed that only
PLP is tightly bound to plasma proteins, the completeness of PLP
extraction from plasma by TCA was calculated to be 97.4%.

It is known that PLP in plasma is bound principally to albumin (17) and that this binding process is time-dependent (18). For this reason, in experiment B, Table 3, the plasma collected from (^{14}C)PN injected rats was incubated for 22 hours at 25^0 before deproteinization with TCA. As shown in Table 3, the calculated recovery of (^{14}C)PLP in this experiment was 96.8%.

In both experiments A and B, about 30% of the counts in the TCA-treated plasma was in the washings of the precipitated protein. This observation could be explained by either a lack of extraction of protein-bound (^{14}C) PLP or mere entrapment of (^{14}C)-labeled B-6 compounds in the interstices of the precipitated protein pellet. In order to distinguish between these possibilities, another experiment was performed by adding ^{3}H$_2$O to plasma before TCA treatment, centrifugation, and washing. The results of this experiment indicates that $23.3 \pm 0.9\%$ of the tritium count was in the washings and the remainder was in the supernatant fraction. These data, therefore, indicate that TCA is effective in extracting PLP from plasma proteins but a significant portion of the extracted PLP remains entrapped in the interstices of the precipitated protein after centrifugation. It should be emphasized that in the procedure for plasma PLP determination, the usual calculation[1] takes this finding into account.

COMPARISON OF PLP ASSAYS BY TYROSINE APODECARBOXYLASE AND BY FLUOROMETRIC ANALYSIS AFTER CHROMATOGRAPHIC SEPARATION

In the course of experiments which examined the metabolism of PN by isolated rat hepatocytes, the PLP content in the cells and medium was analyzed. The analysis was performed by direct assay with tyrosine apodecarboxylase and by fluorometric analysis (13) after chromatographic separation. These experiments provided the opportunity to compare directly in the same sample the two methods of PLP assay. The results shown in Fig. 2 indicate a close agreement between the two methods of PLP assay.

---

[1]In the process of plasma PLP determination, 1.8 ml of plasma is mixed with 0.2 ml of 75% TCA, yielding a final volume of 2.0 ml. After centrifugation and ether extraction of the supernatant fraction, a 0.1 ml aliquot is used for assay. In calculating the plasma PLP concentration, the amount of PLP assayed in the 0.1 ml aliquot is multiplied by a factor 2.0/1.8. This factor explicitly assumes that in the 2 ml of supernatant fraction and protein precipitate, PLP is distributed evenly both in the supernatant fraction and the precipitated protein pellet.

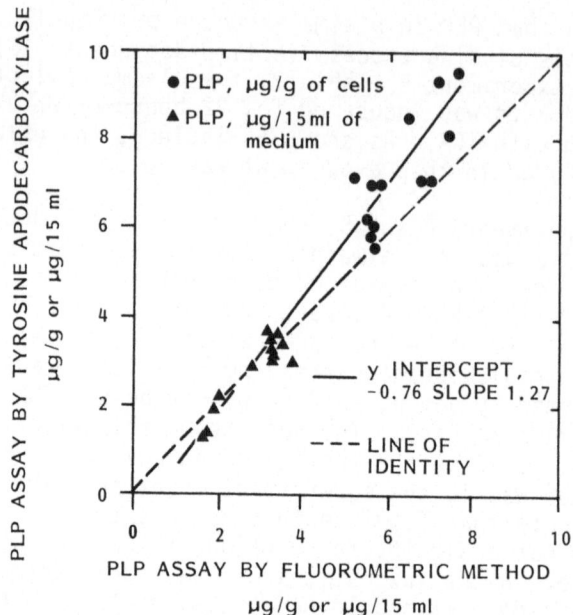

Fig. 2.   Comparison of PLP assayed by tyrosine apodecarboxylase
          and by fluorometric method in cultured cells and in the
          growth medium.

LITERATURE CITED

1. Epps, H. M. R. (1944) Studies on bacterial amino-acid
    decarboxylases. 2. 1(-)-Tyrosine decarboxylase from
    Streptococcus faecalis. Biochem. J. 38, 242-249.
2. Umbreit, W. W., Bellamy, W. D. & Gunsalus, I. C. (1945) The
    function of pyridoxin derivatives: A comparison of natural
    and synthetic codecarboxylase. Arch. Biochem. Biophys. 7,
    185-199.
3. Baddiley, J. & Gale, E. F. (1945) Codecarboxylase function
    of 'pyridoxal phosphate'. Nature 155, 727-728.
4. Sloane-Stanley, G. H. (1949) The use of tyrosine apodecar-
    boxylase of Streptococcus faecalis R for the estimation of
    codecarboxylase. Biochem. J. 44, 567-573.
5. Boxer, G. E., Pruss, M. P. & Goodhart, R. S. (1957) Pyridoxal-
    5-phosphoric acid in whole blood and isolated leukocytes of
    man and animals. J. Nutr. 63, 623-636.
6. Hamfelt, A. (1962) A method of determining pyridoxal phosphate
    in blood by decarboxylation of L-tyrosine-[14]C (U). Clin. Chim.
    Acta 7, 746-748.

7. Maruyama, H. & Coursin, D. B. (1968) Enzymic assay of pyridoxal phosphate using tyrosine apodecarboxylase and tyrosine-1-^{14}C. Anal. Biochem. 26, 420-429.
8. Sundaresan, P. R. & Coursin, D. B. (1970) Microassay of pyridoxal phosphate using L-tyrosine-1-^{14}C and tyrosine apodecarboxylase. Methods in Enzymol. 18, 509-512.
9. Chabner, B. & Livingston, D. (1970) A simple enzyme assay for pyridoxal phosphate. Anal. Biochem. 34, 413-423.
10. Lumeng, L. & Li, T.-K. (1974) Vitamin B-6 metabolism in chronic alcohol abuse: Pyridoxal phosphate levels in plasma and the effects of acetaldehyde on pyridoxal phosphate synthesis and degradation in human erythrocytes. J. Clin. Invest. 53, 693-704.
11. Li, T.-K., Lumeng, L. & Veitch, R. L. (1974) Regulation of pyridoxal 5'-phosphate metabolism in liver. Biochem. Biophys. Res. Commun. 61, 677-684.
12. Lumeng, L., Ryan, M. P. & Li, T.-K. (1978) Validation of the diagnostic value of plasma pyridoxal 5'-phosphate measurements in vitamin B-6 nutrition of the rat. J. Nutr. 108, 545-553.
13. Lumeng, L., Lui, A. & Li, T.-K. (1980) Plasma content of B-6 vitamers and its relationship to hepatic vitamin B-6 metabolism. J. Clin. Invest. 66, 688-695.
14. Peterson, E. A. & Sober, H. A. (1954) Preparation of crystalline phosphorylated derivatives of vitamin B-6. J. Am. Chem. Soc. 76, 169-175.
15. Allenmark, S. & Servenius, B. (1978) Characterization of bacterial L-levo tyrosine decarboxylase EC-4.1.1.25 by iso-electric focusing and gel chromatography. J. Chromatogr. 153, 239-246.
16. Srivastava, S. K. & Beutler, E. (1973) A new fluorometric method for the determination of pyridoxal 5'-phosphate. Biochem. Biophys. Acta 304, 765-773.
17. Lumeng, L., Brashear, R. E. & Li, T.-K. (1974) Pyridoxal 5'-phosphate in plasma: Source, protein-binding and cellular transport. J. Lab. Clin. Med. 84, 334-343.
18. Dempsey, W. B. & Christensen, H. N. (1962) The specific binding of pyridoxal 5'-phosphate to bovine plasma albumin. J. Biol. Chem. 237, 1112-1120.

AN IMPROVED COLORIMETRIC ASSAY FOR PYRIDOXAL PHOSPHATE USING HIGHLY PURIFIED APOTRYPTOPHANASE

Betty E. Haskell

Department of Home Economics
University of Texas
Austin, TX 78712

Methods for the analysis of pyridoxal phosphate, the principal cofactor form of vitamin B-6, have achieved new importance with the demonstration that levels of the coenzyme in serum constitute a useful test of vitamin B-6 nutritional status (1). Enzymic assays are among the most satisfactory for measuring pyridoxal phosphate in biological samples for several reasons: 1) they are highly specific, 2) they permit quantification of pyridoxal phosphate at the level of 10^{-11} moles, and 3) the analyses work well in crude biological extracts without prior isolation or purification.

Enzymic assays for pyridoxal phosphate depend on the ability of this cofactor to restore activity to a purified apoenzyme. In the presence of excess apoenzyme and substrate, the amount of product formed is directly proportional to the amount of pyridoxal phosphate in sample or standard.

It is interesting that the first enzymic assay for pyridoxal phosphate was developed before the structure of this vitamin B-6 coenzyme was known. Umbreit and co-workers in 1945 (2) described a Warburg assay for "codecarboxylase" based on the ability of natural or synthetic coenzyme to restore activity to the apoenzyme of tyrosine decarboxylase. The apoenzyme was isolated from cells of Streptococcus faecalis R grown in a vitamin B-6-deficient medium. At the time this paper was written, it was not known whether phosphate was an integral part of "codecarboxylase" or a contaminant. The tyrosine apodecarboxylase assay for pyridoxal phosphate is widely used today.

This paper deals with an enzymic assay for pyridoxal phosphate which uses a highly purified apotryptophanase from Escherichia coli B/1t7A. The assay depends on the following sequence of reactions:

apotryptophanase ——————————→holoenzyme
                          pyridoxal
                          phosphate

L-tryptophan + water ——————→pyruvic acid + indole + ammonia
                          holoenzyme

                Ehrlich reagent
indole ——————————————————————→absorbance at 570 nm

The assay is specific for pyridoxal phosphate. Other forms
of vitamin B-6, alone or in combination with ATP, have no activity.

The assay quantifies as little as 10 picomoles pyridoxal
phosphate in a final volume of 5.0 ml. Thus, this colorimetric
assay is comparable in sensitivity to methods using radioactive
substrates (3).

An advantage of the apotryptophanase assay is that the apoenzyme is easily obtained pure and free of detectable pyridoxal
phosphate. Isolation of the enzyme can be accomplished in a single
working day. Depending on the care exercised in the final ammonium
sulfate precipitation, the apoenzyme is obtained in crystalline
form (12 units/mg protein) or as a highly active ammonium sulfate
precipitate (0.75 units/mg protein). One unit is the amount of
enzyme that produces 1 micromole of indole per minute at saturating
substrate and pyridoxal phosphate concentrations (4). Both crystalline and non-crystalline preparations usually contain no
detectable pyridoxal phosphate and give excellent results in the
assay described here. The enzyme is stable several months at 4^0
as an ammonium sulfate precipitate or when lyophilized and stored
at 4^0.

The apotryptophanase assay for pyridoxal phosphate is less
sensitive to inhibition by sulfate ion than is the tyrosine
apodecarboxylase assay. Tyrosine apodecarboxylase is inhibited 47%
by 3.3×10^{-3} M sulfate (5). When apotryptophanase was assayed in
the presence of excess (0.6 μg) pyridoxal phosphate, the concentration of ammonium sulfate required to inhibit indole formation by
50% was 0.3 M. Zinc in concentrations up to 12 μM did not interfere
with quantification of pyridoxal phosphate by the apotryptophanase
method. Potassium chloride (0.2 M) or sodium chloride (0.2 M)
inhibited pyridoxal phosphate estimation by the apotryptophanase
method by 9.5% and 12.0% respectively (3).

A disadvantage of the assay is that apotryptophanase of suitable activity and purity is not commercially available. E. coli B/lt7A, a strain constituitive for tryptophanase, is available from American Type Culture Collection (ATCC 27553). Apotryptophanase is isolated from E. coli B/lt7A cells grown under carefully controlled culture conditions which increase the tryptophanase content to approximately 10% of the soluble cellular protein. To retain the genetic characteristics of the strain, cells must be maintained on slants prepared from the following medium: (g/liter) KH_2PO_4, 3.0; $K_2HPO_4 \cdot 3 H_2O$, 9.5; ammonium sulfate, 1.0; calcium chloride$\cdot$2 H_2O, 0.01; ferrous sulfate$\cdot$7 H_2O, 0.1; glucose, 1.0; indole, 0.01; agar, 20 (4).

The apotryptophanase assay described here represents an adaptation of the tryptophanase assay of Morino and Snell (4) to the quantitative determination of pyridoxal phosphate. The assay consists of three separate steps:

1) preincubation of apoenzyme with pyridoxal phosphate
2) incubation of the holoenzyme with substrate
3) colorimetric determination of the product of the reaction

The assay described here is simpler than earlier methods (6-10) in that all three steps are carried out in a single flask.

Regarding step 1, preincubation of apoenzyme with pyridoxal phosphate is necessary to allow reassociation of apoenzyme with cofactor. That 20 minutes is adequate for this purpose as indicated by Fig. 1. It is critical to the success of the assay that samples be protected from light. Dilute solutions of pyridoxal phosphate rapidly lose the ability to restore activity to apotryptophanase when exposed to ordinary laboratory light, but are stable in red light (Table 1).

Regarding step 2, assay of the reconstituted tryptophanase is initiated by adding L-tryptophan. Indole, the product of the reaction, inhibits tryptophanase (6). To minimize product inhibition, the enzyme reaction mixture is layered with toluene which is intended to extract indole from the aqueous phase as it is formed. The assay is linear to about 60 nanomoles of indole.

Regarding step 3, indole is estimated colorimetrically with Ehrlich reagent. Usually, the reagent forms a single phase with the toluene and aqueous layers. Color development is complete in 20 minutes and is stable for 24 hours (10).

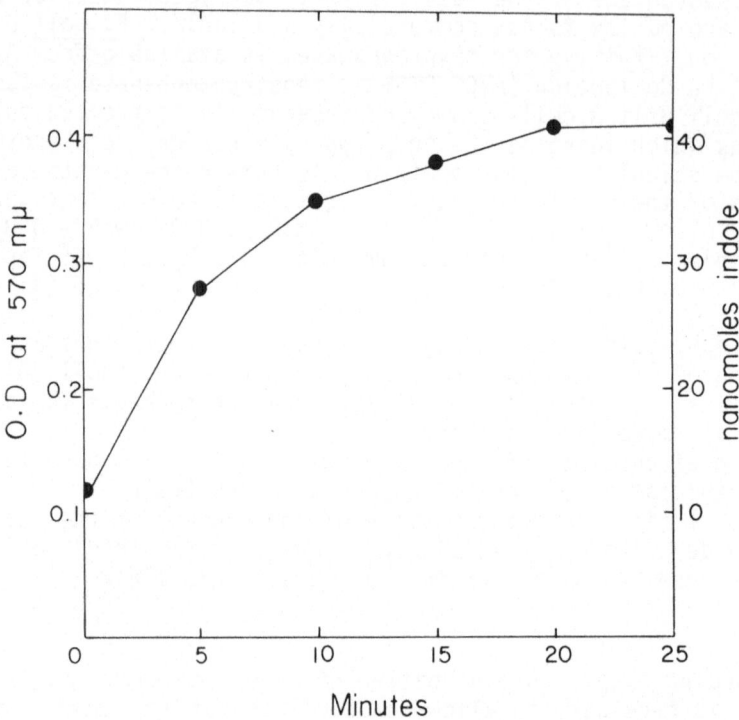

Fig. 1.   Effect of time of preincubation of pyridoxal phosphate
          with apoenzyme on indole formation. Apotryptophanase
          (0.04 units per flask) was incubated at 37° with gentle
          shaking with 120 ng pyridoxal phosphate for varying
          lengths of time prior to addition of substrate. The
          yield of indole was determined colormetrically.

Table 1.   Effect of Light on Stability of 0.1M
           Pyridoxal Phosphate

Time of Preincubation with Apoenzyme	O. D. at 570 nm	
	Red Light	Ordinary Light
min		
20	0.53	0.25
25	0.52	0.20
30	0.54	0.15
35	0.52	0.13
45	--	0.10

Typical standard curves for the assay of pyridoxal phosphate with apotryptophanase are shown (Fig. 2). Depending on time of incubation with substrate (step 2), the assay is suitable for use in the range of 3 to 15 ng or 60 to 140 ng in a final volume of 5.0 ml. For reasons that are not known, the response of the apoenzyme to added pyridoxal phosphate varies from one enzyme preparation to another, and also, it may change as the enzyme ages. Thus, a standard curve should be run daily.

The apotryptophanase assay is satisfactory for use in connection with the assay of two enzymes whose product is pyridoxal phosphate: pyridoxal phosphokinase (ATP: pyridoxal 5'-phosphotransferase EC 2.7.1.35) (9) and pyridoxamine phosphate oxidase (pyridoxamine phosphate: oxygen oxidoreductase deaminating EC 1.4.3.5) (11). It may also be used to measure pyridoxal phosphate in neutralized perchloric acid extracts of tissue prepared as described by Bain and Williams (12). Recovery of pyridoxal phosphate standard added either to enzyme reaction mixtures or to tissue extracts was quantitative (92% to 96.5%) (3).

The colorimetric assay described here is only one of several possible approaches to the use of apotryptophanase in the quantification of pyridoxal phosphate. Tryptophanase is capable of degrading a wide variety of synthetic and natural amino acid substrates. Known substrates include: cysteine, S-alkylcysteine, cysteine sulfinic acid, S-benzylcysteine, serine, beta-chloroalanine, 0-benzylserine and L-alpha, beta-diaminopropionic acid. In the case of each substrate, tryptophanase catalyzes an alpha, beta-elimination reaction to yield pyruvate, ammonia and the beta-substituent (13).

Some substrates which might be adapted to the quantification of pyridoxal phosphate with apotryptophanase are shown in Table 2 (14). Of these assays, only the S-o-nitrophenyl-L-cysteine has been developed (15). This substrate absorbs at 370 nm and the product, o-nitrothiophenolate, absorbs at 470 nm. Thus, either substrate disappearance or product formation forms the basis of a direct spectrophotometric assay.

Using substrate disappearance, Sueller and co-workers (15) assayed pyridoxal phosphate in the range of 1 to 400 picomoles in a final volume of 1 ml. The assay was adapted for quantification of pyridoxamine phosphate by non-enzymatic transamination of pyridoxamine phosphate to pyridoxal phosphate with glyoxalate. Conversion of pyridoxamine phosphate to pyridoxal phosphate was quantitative. To measure pyridoxamine phosphate in the presence of pyridoxal phosphate, the pyridoxal phosphate was inactivated by prior reduction with sodium borohydride to pyridoxine phosphate. Recoveries of pyridoxal phosphate and pyridoxamine phosphate from perchloric acid extracts of rat tissue were quantitative.

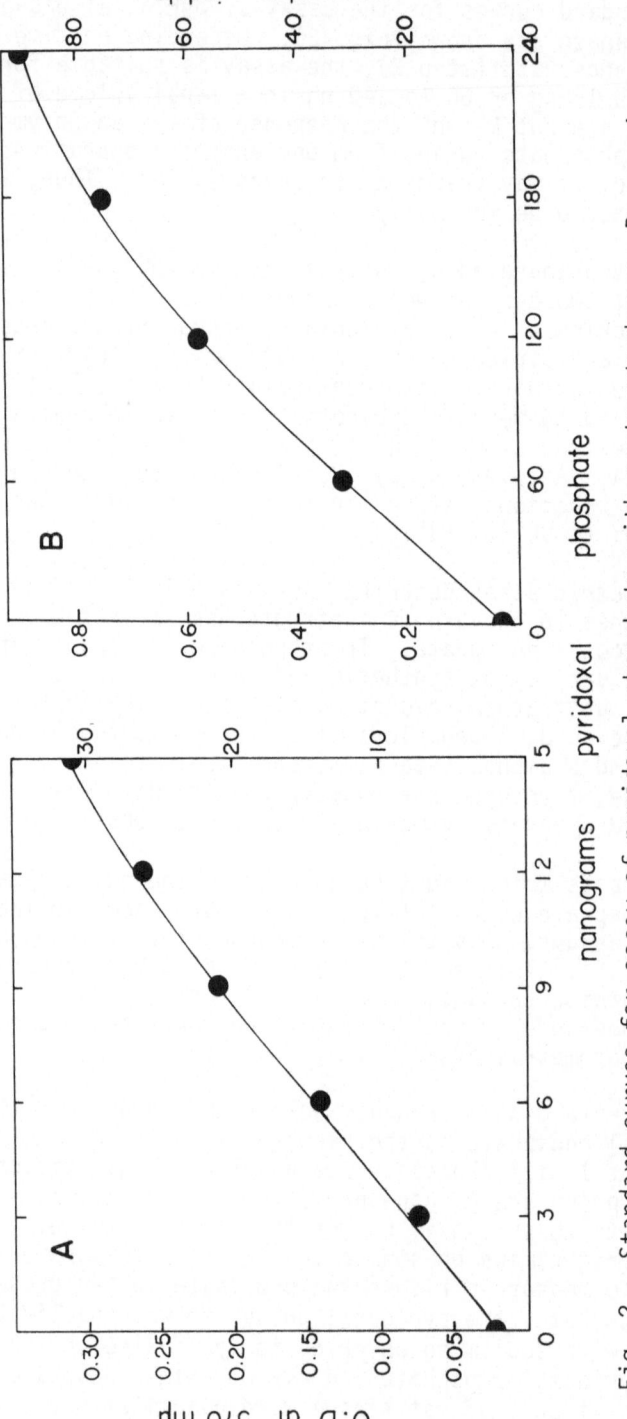

Fig. 2. Standard curves for assay of pyridoxal phosphate with apotryptophanse. By varying the incubation time after additon of substrate, pyridoxal phosphate may be assayed in the range 3 to 15 ng or 60 to 240 ng in a final volume of 5.0 ml. Curve A was incubated 20 minutes after the addition of substrate; Curve B, 3 minutes. The apoenzyme concentration was 0.02 units per flask in Curve A, 0.04 units per flask in Curve B. Color reagents and final volume (5.0 ml) were the same in both cases.

Table 2. Possible Assays for Pyridoxal Phosphate
          Using Apotryptophanase[a]

Substrate	Basis of Assay
S-o-nitrophenyl-L-cysteine	Spectrophotometric Determination (Substrate or Product)
Tryptophan	Pyruvate Formation Coupled to NADH Oxidation via Lactic Dehydrogenase
Beta-chloroalanine	Chloride Analysis (Cl⁻ Electrode or pH Stat)
S-pyridyl-L-cysteine	Spectrophotometric Determination (Pyridinethiol)
Cysteine or S-alkylcysteine	Assay of Mercaptans by Non-Enzymatic Reduction of Dithiopyridines or 5, 5'-dithiobis (2-nitrobenzoic Acid)

[a]Source: Suelter et al., 1976 (14).

An apotryptophanase assay for pyridoxal phosphate based upon pyruvate formation would appear to be feasible but has not yet been developed. Morino and Snell (4) assayed tryptophanase by coupling pyruvate formation to NADH oxidation in the presence of excess lactic dehydrogenase. With tryptophan as substrate, duration of linearity is short because of product (indole) inhibition. With another substrate, the assay might provide another alternative for the quantitation of pyridoxal phosphate with apotryptophanase.

In summary, the possibilities for the use of apotryptophanase in the assay of pyridoxal phosphate would appear to be limited only by biochemical ingenuity in devising suitable substrates.

A detailed working procedure for the colorimetric determination of pyridoxal phosphate with apotryptophanase follows.

REAGENTS

Pyridoxal phosphate standard. For assays in the range of 60 to 240 ng in a final volume of 5.0 ml, prepare a stock solution containing 24.0 mg pyridoxal phosphate in 100 ml H_2O. Dilute 0.1 ml of the stock solution to 10 ml with H_2O to provide a standard solution containing 240 ng in 0.1 ml. For assays in the range 3 to 15 ng, prepare a stock solution containing 15.0 mg pyridoxal phosphate in 100 ml H_2O. Dilute 0.1 ml to 100 ml to provide a standard containing 15 ng in 0.1 ml.

Buffer: 0.12 M potassium dihydrogen phosphate buffer, pH 7.8, containing 0.25 mg bovine serum albumin per milliliter and 0.2 mM reduced glutathione. Prepare fresh daily.

Enzyme: Apotryptophanase is purified from E. coli B/1t7A as previously described (3). The enzyme is dissolved in the buffer described above to provide a solution containing about 10 units of enzyme per ml. Dilute solutions of the apotryptophanase (10 units/ml) are relatively unstable. They retain 85% of their activity when stored at 4° for one week. The apoenzyme is stable for several months when stored as an ammonium sufate precipitate (4°). It retains 85% of its activity for at least 5 months when dissolved in the buffer described above, lyophilized and stored at 4°.

Substrate: 0.02 M L-tryptophan in H_2O.

Color reagent: Solution 1. (5% w/v p-dimethylaminobenzaldehyde in 95% ethanol.) Solution 2. 5 ml concentrated sulfuric acid diluted to 100 ml with n-butanol. Ehrlich reagent is prepared fresh daily by mixing 5 volumes of solution 1 with 12 volumes of solution 2. The stock solutions are stable at room temperature.

PROCEDURE

1. Preincubation. Combine in a 10 ml Erlenmeyer flask 0.3 ml buffer, 1 to 5 microliters enzyme (0.02 units per flask for pyridoxal phosphate concentrations in the range 3 to 15 ng per flask; 0.04 units per flask for pyridoxal phosphate concentrations in the range 60 to 240 ng per flask), 0 to 0.1 ml standard or sample and water to a final volume of 0.4 ml. Layer 1 ml of toluene over the surface of the reaction mixture. Cover the flask with Parafilm and incubate 20 minutes at 37° with gentle shaking.

2. Incubation with substrate. Add substrate (0.1 ml of 0.02 M L-tryptophan). Tip flask so that solution goes under the toluene layer. Incubate 20 minutes for an assay in the 3 to 15 ng range or 3 minutes for an assay in the 60 to 240 ng range.

3. Stop the reaction by adding 3.5 ml Ehrlich reagent. Usually a single phase forms. With some biological samples, the mixture may be turbid. In this case, centrifuge the mixture briefly at low speed and decant the organic phase from a few drops of aqueous residue. The sample is transferred to a 0.5 inch colorimeter tube and the absorbance read at 570 nm in a Bausch and Lomb colorimeter. Duplicate determinations agree within about 3% for assays in the 60 to 240 ng range. In the 3 to 15 ng range, the error is about 7%.

ACKNOWLEDGMENT

The apotryptophanase assay described here was developed in collaboration with Dr. Esmond E. Snell.

LITERATURE CITED

1. Lumeng, L., Ryan, M. P. & Li, T.-K. (1978) Validation of the diagnostic value of plasma pyridoxal 5'-phosphate measurements in vitamin B-6 nutrition of the rat. J. Nutr. 108, 545-553.
2. Umbreit, W. W., Bellamy, W. D. & Gunsalus, I. C. (1945) The function of pyridoxin derivatives: A comparison of natural and synthetic codecarboxylase. Arch. Biochem. 7, 185-199.
3. Haskell, B. E. & Snell, E. E. (1972) An improved apotrypto-phanase assay for pyridoxal phosphate. Anal. Biochem. 45, 567-576.
4. Morino, Y. & Snell, E. E. (1970) Tryptophanase (Escherichia coli B). In: Methods in Enzymology (Tabor, H. & Tabor, C. W., eds.), vol. 17A, pp. 439-447, Academic Press, New York.
5. Sloane-Stanley, G. H. (1949) The use of the tyrosine apodecarboxylase of Streptococcus faecalis R for the estimation of codecarboxylase. Biochem. J. 44, 567-573.
6. Gunsalus, I. C., Galeener, C. C. & Stamer, J. R. (1955) Tryptophan cleavage. Tryptophanase from E. coli. In: Methods in Enzymology (Colowick, S. P. & Kaplan, N. O., eds.), vol. 2, pp. 238-242, Academic Press, New York.
7. Pardee, A. B. & Prestidge, L. S. (1961) The initial kinetics of enzyme induction. Biochem. Biophys. Acta 49, 77-88.
8. Wada, H., Morisue, T., Sakamoto, Y. & Ichihara, K. (1957) Quantitative determination of pyridoxal phosphate by apotrypto-phanase of Escherichia coli. J. Vitaminol. (Japan) 3, 183-188.
9. McCormick, D. B., Gregory, M. E. & Snell, E. E. (1961) Pyri-doxal phosphokinases. I. Assay, distribution, purification and properties. J. Biol. Chem. 236, 2076-2084.

10. Gailani, S. (1965) Pyridoxal phosphate determination in
     isolated leucocytes and tissue by E. coli apotryptophanse.
     Anal. Biochem. 13, 19-27.
11. Wada, H. & Snell, E. E. (1961) The enzymatic oxidation of
     pyridoxine and pyridoxamine phosphates. J. Biol. Chem. 236,
     2089-2095.
12. Bain, J. A. & Williams, H. L. (1970) Concentrations of B-6
     vitamers in tissue and tissue fluids. In: Inhibition in the
     Nervous System and Gamma-aminobutyric Acid (Roberts, E., ed.),
     pp. 275-293. Macmillan (Pergamon), New York.
13. Snell, E. E. (1975) Tryptophanase: Structure, catalytic
     activities, and mechanism of action. Adv. in Enzymol. 42,
     287-333.
14. Suelter, C. H., Wang, J. & Snell, E. E. (1976) Direct
     spectrophotometric assay of tryptophanase. FEBS Lett. 66,
     230-232.
15. Suelter, C. H., Wang, I. & Snell, E. E. (1976) Application
     of a direct spectrophotometric assay employing a chromogenic
     substrate for tryptophanase to the determination of pyridoxal
     and pyridoxamine 5'-phosphates. Anal. Biochem. 76, 221-232.

SIMPLE ASSAY FOR FEMTOMOLES OF PYRIDOXAL AND PYRIDOXAMINE

PHOSPHATES

Bob In-yu Yang, Ashok K. Sawhney, Ronnie C. Pitchlyn
and Peter M. Peer

Department of Chemistry, College of Arts & Sciences
and the School of Medicine
University of Missouri-Kansas City
Kansas City, MO   64110

In recent years, there has been a renewed interest in vitamin B-6, sparked in part by the discoveries that several population groups are only marginally sufficient in the vitamin. These include alcoholics (1), pregnant women (2,3), females on oral contraceptive agents (3,4), and senior citizens (1,5-7). Of the various methods devised to indicate the nutritional status of vitamin B-6, measurement of plasma levels of pyridoxal 5'-P is being employed with increasing frequency. Pyridoxal 5'-P concentration in human blood correlates with the urinary excretion of xanthurenic acid (8), and enzyme activity and coenzyme saturation of erythrocyte aspartate aminotransferase (9). In rats, plasma pyridoxal 5'-P bears close relation to pyridoxine intake, growth, erythrocyte aspartate, and alanine aminotransferase activities and muscle store of the vitamer (10). Assay of pyridoxal 5'-P is best carried out by enzymatic means because they offer high specificity and sensitivity. Currently available protocols involve the use of the apoenzyme of tyrosine decarboxylase (11-13), tryptophanase (14,15), wheat germ and yeast aspartate aminotransferase (6,16), D-serine dehydratase (17), phosphorylase b (18), and γ-cyanoaminobutyric acid synthetase (19). The apotryptophanase assay (14), while offering such advantages as apoenzyme stability and ease of preparation, suffers from susceptibility to inhibition by the reaction product indole (20). Furthermore, the assay is discontinuous, requiring termination of the reaction. These disadvantages are obviated by substituting a chromogenic substrate for tryptophan (15). However, the molar absorptivity is low. And unlike tryptophan, the chromogenic substrate cannot be obtained commercially, but must be synthesized. Other continuous assays, e.g., those based on wheat germ and yeast aspartate aminotransferase and D-serine dehydratase and stop assays,

e.g., those based on phosphorylase b and γ-cyanoaminobutyric acid
synthetase, display low sensitivity resulting from low specific
activity of the holoenzyme and high residual activity in the apoenzyme. At present, the apotyrosine decarboxylase assay appears
to be most popular, apparently because of its sensitivity derived
from the use of $(1-^{14}C)$-tyrosine, and the commercial availability
of the enzyme in crude form. In the most recent version of this
assay, the sensitivity is placed at 50 pg of pyridoxal 5'-P (13).
To date, aspartate aminotransferase from pig hearts has not been
systematically examined for its suitability in assaying physiologically active forms of vitamin B-6. Huntly and Metzler (21) used
pig heart apoaspartate aminotransferase to identify pyridoxamine
5'-P.

In this report, we describe a highly sensitive spectrophotometric assay for pyridoxal 5'-P as well as pyridoxamine 5'-P,
employing the pig heart enzyme prepared in our laboratory or
purchased commercially and using non-radioactive substrates.

MATERIALS

Pyridoxal 5'-P, pyridoxamine 5'-P, and pig heart malate dehydrogenase were obtained from Sigma Chemical Company or Calbiochem-
Behring Corporation. Sodium dihydrogen phosphate was from Fisher
Scientific Company. L-glutamic acid, L-aspartic acid[1], α-keto-
glutaric acid, β-NADH, ammonium sulfate (Grade III), Tris, and
Sephadex G-25-40 gel filtration resin were purchased from Sigma
Chemical Company. Sodium borohydride and sodium cyanoborohydride
were from Aldrich Chemical Company. All other reagents were of the
highest purity available. Male rats, of the Sprague-Dawley strain,
were purchased from Sasco Incorporated, Omaha, Nebraska.

METHODS

Purification of Holoaspartate Aminotransferase

Aspartate aminotransferase prepared in this laboratory was
considerably more active than commercial lots. The holoenzyme was
purified according to Yang and Metzler (22) based on the original
protocols of Jenkins et al. (23) and Martinez-Carrion et al. (24).

---

[1]L-aspartic acid obtained from several other sources caused deviation from linearity in the spectrophotometric assay of aspartate
aminotransferase activity. The deviation was particularly pronounced when low rates were being measured as in the determination
of residual aminotransferase activity in the apoenzyme.

Pig hearts were ground up, heat treated, fractionated with ammonium sulfate, and chromatographed on hydroxyapatite and carboxymethyl-Sephadex. This procedure yielded the α-subform of the holoenzyme with a specific activity of approximately 250 μmol/min/mg at 22°.

Preparation of Apoaspartate Aminotransferase

Holoenzyme prepared as described above or procured commercially was suitable for the purpose. One ml of holoaspartate aminotransferase containing no less than 10 mg of protein was used. Dilute commercial lots were precipitated with a saturated ammonium sulfate solution and the protein dissolved in a minimal amount of 50 mM Tris buffer, pH 8.3, to yield a concentrated enzyme solution as the starting material. The resolution procedure was that of Scardi et al. (25) as modified by Furbish et al. (26). Into a 500 ml Erlenmeyer flask was introduced 1 ml of holoenzyme. Twenty-four ml of 0.2 M L-glutamate at pH 8.3 were added to convert the holoenzyme to its pyridoxamine 5'-P form. After 5 minutes, 25 ml of 1.0 M sodium phosphate buffer at pH 4.8 were added. The pH of the mixture was 5.0. The flask was then placed in a 30° water bath and incubated for 30 minutes. Protein was precipitated by the addition of 150 ml of saturated ammonium sulfate solution. The precipitate was collected by centrifugation and taken up in 0.5 ml of the Tris buffer. The entire process was repeated a second time. The dissolved protein precipitate was clarified by centrifugation and applied to a 1.0 x 20 cm Sephadex G-25-40 gel filtration column which had previously been equilibrated with the Tris buffer. The column was eluted with the same buffer to yield apoaspartate aminotransferase of approximately 10^{-4}M in concentration (mol wt apoenzyme = 46,300).

Enzyme Reconstitution

Reformation of catalytically active aspartate aminotransferase was done by mixing 10^{-4}M apoenzyme in 50 mM Tris buffer, pH 8.3, with 50-fold molar excess of an aqueous solution of pyridoxal 5'-P approximately 10^{-2}M in concentration. Following a 30-minute incubation period at room temperature, the mixture was diluted in two steps with 50 mM Tris buffer, pH 8.3, to yield a solution that was 1.0×10^{-7}M in enzyme. Fifty μl of this solution was then assayed to obtain enzyme specific activity.

Enzyme Assay

Aspartate aminotransferase activity was measured, after coupling to malate dehydrogenase, by spectrophotometrically monitoring the disappearance of NADH at 340 nm. The composition of the assay mixture was essentially that of Okamoto and Morino (27). To a semi-micro cuvette was transfered 1.0 ml of a mixture containing

10 μmol of L-aspartate, 0.1 μmol of NADH, 10.5 units of malate dehydrogenase and 100 μmol of Tris, pH 8.3. Ten μl of 0.3M α-keto-glutarate were then added.[2] The reaction was initiated by the introduction of 50 μl of 1.0×10^{-7} M aspartate aminotransferase which was either the holoenzyme or the apoenzyme in the absence of any cofactor, partially saturated with a cofactor or reconstituted with excess pyridoxal 5'-P. The rate of the reaction was followed in a Varian Cary 1501 UV-visible absorption spectrophotometer with its full-scale deflection set at 0.1 absorbance unit and with chart speed fixed at 5.91 s to 24.61 min/cm. All assays were performed at room temperature, i.e., 22 ± 2^0. Enzyme specific activity was defined as μmoles of products formed per min per mg of enzyme (μmol/min/mg), using 46,300 as the latter's molecular weight (28).

Determination of Enzyme Residual Activity

Residual aminotransferase activity in the apoenzyme was calcu-lated from the coupled transamination rate measurement using 50 μl of 1.0×10^{-7} M apoaspartate aminotransferase in the assay described above.

Determination of Protein Concentration

The concentration of both the holo and apoaspartate amino-transferase was determined spectrophotometrically, using molar absorptivity at 280 nm of 6.55×10^4 and 6.36×10^4 cm^{-1} M^{-1} (26) respectively. Commercial enzyme preparations, which usually con-tained various stabilizing agents, were eluted from a Sephadex G-25-40 column, in 50 mM Tris, pH 8.3, prior to the measurement of holoenzyme activity and protein concentration.

Determination of Coenzyme Concentration

Stock solutions of pyridoxal 5'-P and pyridoxamine 5'-P of approximately 10^{-2} M were prepared by dissolving the solid chemicals in water. The exact concentration of each coenzyme was determined spectrophotometrically following a 100-fold dilution of the stock solution. The molar absorptivity used was 6600 cm^{-1} M^{-1} in 0.1 N NaOH at 388 nm for pyridoxal 5'-P and 8300 cm^{-1} M^{-1} in 0.1 M sodium phosphate buffer, pH 7.0 at 325 nm for pyridoxamine 5'-P (29).

---

[2]Addition of α-ketoglutarate immediately before assaying prevented the slow but significant oxidation of NADH in the absence of aspartate aminotransferase.

Dilution of Coenzymes

Stock solutions of pyridoxal 5'-P and pyridoxamine 5'-P were diluted as much as 5×10^7-fold. This was done by serial dilution, up to five steps. Distilled and deionized water which had been repeatedly deaerated and stored under nitrogen gas was used in these dilutions. Exposure of coenzyme solutions to laboratory light was minimized.

Establishment of Standard Curves

Apoaspartate aminotransferase at 2.0×10^{-7}M in 50 mM Tris buffer, pH 8.3, was mixed with an equal volume of either pyridoxal 5'-P or pyridoxamine 5'-P ranging in concentration from 2×10^{-10}M to 1×10^{-7}M. Following 30 minutes of incubation at room temperature, 50 μl of the mixture were assayed for the aminotransferase activity. Standard curves were obtained by expressing enzyme specific activity as a function of the amount of coenzymes added.

Care of Animals

Rats weighing approximately 250 g were purchased and fed ad libitum Purina Rodent Lab Chow No. 501 which contained 6 mg/kg of pyridoxine. The rats were housed individually in wire bottom cages in the University Laboratory Animal Center which is accredited by the American Association of Laboratory Animal Care. Regulated lighting of 12-h light and 12-h dark schedule was provided. At least one week was allowed for acclimation before the animals were used.

Preparation of Plasma and Tissue Extracts

The rats were fasted overnight and killed by carbon dioxide asphyxiation. Blood was collected from the aorta with a needle and syringe, transfered to a tube containing 0.1 ml of 0.2 M EDTA, pH 7.4, and centrifuged at 600 x g for 20 minutes. The resulting plasma was processed by two different methods. In the acid extraction method, 0.5 ml of the plasma was mixed with 50 ml of 75% (w/v) trichloroacetic acid and centrifuged to remove precipitated proteins (1). To 50 μl aliquots of the deproteinized supernatant were added 950 μl of 50 mM Tris buffer, pH 8.3. This diluted solution was assayed for its pyridoxal 5'-P and pyridoxamine 5'-P content. In the base extraction method, 0.5 ml of plasma was added to 50 ml of 0.10 N sodium hydroxide and the mixture was allowed to stand for 30 minutes at 4^0. To 5 ml of the mixture were added 250 μl of 2.0 N hydrochloric acid and 5.25 ml of 50 mM Tris buffer, pH 8.3. The neutralized and diluted solution was then assayed.

Preparation of Liver Extract

Liver samples were processed according to two procedures. In
the first, approximately 1 g of liver was placed in 100 ml of 80 mM
phosphate buffer, pH 7.4, and homogenized.[3] The homogenate was made
7.5% in trichloroacetic acid (10) and diluted 4-fold with water. The
mixture was allowed to stand at 4^0 for 30 minutes and centrifuged.
The deproteinized supernatant was diluted 50-fold with the Tris
buffer and assayed. In the second procedure, the liver was homogenized instead in 0.1 N NaOH and allowed to stand at 4^0 for 30
minutes. Aliquots were then made 0.1 N in excess hydrochloric acid
by addition of a 0.5 N solution, diluted 4-fold with water and
again permitted to stand for 30 minutes. Small amounts of precipitate were removed by centrifugation. The supernatant was diluted
50-fold with the Tris buffer and assayed.

Preparation of Brain Extract

Metaphosphoric acid and sodium hydroxide were used to liberate
the cofactors. The metaphosphoric acid procedure was carried out
according to Lumeng et al. (10). The sodium hydroxide treatment
for liver samples was also employed to prepare brain extract. Whole
brains were divided along the midline with one-half being used for
each method.

Preparation of Saliva and Urine

Human saliva, 950 μl in volume, was mixed with 50 μl of 2.0 N
sodium hydroxide and allowed to stand at room temperature for 30
minutes. Following addition of 50 μl of 2.0 N hydrochloric acid,
the sample was centrifuged to remove cell debris and protein
precipitate. The supernatant was assayed. Human urine was processed identically except that twice as much sodium hydroxide and
hydrochloric acid were used.

Reduction of Pyridoxal 5'-P

Pyridoxal 5'-P solutions were reduced by addition of 1.25 N
sodium borohydride in 1.0 N sodium hydroxide and 2.0 N sodium
hydroxide so that the reaction mixture contained 2.5 mM sodium borohydride and 1.5 mM sodium hydroxide. Fiften minutes later, 2.0 N
hydrochloric acid was added to neutralize the sodium hydroxide. To
this reaction mixture was introduced 0.1 volume of acetone and 10
minutes were allowed to permit total destruction of the reductant.
The solution so treated was assayed with apoaspartate aminotransferase.

---

[3] Du Pont Sorvall Omni-Mixer, set at top speed for 45 s.

Reduction of Apoaspartate Aminotransferase

Apoenzyme in 50 mM Tris buffer, pH 8.3, was made 40 mM in sodium cyanoborohydride, which had been recrystallized in acetonitrildichloromethane (30), by addition of a 1 M aqueous stock solution. Reduction was allowed to proceed for 2 hours at 4⁰. The protein was precipitated by addition of 3 volumes of saturated ammonium sulfate and collected by centifugation. The reduced apoenzyme was taken up in a minimum amount of the Tris buffer and eluted from a gel-filtration column (26).

Treatment of Data

All values reported were the mean of at least three determinations. For the calibration curves, each determination began with concentrated apoenzyme and cofactor, each of which was serially diluted as required. Standard deviation was calculated for all values.

RESULTS

Activities of Aspartate Aminotransferase

The holoenzyme prepared in this laboratory was consistently highly active (Table 1). It could be readily resolved to yield apoenzyme of very low residual activity. Upon reconstitution with excess pyridoxal 5'-P, the enzyme was nearly fully activated. The low residual and high reconstituted activities afforded the remarkable sensitivity characteristic of this assay. Commercial holoenzyme preparations, as exemplified by that supplied by Calbiochem-Behring Corp., also share similar characteristics (Table 1). All commercial lots examined displayed lower holo- and reconstituted activities and higher residual activity.

Stability of Apoenzyme

For apoaspartate aminotransferase to be of utility, stability during storage would be a prerequisite. As prepared in 50 mM Tris buffer, pH 8.3, and kept at 4⁰, the apoenzyme remained no less than 70% reconstitutible after one month (Table 2). No stabilizing agents of any kind were needed to obtain such stability.

Table 1. Activities of Holo-, Apo-, and Reconstituted Aspartate Aminotransferase

Enzyme Form	Specific Activity		
	Preparation I[a]	Preparation II[a]	Preparation III[b]
		μmol/min/mg	
Holo	237 ±13 (100 %)	220 ± 8 (100 %)	160 ±8 (100 %)
Apo	0.43± 0.06 (0.2%)	0.47± 0.02 (0.2%)	0.69±0.06 (0.4%)
Reconstituted	221 ±14 (93 %)	220 ±13 (100 %)	129 ±1 (80 %)

[a]Starting with holoenzyme prepared in this laboratory.
[b]Starting with holoenzyme purchased from Calbiochem-Behring Corp.

Time Course of Recombination

Binding of pyridoxal 5'-P by apoaspartate aminotransferase was approximately 90% complete 5 minutes following the mixing of apo-enzyme and the cofactor (Fig. 1). Similar results were obtained using apoenzyme prepared from commercially acquired holoenzyme. For the sake of completeness, all recombinations in this study were allowed to proceed for 30 minutes, unless otherwise specified.

Table 2. Stability of Apoaspartate
Aminotransferase[a]

Time	Specific Activity After Reconstitution[b]
day	μmol/min/mg
1	220 $\pm$ 13
21	183 $\pm$ 8
35	153 $\pm$ 7
58	117 $\pm$ 4

[a]Apoenzyme concentration, 1.02 x 10^{-4}M (mol wt apoenzyme = 46,300).
[b]Fifty-fold molar excess of 9.03 x 10^{-3}M pyridoxal 5'-P added.

Standard Curves for Pyridoxal 5'-P and Pyridoxamine 5'-P

The gain in the activity of the enzyme was directly related to the amount of either cofactor added. This was true for the apoenzyme prepared in this laboratory (Figs. 2 and 3) as well as similar prep-arations from several commercially available holoaspartate amino-transferases (Fig. 4). As shown in Figs. 2 and 3, linearity of the standard curves existed not only in the range of 50 to 500 fmol but could be extended to 2500 fmol (insets). Apoaspartate aminotrans-ferase of commercial origins afforded a similar range of linear response although the gain in enzyme activity for a given amount of cofactor added was usually somewhat less (Fig. 4). This reflected the fact the commercially available holoenzyme preparations invari-ably had lower specific activity than those purified in this laboratory. However, commercial lots appeared adequate for nearly all the assays in this study.

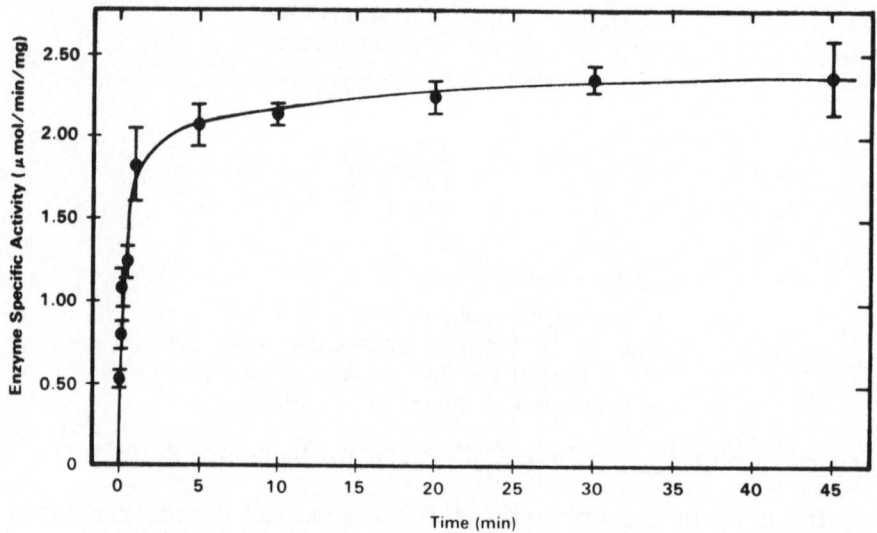

Fig. 1.   Time course of recombination of apoaspartate aminotransferase with pyridoxal 5'-P. Equal volumes of 2.0×10^{-7}M
apoenzyme and 2.0×10^{-9}M cofactor were mixed. Fifty μl
aliquots were assayed at various times. Mean ± SD are
reported for each value.

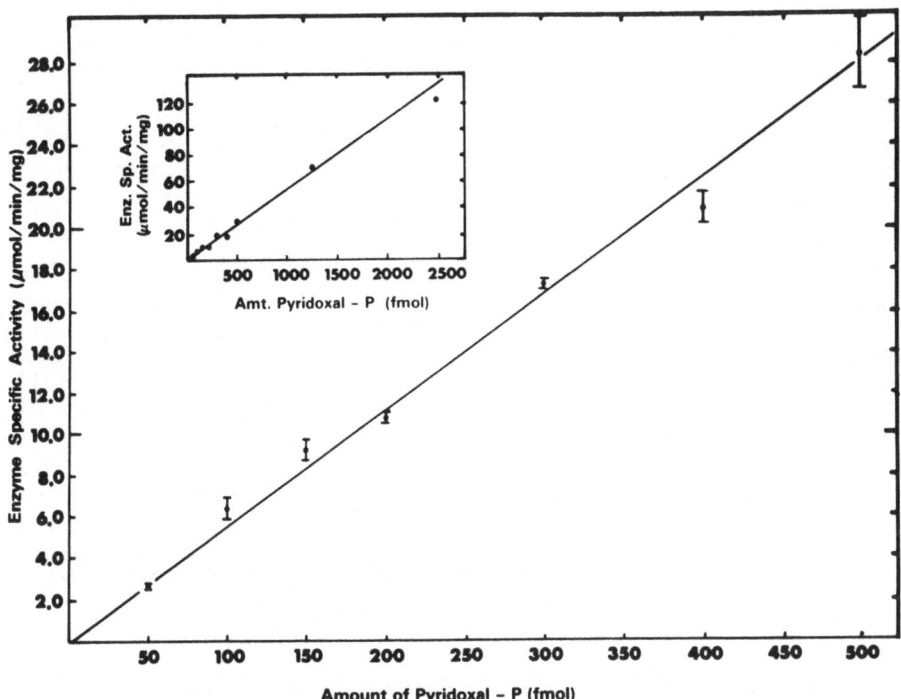

Fig. 2. Standard curve for pyridoxal 5'-P determination using
apoenzyme derived from holoaspartate aminotransferase
prepared in this laboratory. The actual rate measured
for 50 fmol of pyridoxal 5'-P was 5.8 x 10^{-3} absorbance
unit/min of which 2.1 x 10^{-3}/min was due to residual
activity in the apoenzyme. Residual activity has been
subtracted from all the values shown.

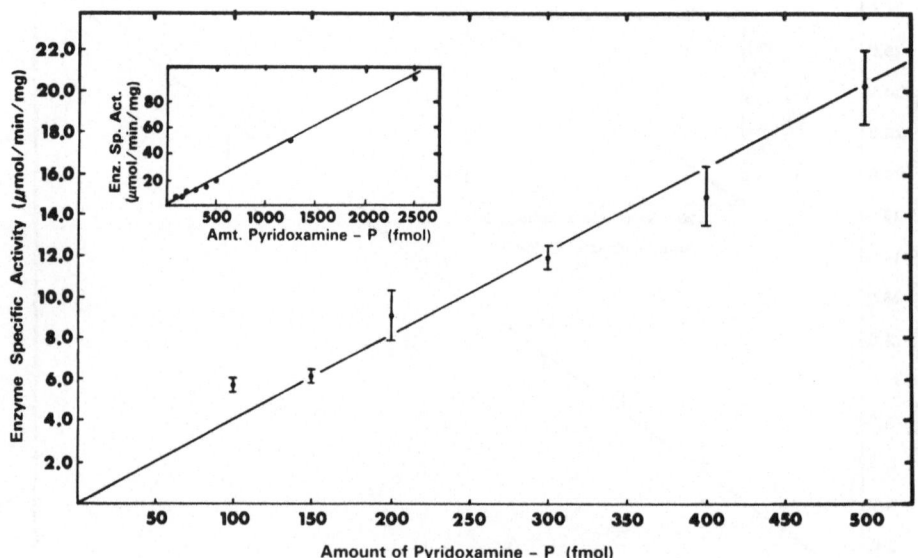

Fig. 3.   Standard curve for pyridoxamine 5'-P determination using
          apoenzyme derived from holoaspartate aminotransferase
          prepared in this laboratory. The actual rate measured
          for 100 fmol of pyridoxamine 5'-P was 7.8 x 10^{-3} absorbance
          unit/min of which 2.1 x 10^{-3}/min was due to residual
          activity in the apoenzyme. Residual activity has been
          substracted from all values shown.

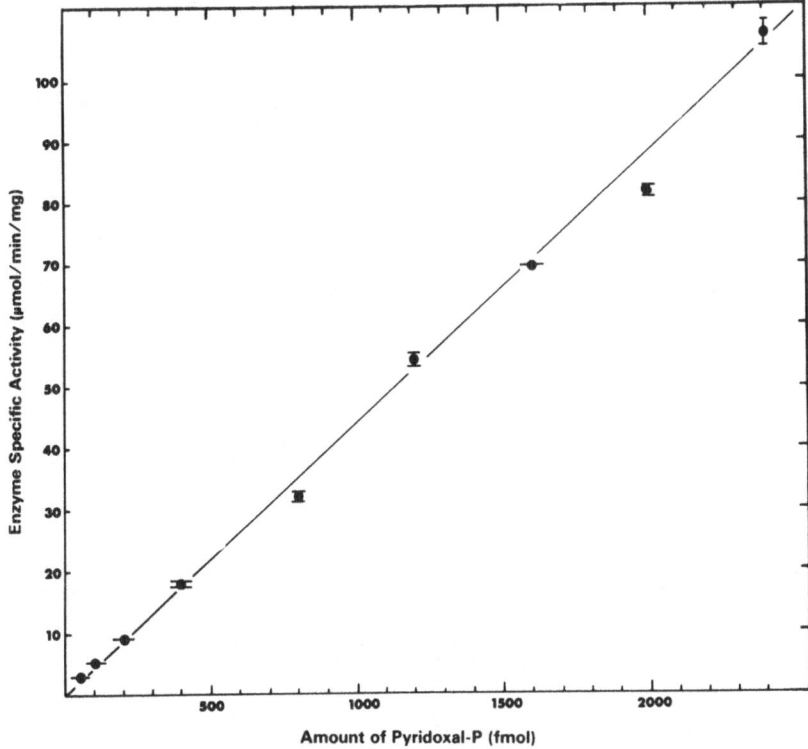

Fig. 4. Standard curve for pyridoxal 5'-P determination using apo-
         enzyme derived from holoaspartate aminotransferase pur-
         chased from Calbiochem-Behring Corp. The actual rate
         measured for 50 fmol of pyridoxal 5'-P was 5.0×10^{-3}
         absorbance unit/min of which 0.95×10^{-3}/min was due to
         residual activity. Residual activity has been subtracted
         from all values shown.

Standard Curve for Small Quantities of Pyridoxal 5'-P

To determine the lowest detection limit for pyridoxal 5'-P
using apoaspartate aminotransferase, a standard curve for 5 to 50
fmol of the cofactor was obtained (Fig. 5). It is apparent that
amounts of pyridoxal 5'-P as low as 5 fmol (1.2 pg) could be
satisfactorily determined. For such determinations, the residual
activity of the apoenzyme must necessarily be very low.

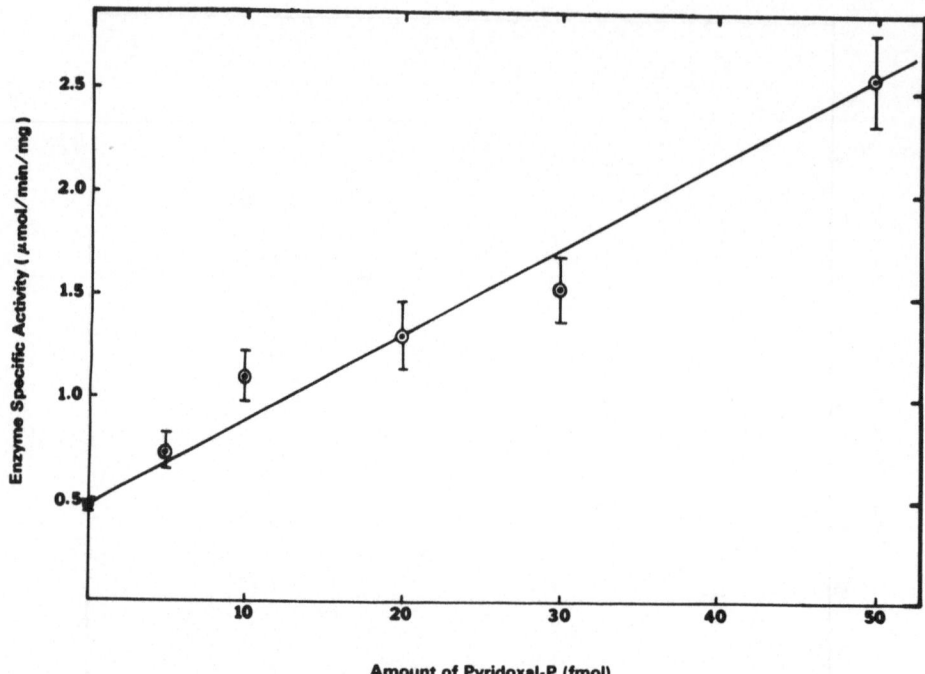

Fig. 5. Standard curve for 5-50 fmol of pyridoxal 5'-P. The
apoenzyme employed was obtained from holoenzyme prepared
in this laboratory. All values shown included the
residual activity which was indicated by the point at
0 fmol of the cofactor. Actual rate measured for the
residual activity was $6.5 \pm 0.3 \times 10^{-4}$ absorbance unit/
min.

Pyridoxal 5'-P and Pyridoxamine 5'-P Content of Rat Plasma and Tissues

The cofactor concentration measured from these animal sources
depended greatly on the method of extraction. When rat plasma and
liver were extracted with trichloroacetic acid and brain with metaphosphoric acid essentially according to the methods of Lumeng et
al. (10), considerably lower values were obtained for their pyridoxal 5'-P and pyridoxamine 5'-P content (data not shown) compared
to those resulted from 0.1 N sodium hydroxide extraction (Table 3).
This difference appeared particularly prominent when plasma values
of this report were compared with literature results obtained
through acid extraction, the former being up to 6-fold as much as
the latter. The cause for this discrepancy is yet unclear.
Whereas 30 minutes were shown to be sufficient time for the nearly
complete recombination of authentic pyridoxal 5'-P and the apoenzyme
(Fig. 1), the cofactors of biological origins presented different

Table 3. Pyridoxal 5'-P and Pyridoxamine 5'-P
          Content of Rat Plasma, Liver, and Brain

Source	Blood Plasma	Liver	Brain
	ng/ml	µg/g	µg/g
This Report[a]			
30 min	160 + 40	19 + 2	5.2 + 0.6
60 min	250 + 50	21 + 2	6.7 + 0.5
120 min	350 + 70	24 + 4	8.0 + 1.0
Literature			
1[b]	47[d] - 64[e]	-	1.5[d,e]
2[c]	-	11.6	4.8

[a]Number of rats, 6; weight of rats, 288 + 20 g.
[b]Lumeng et al. (10); values excluding pyridoxamine
  5'-P.
[c]Suelter et al. (15); values including pyridoxamine
  5'-P.
[d]Values from rats fed 12 µg/day of pyridoxine.
[e]Values from rats fed 24 µg/day of pyridoxine.

time courses (Table 3). Blood plasma provided active vitamers to
the apoenzyme long past the usual 30 minute incubation period.
Brain extract also continued to liberate the cofactors for no less
than 2 hours. Of the three sources examined, liver appeared to
yield all available cofactors within 30 minutes.

Pyridoxal 5'-P and Pyridoxamine 5'-P Content of Human Saliva and Urine

While plasma content of pyridoxal 5'-P constitutes a valid
indicator of the nutritional status of vitamin B-6, a noninvasive
method would still be desirable. As a first step in the search for
such protocols, human saliva and urine were examined for the presence
of pyridoxal 5'-P and pyridoxamine 5'-P. Although none were detected
in urine (Table 4), low but significant concentrations were measured
in saliva. It should be noted that such small quantities of the
vitamers would probably have escaped detection by the less sensitive
assays currently in use. With the apoaspartate aminotransferase
assay, considerable precision accompanied the measurements.

Table 4.   Pyridoxal 5'-P and Pyridoxamine 5'-P in Human
           Saliva and Urine[a]

Sample	Actual Rate Measured	Specific Activity	Content of Vitamers in Original Fluid
	10^3 x Δ A/min	μmol/min/mg	ng/ml
Buffer[b]	2.11 ± 0.04	-	-
Urine[b]	2.33 ± 0.22	-	0
	2.17 ± 0.44	-	0
Saliva[c]	1.73 ± 0.18	1.27 ± 0.13	0.26 ± 0.021[d]

[a]Saliva and urine samples from one of the authors (BIY).
[b]Both fluids assayed with the same batch of apoenzyme.
[c]Assayed with a different batch of apoenzyme; same as
  that used in obtaining the standard curve for 5-50 fmol
  of pyridoxal 5'-P (Fig. 5).
[d]Value obtained by interpolation in Fig. 5.

Standard Curve for Differential Determination of Pyridoxal 5'-P
and Pyridoxamine 5'-P

     Inspection of Fig. 6 revealed that the sum of the slopes of the
pyridoxal 5'-P and pyridoxamine 5'-P curves closely approximated,
i.e. amounting to 94%, the slope of the standard curve for
pyridoxal 5'-P plus pyridoxamine 5'-P. As expected, addition of
sodium borohydride to mixtures of pyridoxal 5'-P and pyridoxamine
5'-P destroyed the great majority of the pyridoxal 5'-P, the slope
of the resulting curve being 117% of that of the standard curve for
pyridoxamine 5'-P. These results suggested that pyridoxal 5'-P and
pyridoxamine 5'-P might be differentially determined in samples
containing both vitamers.

DISCUSSION

     In this study, pig heart apoaspartate aminotransferase has
been shown to be highly suitable for the determination of pyridoxal 5'-P and pyridoxamine 5'-P. In preliminary investigation, it
was found that the apoenzyme remained greater than 80% reconstitutible after seven freeze-thaw cycles in and out of a dry ice-
acetone bath. This suggests that the apoenzyme may be conveniently
shipped and stored for long-term use.

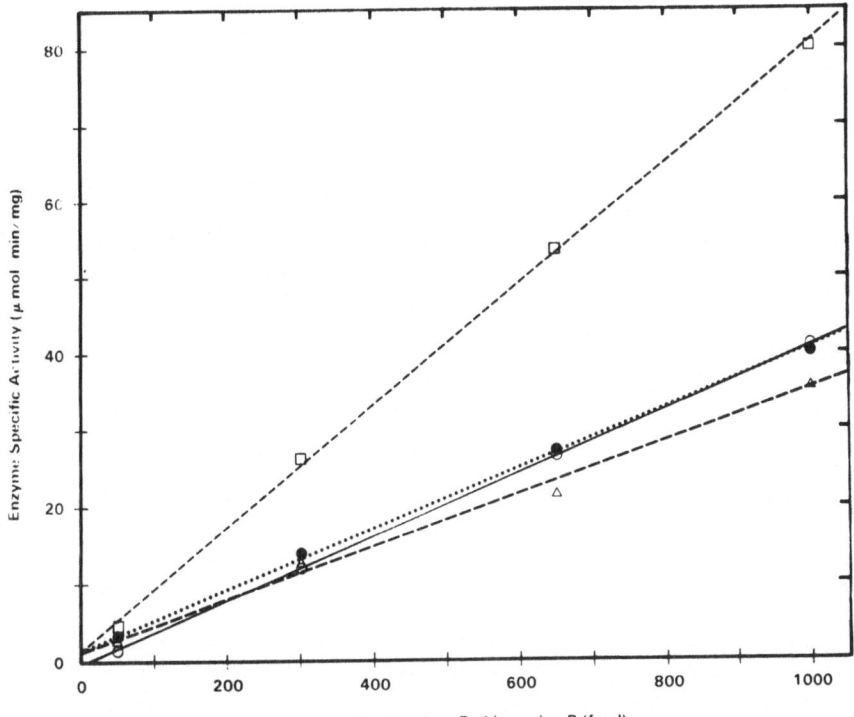

Fig. 6. Standard curve for differential determination of
         pyridoxal 5'-P and pyridoxamine 5'-P. □-----□ ,
         pyridoxal 5'-P plus pyridoxamine 5'-P curve, with
         abscissa indicating the amount of each of the two
         vitamers; ●······● , pyridoxal 5'-P plus pyridoxamine
         5'-P curve following sodium borohydride reduction;
         O——O, pyridoxal 5'-P curve; △－－－△ , pyridoxamine
         5'-P curve. Each curve was fitted by the linear
         regression least squares method.

        Apoaspartate aminotransferase prepared from some commercially
supplied holoenzyme preparations tended to retain more than 0.2%
residual activity. Since high residual activity leads to decreased
sensitivity of the assay, attempts were made to reduce the residual
activity following the usual resolution procedure. Treatment with
recrystallized sodium cyanoborohydride appeared to accomplish this
purpose. In one case, such treatment reduced the residual activity
from 1.1 ± 0.2 to 0.27 ± 0.05 μmol/min/mg. However, two and five
days later, the specific activity rose to 0.52 ± 0.06 and 0.54 ±
0.04 μmol/min/mg, respectively. There had not been excessive exposure of the apoenzyme to light. Neither pyridoxal 5'-P nor pyridoxamine 5'-P had been introduced. Thus, the light facilitated

mechanism for regenerating underivatized apoenzyme (31) appeared not to be responsible for the gain in residual activity. Further exploration in this subject is underway.

An unresolved problem in this study is the apparent slow release of the cofactors by such materials as plasma and brain (Table 3). More rigorous extraction methods, e.g., treatment with hot 1 N sodium hydroxide (32), may speed up the liberation of pyridoxal 5'-P and pyridoxamine 5'-P. It is to be noted that the 0.1 N sodium hydroxide used in this study already extracted considerably more of the vitamers, as assayed by the apoaspartate aminotransferase method, than previously reported for all the biological materials examined.

ACKNOWLEDGMENTS

This work was supported by the United States Department of Agriculture Grant SEA 5901-0410-9-030-0 and by the United States Public Health Service Grant GM-27280.

LITERATURE CITED

1. Lumeng, L. & Li, T.-K.   (1974) Vitamin B-6 metabolism in chronic alcohol abuse: Pyridoxal phosphate levels in plasma and the effects of acetaldehyde on pyridoxal phosphate synthesis and degradation in human erythrocytes. J. Clin. Invest. 53, 693-704.

2. Shane, B. & Contractor, S. F.   (1975) Assessment of vitamin B-6 status. Studies on pregnant women and oral contraceptive users. Am. J. Clin. Nutr. 28, 739-747.

3. Lumeng, L., Cleary, R. E., Wagner, R., Yu, P.-L. & Li, T.-K. (1976) Adequacy of vitamin B-6 supplementation during pregnancy: A prospective study. Am. J. Clin. Nutr. 29, 1376-1383.

4. Lumeng, L., Cleary, R. E. & Li, T.-K. (1974) Effect of oral contraceptives on the plasma concentrations of pyridoxal phosphate. Am. J. Clin. Nutr. 27, 326-333.

5. Hamfelt, A. (1964) Age variation of vitamin B-6 metabolism in man. Clin. Chim. Acta 10, 48-54.

6. Walsh, M. P. (1966) Determination of plasma pyridoxal phosphate with wheat germ glutamic-aspartic apotransaminase. Am. J. Clin. Path. 36, 282-285.

7. Jacobs, A., Cavill, I.A.J. & Hughes, J.N.P. (1968) Erythrocyte transaminase activity: Effect of age, sex, and vitamin B-6 supplementation. Am. J. Clin. Nutr. 21, 502-507.

8. Hamfelt, A. (1967) Enzymatic determination of pyridoxal phosphate in plasma by decarboxylation of L-tyrosine-[14]C (U) and a comparison with the tryptophan load test. Scan. J. Clin. Lab. Invest. 20, 1-10.

9. Hamfelt, A. (1967) Pyridoxal phosphate concentration and aminotransferase activity in human blood cells. Clin. Chim. Acta 16, 19-28.
10. Lumeng, L., Ryan, M. P. & Li, T.-K. (1978) Validation of the diagnostic value of plasma pyridoxal 5'-phosphate measurements in vitamin B-6 nutrition of the rat. J. Nutr. 108, 545-553.
11. Chabner, B. & Livingston, D. (1970) A simple enzymatic assay for pyridoxal phosphate. Anal. Biochem. 34, 413-423.
12. Sundaresan, P. R. & Coursin, D. B. (1970) Microassay of pyridoxal phosphate using L-tyrosine-1-^{14}C and tyrosine apodecarboxylase. Methods Enzymol. 18A, 509-512.
13. Bhagavan, H. N., Koogler, J. M., Jr. & Coursin, D. B. (1976) Enzymatic microassay of pyridoxal-5'-phosphate using L-(1-^{14}C) tyrosine. Internat. J. Vit. Nutr. Res. 46, 160-164.
14. Haskell, B. E. & Snell, E. E. (1972) An improved apotryptophanase assay for pyridoxal phosphate. Anal. Biochem. 45, 567-576.
15. Suelter, C. H., Wang, J. & Snell, E. E. (1976) Application of a direct spectrophotometric assay employing a chromogenic substrate for tryptophanase to the determination of pyridoxal and pyridoxamine 5'-phosphates. Anal. Biochem. 76, 221-232.
16. Holzer, H. & Gerlach, U. (1963) Pyridoxal phosphate determination with apotransaminase from Brewers yeast. In: Methods of Enzymatic Analysis (Bergmeyer, H. U., ed.), pp. 606-609, Academic Press, New York.
17. Worland, S. T. & Shafer, J. A. (1980) A convenient lactic dehydrogenase-coupled assay for determing pyridoxal 5'-phosphate in plasma. Anal. Biochem. 103, 323-330.
18. Hines, J. D. & Love, D. S. (1969) Determination of serum and blood pyridoxal phosphate concentrations with purified rabbit skeletal muscle apophosphorylase. J. Lab. Clin. Med. 73, 343-349.
19. Abe, K. & Ressler, C. (1979) Enzymatic determination of pyridoxal 5'-phosphate with γ-cyanoaminobutyric acid aposynthase. Internat. J. Peptide Protein Res. 13, 102-105.
20. Newton, W. A., Morino, Y. & Snell, E. E. (1965) Properties of crystalline tryptophanase. J. Biol. Chem. 240, 1211-1218.
21. Huntly, T. E. & Metzler, D. E. (1968) The reaction of α-methylglutamate with glutamic acid decarboxylase. In: Symposium on Pyridoxal Enzymes, pp. 81-84. Maruzen, Tokyo.
22. Yang, B. I. & Metzler, D. E. (1979) Pyridoxal 5'-phosphate and analogs as probes of coenzyme-protein interaction. Methods Enzymol. 62D, 528-551.
23. Jenkins, W. T., Yphantis, D. A. & Sizer, I. W. (1959) Glutamic aspartic transaminase: Assay, purification and general properties. J. Biol. Chem. 234, 51-57.

24. Martinez-Carrion, M., Turano, D., Chiancone, E. Bossa, F.,
    Giartosio, A., Riva, F. & Fasella, P. (1967) Isolation and
    characterization of multiple forms of glutamate-aspartate
    aminotransferase from pig heart. J. Biol. Chem. 242, 2397-
    2409.
25. Scardi, V., Scotto, P., Saccarino, M. & Scarano, E. (1963)
    The binding of pyridoxal 5'-phosphate to aspartate aminotrans-
    ferase of pig heart. Biochem. J. 88, 172-175.
26. Furbish, F. S., Fonda, M. L. & Metzler, D. E. (1969) Reactions
    of apoaspartate aminotransferase with analogs of pyridoxal
    phosphate. Biochemistry 8, 5169-5180.
27. Okamoto, M. & Morino, Y. (1973) Affinity labeling of aspartate
    aminotransferase isozymes by bromopyruvate. J. Biol. Chem.
    248, 82-90.
28. Ovchinnikov, Yu. A., Egorov, C. A., Adlanova, N. A.,
    Feigina, M. Yu., Lipkin, V. M., Abdulaev, N. G., Grishin, E. V.,
    Kiselev, A. P., Modyanov, N. N., Braunstein, A. E., Polyanovsky,
    O. L. & Nosikov, V. V. (1973) The complete amino acid sequence
    of cytoplasmic aspartate aminotransferase from pig heart.
    FEBS Lett. 29, 31-34.
29. Peterson, E. A. & Sober, H. A. (1954) Preparation of crys-
    talline phosphorylated derivatives of vitamin B-6. J. Am.
    Chem. Soc. 76, 169-175.
30. Jentoft, N. & Dearborn, D. G. (1979) Labeling of proteins
    by reductive methylation using sodium cyanoborohydride. J.
    Biol. Chem. 254, 4359-4365.
31. Ritchey, J. M., Gibbons, I. & Schachman, H. K. (1977)
    Reactivation of enzymes by light-stimulated cleavage of
    reduced pyridoxal 5'-phosphate-enzyme complexes. Biochemistry
    16, 4584-4590.
32. Uchida, T. & O'Brian, R. D. (1964) The effects of hydrazines
    on pyridoxal phosphate in rat brain. Biochem. Pharmacol. 13,
    1143-1150.

CHEMICAL ANALYSIS OF PYRIDOXINE VITAMERS

K. Dakshinamurti and M. S. Chauhan

Department of Biochemistry, Faculty of Medicine
University of Manitoba
Winnipeg, Canada, R3E 0W3

The metabolic function of vitamin B-6 is related to the role of pyridoxal phosphate as the coenzyme of over 50 enzymes. Most are involved in catabolic reactions of various amino acids. Other pyridoxal phosphate-dependent enzymes are glycogen phosphorylase and dihydrosphingosine synthetase. There is increasing recognition of the vital role of pyridoxine in the development and maintenance of the integrity of the nervous system. Both the metabolism of neurotransmitters and the process of myelination are affected in pyridoxine deficiency. There is much evidence that even a moderate deficiency of vitamin B-6 is deleterious. The need for an increased requiremnt of this vitamin under certain normal physiological conditions and the occurrence of iatrogenic deficiency are also well recognized. Yet, the assessment of the vitamin B-6 status of various population groups has been excluded in most national nutritional surveys in view of technical difficulties. The assessment is complicated as vitamin B-6 exists as pyridoxine (PN), pyridoxal (PL), pyridoxamine (PM) as well as their phosphorylated derivatives. In the assessment of the vitamin B-6 status of an individual, the concentrations of the various vitamers should be taken into consideration.

Several chemical (1-19), microbiological (20-26), and enzymatic (27-31) methods are available for the determination of these vitamers. Each method has its special advantages and limitations. Newer methods have been published since the reviews by Storvick (7,32). Currently available chemical methods will be reviewed with respect to their sensitivity and specificity. As the levels of the vitamers vary considerably in various tissues, a method capable of determining 100 pg to 10 ng of these compounds would have biological application.

GENERAL PROBLEMS IN THE ASSAY OF B-6 VITAMERS

The assay of vitamin B-6 vitamers in biological materials is
generally unsatisfactory and difficult as all forms are photosensi-
tive and heat labile. The polyfunctional nature of the various
molecules creates further problems in the development of an efficient
and reliable assay procedure. Functional groups like hydroxy,
phenolic, and amino groups react without discrimination with the
usual reagents like disyl chloride, dansyl chloride, acetic anydride,
trimethylsilyl chloride, or trifluoroacetyl chloride, and form mono-,
bis, and tris-products in the reactions mixture. The specificity
of these reactions is thus lost and a wide scatter in assay results
occur. Thus, the development of a method which can offer specificity,
sensitivity, reliability, and ease of operation for all the vitameric
forms in a limited amount of biological material is a real challenge.

Two approaches, each with its own advantage and limitation,
have been used. The first involves separation of the various B-6
forms on suitable resin columns followed by their derivatization
under optimal reaction conditions. Derivatization, further, would
stablilize the vitamers which are sensitive to radiation in both
the ultraviolet and visual range. This is the method of choice in
an assay which includes all vitamers. In the second approach,
derivatization is achieved first followed by purification and assay
of the desired derivatives. This approach is useful for the assay
of individual vitamers. It is obvious that in the same reaction a
single reagent cannot react optimally with all the vitamers which
carry different functions at the 4-position and which are capable
of existing in different ionic forms under acidic, basic, and
neutral conditions (Figs. 1,2,3).

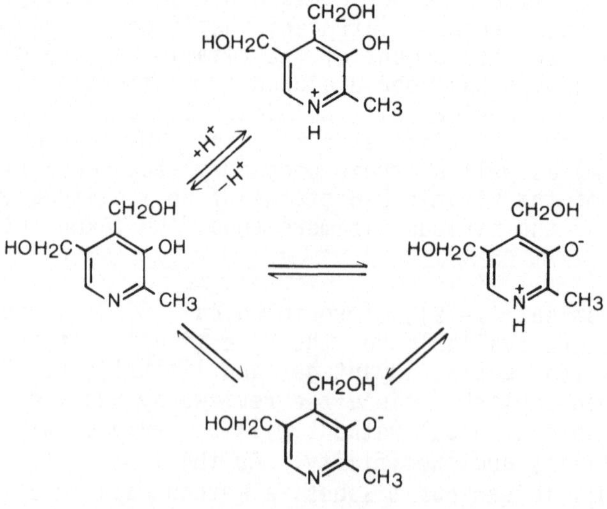

Fig. 1. Dissociable forms of pyridoxine.

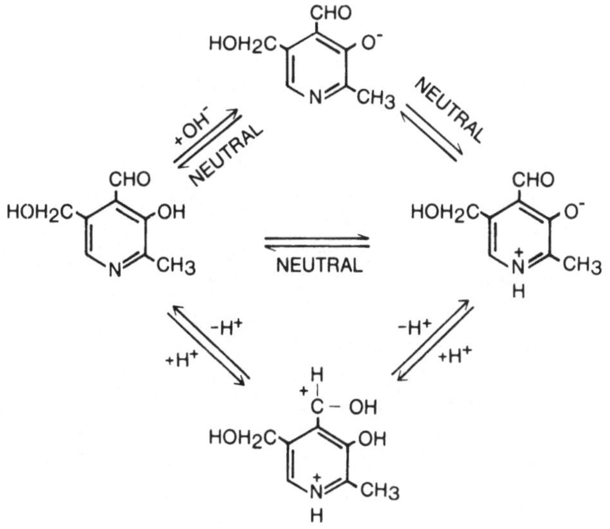

Fig. 2.   Dissociable forms of pyridoxal.

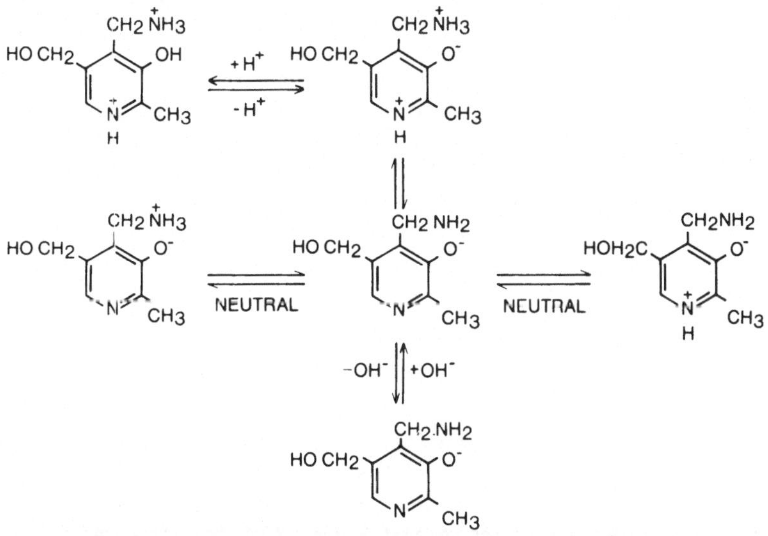

Fig. 3.   Dissociable forms of pyridoxamine.

EXTRACTION OF B-6 VITAMERS FROM BIOLOGICAL MATERIAL

Common to all assay methods is the need for a complete extraction of the vitamers from biological material. The majority of extraction procedures deal with serum or whole blood and can be used for other tissues with little or no modification. Tissue proteins are removed by precipitation with either acetone, ethanol, methanol, perchloric acid, or trichloracetic acid. Organic solvents are removed and an aqueous extract is used as such or after further separation for B-6 vitamer analysis. Perchloric acid is removed easily as the potassium salt. In extractions using trichloroacetic acid (TCA), the protein-free supernatant is extracted with ether or ether containing 2% trioctylamine to remove TCA. Extraction with perchloric or trichloroacetic acid at room temperature is superior to extraction with organic solvents. This is partly due to the conversion of the pyridine bases to quarternary ammonium salts. In addition, the presence of polar groups and the zwitterionic nature of these molecules make them more soluble in water than in organic solvents.

The procedures mentioned above extract the non-covalently bound forms of the vitamers from the biological material. The extraction of the covalently bound vitamin B-6 form is carried out under more drastic hydrolytic conditions which could create further problems of polymerization or condensation of the vitamers with free amino acids or other constituents of the hydrolysate. Furthermore, pyridoxal phosphate or pyridoxamine phosphate can hydrolyze to pyridoxal and pyridoxamine respectively (32). The use of semicarbazide in releasing the covalently bound PL and PLP by "trans-schiffization" will be discussed later.

Further separation of PN, PL, PM, and their phosphorylated derivatives can be carried out using ion exchange column (8,9,20) or thin layer (33) chromatography. Electrophoretic separation (34, 35) has also been reported.

ANALYTICAL TECHNIQUES

Native State Fluroescence

Duggan and Udenfriend (19) were the first to use the native fluorescence of pyridoxine, pyridoxal, and pyridoxamine to determine the amounts present in simple solutions of these compounds. This method was extended by Coursin and Brown (3) for the determination of the vitamers in whole blood. Treatment of the acetone extract of blood with H_2O_2 and uv irradiation were used for the differential identification rather than the differential assay of the

vitamers by these authors. According to these authors, uv irradiation for 3-5 minutes completely destroys PN, PM, and PL. The
products formed by oxidation with H_2O_2 or treatment with uv radiation
have not been defined. The possibility of incomplete reaction
resulting in some unchanged starting material being present along
with the product has also not been considered by them. Heyl et al.
(36) have identified 3,4 dihydroxy 2-methyl 5-hydroxymethylpyridine
as a product of oxidation of pyridoxal with H_2O_2. Its emission
maxima is in the same wavelength region as pyridoxal. The formation
of other products like N-oxide cannot be ruled out. The effect of
H_2O_2 and uv irradiation on the contaminants in the acetone extract
and their subsequent interference in the fluorescence yield of
these vitamers cannot be assessed in this type of experimental
setup without proper blanks. In view of these considerations, it
is highly improbable that this method could yield reliable data
when applied to the acetone extract of serum which contains a
mixture of fluorescent and nonfluorescent contaminants. Further
purification of the acetone extract seems to be a necessary
preliminary step.

Table 1. Native State Fluorescence Maxima of B-6
          Vitamers

Vitamers	pH	Excitation	Emission
		nm	nm
Pyridoxine	6-7	340	400
Pyridoxal	6-7	330	385
Pyridoxamine	6-7	335	400
Pyridoxamine 5'-phosphate	6-7	330	385

Loo and Badger (9) have used such an approach to assay B-6
vitamers in rat brain. The vitamers were separated on an Amberlite
column. PN, PL, PM, and PMP were determined fluorometrically in the
native state. The exitation and emission maxima are given in Table
1. Pyridoxal phosphate was determined as the cyanohydrin derivative
after a further purification on a Dowex-1 column. This will be
discussed in the next section. The determination of B-6 vitamers
through their native fluorescence, although convenient and time-
saving, is not without its defects. All B-6 vitamers are photo-
sensitive and the extent of the photodecomposition of each in a
sample is not uniform. The use of proper blanks as well as filters
which can mask the absorption due to contaminants in the various
eluates can improve this method considerably.

Methods Based on Fluorescence of Derivatives

Ultraviolet irradiation of B-6 vitamers leads to decomposition of these compounds. The method based on the native fluorescence of B-6 vitamers might not yield accurate data as the rates and extent of this decomposition vary. Hence the various attempts to convert these labile compounds to stable derivatives.

Cyanohydrin method. Bonavita (4) employed the fluorescent characteristics of the cyanohydrin of pyridoxal and pyridoxal phosphate for the assay of these compounds in blood. Reaction of PL and PLP with KCN results in the saturation of the double bond in the 4-position according to the equation (Fig. 4) where R represents the pyridine ring of PL or PLP. Cyanohydrin formation is simple in operation and specific for the 4-formyl group. Also, pyridoxal and pyridoxal phosphate could be determined in the presence of each other when the concentration of pyridoxal in the mixture is not too high. Pyridoxal cyanohydrin yields maximum fluorescence at pH 10 while pyridoxal phosphate responds at pH of 3.5. The conversion of PL and PLP to the cyanohydrins is quantitative and the method is sensitive in the concentration range 10 ng/ml.

Semicarbazone method. Semicarbazide reacts with pyridoxal or its phosphate to give a highly fluorescent semicarbazone (Fig. 5). This procedure has been applied to whole blood, red cells, and plasma (15). Semicarbazide reacts not only with free PL and PLP but is also capable of breaking the Schiff base of PLP with amino groups of proteins by "trans-schiffization" reaction (37). Thus both free and protein-bound pyridoxal phosphate can be estimated. This method compares well with the cyanohydrin method in sensitivity and specificity for the aldehyde group. However, it suffers from the disadvantage that PL and PLP cannot be measured in the presence of each other due to their fluorescence overlap (15). Prior separation of PL from PLP would exclude mutual interference in the assay. Other metabolites like glyceraldehyde, its phosphate, pyruvic acid, phosphoenolpyruvate, and several sugars do not interfere in the determination of PLP.

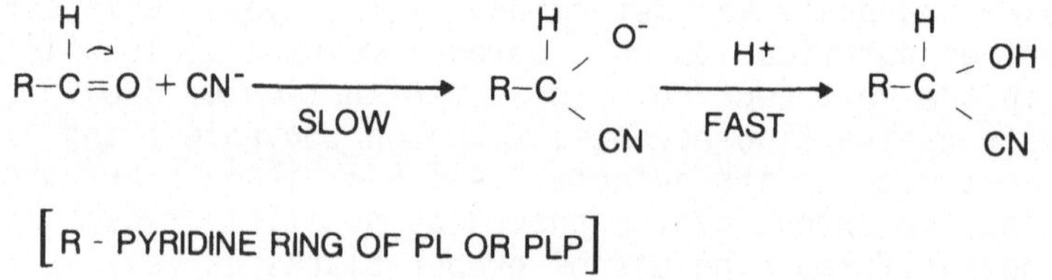

$$R-\overset{\overset{\displaystyle H}{|}}{C}=O + CN^- \xrightarrow[\text{SLOW}]{} R-\overset{\overset{\displaystyle H}{|}}{C}\overset{O^-}{\underset{CN}{}} \xrightarrow[\text{FAST}]{H^+} R-\overset{\overset{\displaystyle H}{|}}{C}\overset{OH}{\underset{CN}{}}$$

[R - PYRIDINE RING OF PL OR PLP]

Fig. 4. Formation of cyanohydrin of PL and PLP.

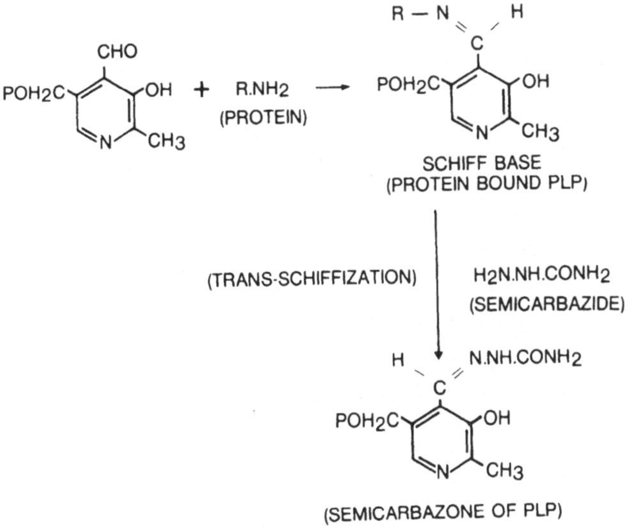

Fig. 5.   Formation of semicarbazone of PLP.

Isobenzofuran method.   This method (14) is based on the reaction
of 2-chlorosulfophenyl-3-phenylindanone. The product, on treatment with sodium ethoxide undergoes rearrangement to a highly
fluorescent diphenylisobenzofuran derivative (Fig. 6). Pyridoxal
gives one product while two products (mono- and bis-) are isolated
from pyridoxamine. The separation of the products is achieved by
thin-layer chromatography on silica gel plates. The yellowish
green fluorescence of these products is measured at 478 nm for the
PL derivative and at 480 nm for the PM derivative when the sodium
ethoxide solution of these compounds is excited at 410 nm.

The procedure is very sensitive and can measure up to 2 ng/ml
of PL. Its use for determination of PM is questionable as both
the mono- and bis-products are formed. The conditions for optimal
formation of one or the other product is not known. The relative
molar fluorescence intensities of these compounds are also not
known. 1-p-Chlorosulfophenyl 3-phenylindanone cannot discriminate
between amino and phenolic groups.

Methyl anthranilate method. This method (17,18) is based on
the reductive amination of PL or PLP with methyl anthranilate and
sodium cyanoborohydride at pH4.5 to 5.0 and 35-38°. Methyl-N-
pyridoxylanthranilate and methyl-N-pyridoxal phosphate-4-anthranilate
are formed from PL and PLP respectively (Fig. 7). The amine product is highly fluorescent and can measure pyridoxal in the range
1-10 ng/ml (Fig. 8). The amine product formed from PLP is hydrolyzed
with alkaline phosphatase before fluorescence determination. The

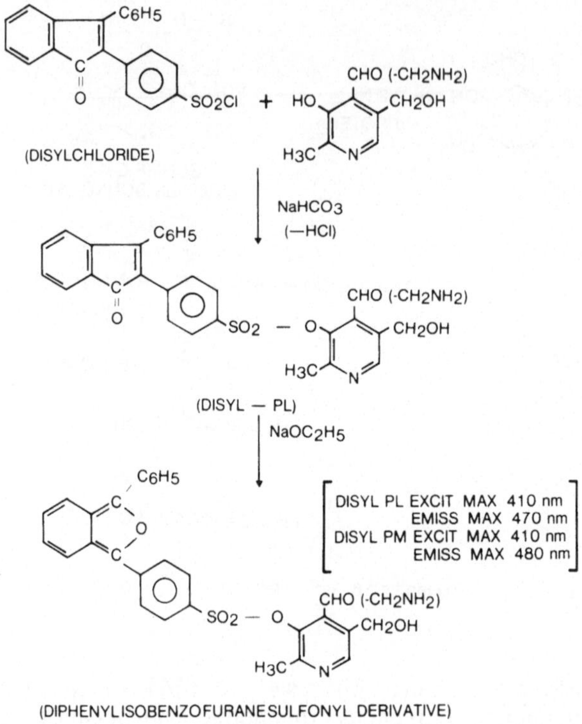

Fig. 6.   Isobenzofurane derivatives of PL and PM.

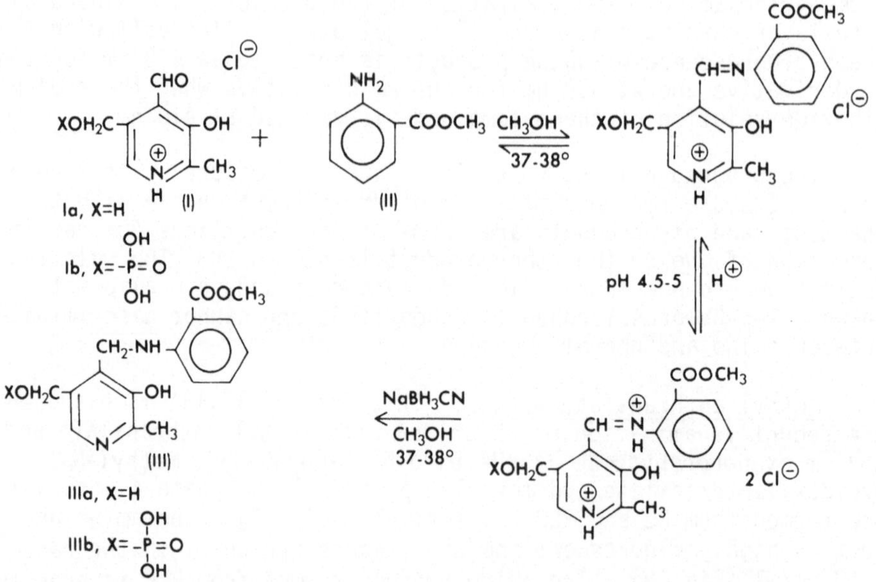

Fig. 7.   Methyl-N-pyridoxylanthranilate of PL and PLP.

purity of the product is based on the combination of column and thin-layer chromatography to get rid of impurities and extra fluorophores. This method is specific for the aldehyde form. PL and PLP can be determined from the same reaction. Interference from impurities is practically absent. All these methods used to form the stable fluorescent derivatives of PL and PLP can be applied for the determination of other B-6 vitamers like PN, PM, and PMP after their conversion to the aldehyde form. The procedures for this will be discussed in a later section.

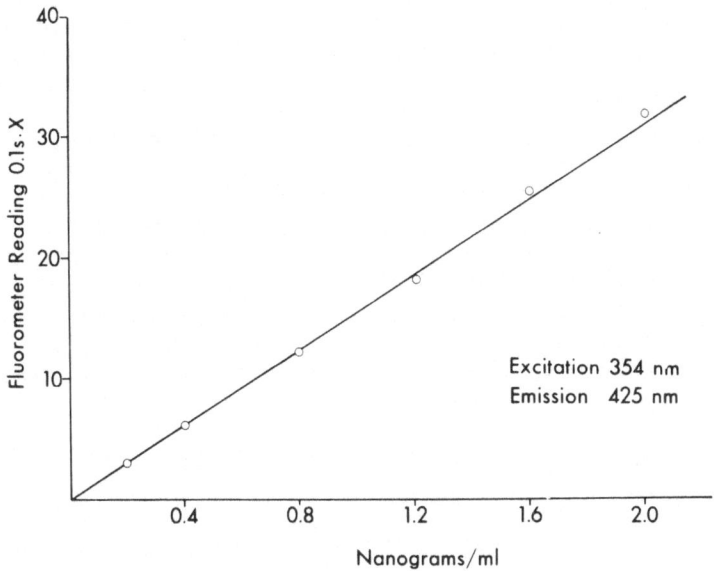

Fig. 8.   Calibration curve for methyl-N-pyridoxylanthranilate.

For the assay of pyridoxal and pyridoxal phosphate in serum, the following stock solutions in absolute methanol were prepared: methylanthranilate = 1 mg/ml; sodium cyanoborohydride = 1 mg/ml. Serum (5 ml) and acetone (25 ml) were stirred for 30 minutes at room temperature in a 100 ml conical flask protected from light. The solution was centrifuged on a clinical centrifuge and the supernatant collected. The residue was treated with acetone (10 ml) and the solution centrifuged again. The combined supernatant was stripped of the organic solvent at 38-40° on a rotary evaporator under reduced pressure. The dry residue was treated with acetone (5 ml) and the solution filtered on a Buchner's funnel. The acetone was completely removed as before and the residue treated with absolute methanol (1 ml) and the solution was filtered. Methylanthranilate (250 µl) was added to the filtrate and the solution brought to pH 4.5-5.0 with methanolic HCl. The reaction mixture was warmed to

37-38° in a water bath for 7 minutes and then sodium cyanoborohydride solution (50 μl) was added while swirling the solution. It
was kept at 37-38° for an additional 15 minutes while the pH of
the solution was maintained at 4.5-5.0 with methanolic HCl. The
pH was then brought to 2 with methanolic HCl and the solvent removed
under reduced pressure taking care that the temperature of the water
bath did not exceed 38°. The residue was treated with water (1 ml)
and the pH of the solution adjusted to 2 with 5 N HCl if necessary.
The pH of the solution was then brought to 8.0-8.5 with sodium
bicarbonate and the aqueous solution extracted with methylene
chloride (4x5 ml). The aqueous solution was saved for pyridoxal
phosphate assay (see below) while the combined organic extract was
stripped of the solvent. The residue was dissolved in chloroform
and chromatographed over a silica gel column (0.5 mm x 15 cm) containing 350 mg of silica gel. It was eluted first with chloroform
(10 ml) to get rid of the unreacted methylanthranilate and then
with a mixture of chloroform and methanol (9:1, v/v, 5 ml) to obtain
methyl-N-pyridoxylanthranilate. The organic solvent was removed
and the residue rechromatographed over a silica gel plate (0.25 mm
x 20 x 20 cm) with a mixture of chloroform and methanol (9:1 v/v)
along with the standard. The methyl-N-pyridoxylanthranilate spot
was scraped off the plate and eluted with a mixture of chloroform
and methanol (9:1, v/v, 10 ml). The organic solvent was removed
and the residual methyl-N-pyridoxylanthranilate was dissolved in
absolute ethanol and assayed fluorometrically. An adjacent equivalent area of the silica gel plate was eluted with the solvent to
provide the blank.

For the assay of pyridoxal phosphate, the above-mentioned
aqueous solution was brought to pH 10.4 with a few drops of 0.1 M
sodium carbonate solution. Alkaline phosphatase (2 units) was added
and the solution incubated at 38° for 1 hour. It was then extracted
with methylene chloride as before. The organic solvent was removed
and the residue was chromatographed on a silica gel plate as before
along with the standard methyl-N-pyridoxylanthranilate (Fig. 9).
Elution and fluorometric assay are performed as described above.

Pyridoxic acid lactone method. This is one of the older methods
for the determination of pyridoxine (1,38). Pyridoxine is oxidized
with potassium permanganate to 4-pyridoxic acid which is converted
into the lactone with hydrochloric acid (Fig. 10). In this procedure, the excess KMnO$_4$ used in the first reaction is destroyed
with hydrogen peroxide. Pyridoxal is also oxidized to 4-pyridoxic
acid under the above reaction conditions (39). Thus, separation
of PN and PL before oxidation is essential for differential assay.
KMnO$_4$ and H$_2$O$_2$ are fairly general oxidizing agents under acidic,
basic, and neutral conditions (40). In order to achieve specificity with these reagents, the use of reproducible conditions and

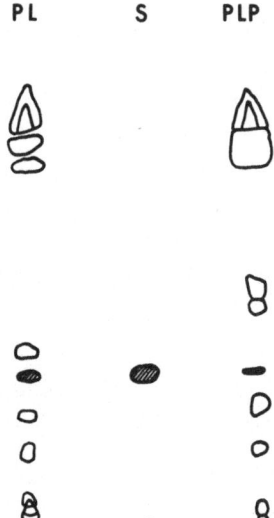

Fig. 9. A "typical" thin-layer chromatogram of derivative from serum.

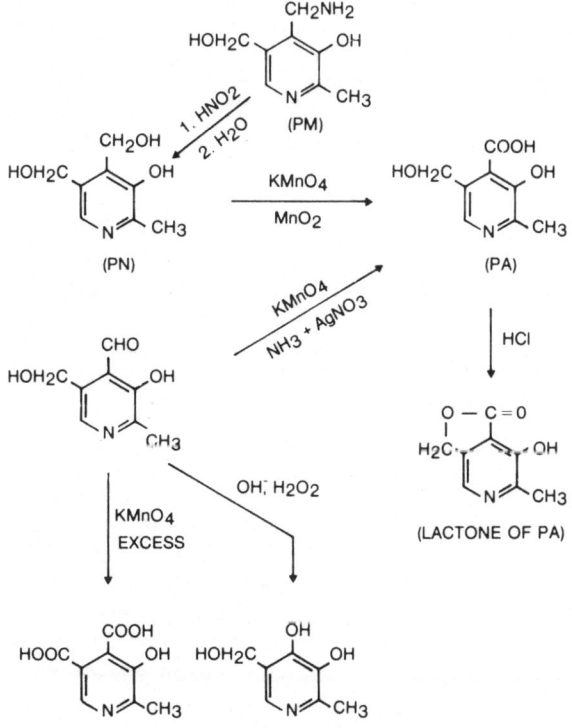

Fig. 10. Formation of PA lactone and side reactions.

equivalent amounts of the reagents is extremely important. Excess oxidizing agents can lead to side reactions. H_2O_2 reacts with PL to give 3,4-dihydroxy 5-hydroxy-methyl 2-methylpyridine. As pointed out earlier, the formation of N-oxide cannot be ruled out. The effect of these products on the fluorescence yield has not been investigated. Furthermore, the direct oxidation of pyridoxine produces the lactone in poor yield (32,39). Moreover, this procedure requires special treatment for the preparation of the blank since lactone formation occurs even at room temperature with hydrochloric acid. Ammoniacal silver nitrate (38) and manganese dioxide (39) are better and more specific oxidizing agents than $KMnO_4$ and do not require further treatment with H_2O_2.

Determination of pyridoxamine. Lactone method--pyridoxamine is diazotised with potassium nitrite and dilute sulfuric acid at 0-4^0 and the diazonium salt is decomposed by heating at 100^0 for 10 minutes (2,38). Pyridoxine is then converted to the lactone of pyridoxic acid as described in the section on pyridoxic acid lactone method.

The conversion of pyridoxamine to pyridoxine proceeds with a low (40-50%) yield due to side reactions. Addition of urea to destroy the excess nitrous acid may improve the yield. Dilute HCl should not be used in the diazotisation reaction as Cl$^-$ can substitute for the OH$^-$. The conversion of pyridoxine to pyridoxic acid is not quantitative, as discussed in the section on pyridoxic acid lactone method. Thus, the overall yield of the product from pyridoxamine is low (32).

Transamination--the transamination of pyridoxamine to pyridoxal in the presence of glyoxylic acid and catalytic amounts of potassium aluminum sulfate proceeds at pH 5 (Fig. 11). Product yields up to 70% have been reported (41). Addition of potassium cyanide to the reaction mixture produces the cyanohydrin of pyridoxal which is measured fluorometrically. This procedure has been used to determine PM content of food stuffs (6).

We recently found (42) that the addition of MnO_2 to the reaction mixture improves by 20-25% the yield of the PL cyanohydrin (Fig. 11). Manganese dioxide seems to reduce the possibility of Schiff base formation as a side reaction. It oxidizes any glycine produced in the reaction to glyoxal. Thus, Schiff base formation between pyridoxal and glycine and between glycine and glyoxal is avoided to a great extent. In addition, direct oxidation of PM to PL is facilitated by MnO_2. This modification has enabled us to measure pyridoxamine levels in serum which was not possible by earlier methods.

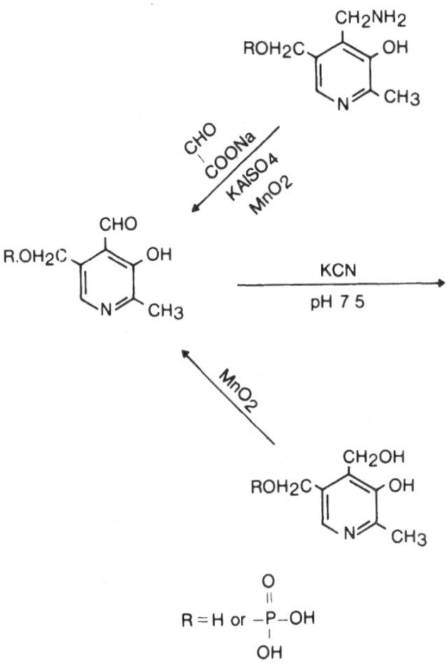

Fig. 11. Conversion of PN and PM to PL and assay as cyanohydrin.

Method for the simultaneous assay of all B-6 vitamers in biological material. We have combined the advantages of a preliminary separation of B-6 vitamers on an ion exchange column with the specificity and simplicity of the cyanohydrin reaction to estimate PN, PL, PM, and the phosphates of PL and PM in biological material like serum, whole blood, or a tissue extract. In this procedure, pyridoxine is oxidized to PL. Pyridoxamine and pyridoxamine phosphate are transaminated (see above) quantitatively to PL. The final reaction is the formation of PL-cyanohydrin which is quantitative. The reactions are specific with no side reactions. Interference due to contaminants is eliminated since the sample and the blank are treated exactly in the same manner except for the addition of KCN. This method has been applied to normal and hemolyzed serum samples with complete recoveries of internal standards. Bile pigments also do not interfere with the assay.

For the extraction of B-6 vitamers from serum, human serum (5 ml) was diluted with 0.2 M sodium acetate buffer pH 4 (25 ml) and 20% trichloroacetic acid (10 ml) added. The mixture was stirred at room temperature for 30 minutes and centrifuged. The supernatant was extracted with peroxide-free diethyl ether containing 5% n-octylamine (3 x 75 ml) to remove trichloroacetic acid. The addition of n-octylamine to ether was found to eliminate completely trichloroacetic acid from the aqueous extract and also convert various pyridinium salts to their respective bases. The combined ethereal extract was washed with water (2 x 5 ml) and the ether discarded. The combined washing was added to the aqueous extract and the aqueous solution evaporated to dryness under reduced pressure on a rotary evaporator. The temperature of the water bath during distillation was not allowed to exceed 40°. The residue was extracted with water (1 ml) and the solution applied to a 2.5 ml Amberlite column.

The method used for the separation of PLP, PMP, PL, PN, and PM was that of Loo and Badger (9) with some modifications.

PLP, PMP, PL, PN, and PM were separated on a sulfonated Amberlite resin. The resin in the Na$^+$-form was equilibrated to pH 3.5 with 0.01 M sodium acetate buffer and packed to 2.5 cm length in a glass column (0.8 mm x 150 cm) with a reservoir of 40 ml capacity with the same buffer. Serum extract (1.0 ml) containing all the B-6 vitamers was applied to the top of the column and the column eluted with 9 ml of water. The effluent containing PLP was collected and held for the assay.

The column was then successively eluted with 0.01 M sodium acetate pH 3.5 (5.0 ml), 0.1 M sodium acetate pH 4 (15.0 ml), and 0.1 M sodium acetate pH 5.0 (15.0 ml). The last fraction contained PMP which was converted into PLP-CN (cyanohydrin derivative of pyridoxal phosphate) derivative at the time of its assay.

Further elution of the column with 0.1 M phosphate buffers, pH 6.0 (12.5 ml) and pH 6.5 (12.5 ml) yielded PL and PN, respectively. PM was finally obtained with 0.1 M Na_2HPO_4 (25.0 ml). The flow rate through the column was maintained at 0.5 ml/min. All extractions and separations were carried out in subdued light and at room temperature.

For recoveries of PLP, PMP, PL, PN, and PM from their standard mixtures, 2.5 ml fractions were collected to check complete elution of each component. The chromatographic separation of B-6 vitamers is described in Fig. 12. A clear separation of PLP, PMP, PL, PN, and PM from a standard mixture of the B-6 vitamers added to serum or serum extract prior to chromatography was in the range 90-96%.

PL and PLP were determined fluorometrically as their cyanohydrin derivatives. PM, PMP, and PN were all converted to the aldehyde form and determined as the cyanohydrin derivatives. All fluorometric measurements were made using an Aminco-Bowman spectrophotofluorometer.

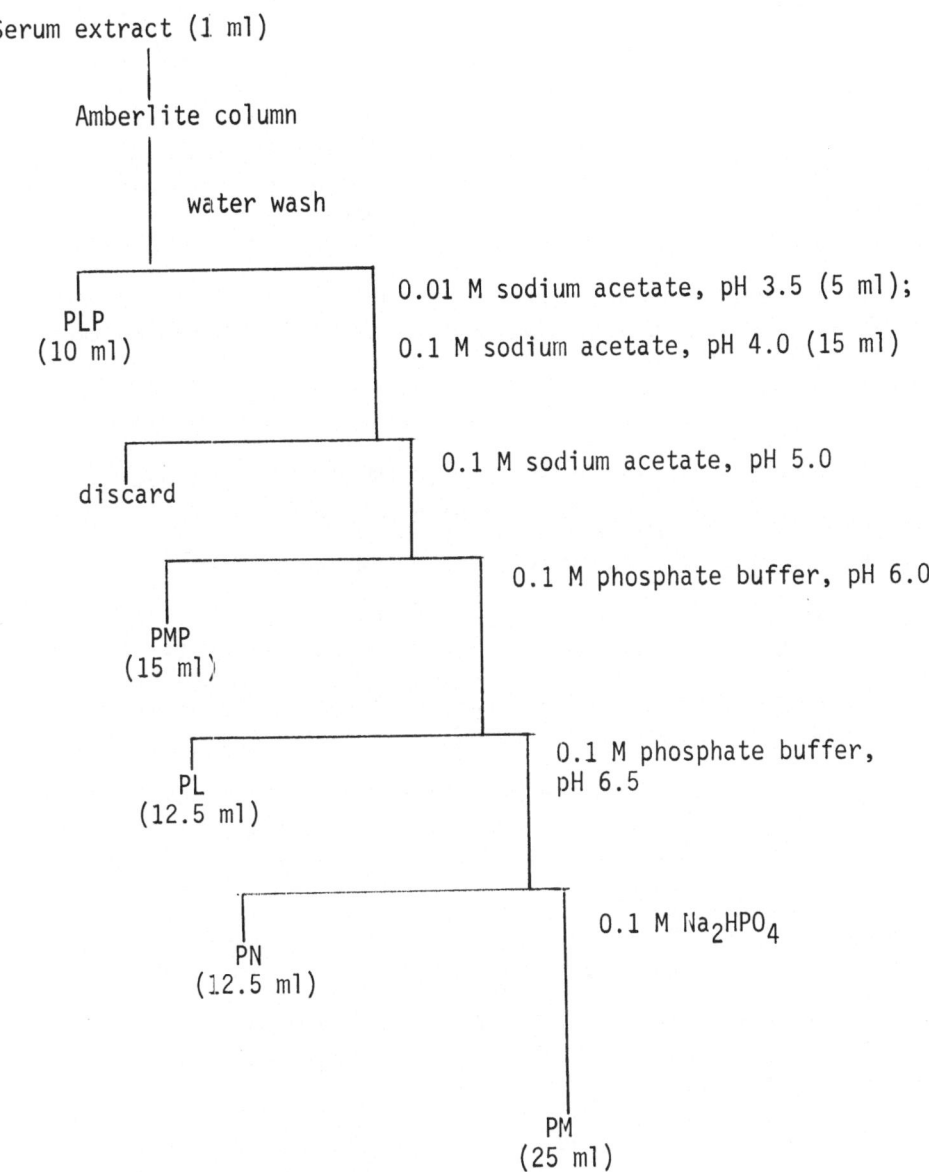

Fig. 12.   Chromatographic separation of B-6 vitamers.

The PL elute was brought to pH 7.5 with 5 N NaOH. To 5.0 ml aliquots of this solution were added 50 μl of 0.1 M potassium cyanide and water, respectively, for the preparation of the samples and the blank. Both the solutions were incubated at 50° for 2 hours and brought to pH 10 with 5 N NaOH. The fluorescence intensity of PL-CN (cyanohydrin derivative of pyridoxal) was measured at 436 nm emission when excited at 358 nm.

0.2 M sodium phosphate buffer, pH 7.5 (10 ml) was added to the PLP elute. PLP-CN and the blank were prepared as described for PL and adjusted to pH 3.5 with dilute phosphoric acid. The fluorescence was read at 420 nm with excitation at 315 nm.

PM and PMP were determined as PL-CN and PLP-CN derivatives, respectively. The quantitative conversion of PM and PMP to the corresponding aldehydes was brought about by a combination of transamination and oxidation reactions using sodium glyoxalate, potassium aluminum sulfate, and manganese dioxide in the same reaction.

For the preparation of PL-CN from PM, the amine eluate was adjusted to pH 5.0 with glacial acetic acid and 0.1 mM sodium glyoxalate (50 μl), 0.01 mM potassium aluminum sulfate (50 μl), and magnanese dioxide (30 mg) were added. The reaction mixture was heated at 100° for 30 minutes with vigorous stirring. The solution was cooled and centrifuged to remove manganese dioxide. The pH of the solution was brought to 7.5 with 5 N NaOH. Aliquots of this solution were used for the preparation of PL-CN and the blank was as described at the top of this page for the estimation of PL. 10 N NH_4OH solution was used for pH adjustment.

For the preparation of PLP-CN from PMP, PMP was converted into PLP and then into PLP-CN, by the procedure described above. The pH of PLP-CN was adjusted to 3.5 for fluorescence measurements.

The PN eluate was brought to pH 4.5 with acetic acid and manganese dioxide (30 mg) was added. The reaction mixture was heated at 100° for 30 minutes with vigorous stirring, cooled to room temperature, centrifuged, and the supernatant adjusted to pH 7.5 with 5 N NaOH. Aliquots of this solution were used for the preparation of PL-CN and the blank. 10 N NH_4OH solution was used for pH adjustments.

Our values for the concentrations of PL, PLP, PM, and PMP in serum are given in Table 2 and compared with those reported in the literature (8,13,14,18,24,28,29,44,45,47).

Table 2. Serum and Whole Blood PLP, PMP, PL, PN, and PM Concentration

PLP Mean±S.D. (ng/ml)	PLP Range	PMP Mean±S.D. (ng/ml)	PMP Range	PL Mean±S.D. (ng/ml)	PL Range	PN Mean±S.D. (ng/ml)	PM Mean±S.D. (ng/ml)	PM Range	No. of observations	Method
17.8±2.7	13.6-23.0	3.7±0.7	2.1-4.9	42.0±8.4	28.5-60.8	N.M.	27.6±6.4	15.6-34.2	27	present method (S-F)
9.9±1.9	7.9-14.2	-	-	38.3±8.1	25.3-55.1	-	-	-	20	Chauhan & Dakshinamurti (18) (S-F)
15.9	6.3-26.5	-	-	16.4	6.7-17.0	-	-	-	5	Takanishi et al. (13) (S-F)
10.0±6.5	-	-	-	-	-	-	-	-	18	Hamfelt (46) (S-E)
34.3	-	31.7	-	28.6	-	-	33.7	-	?	Contractor & Shane (8) (W-F)
-	-	-	-	53.0	11.0-147.0	-	35.0	7.0-96.0	16	Durko et al. (14) (S-F)
34.9±9.3	-	-	-	-	-	-	-	-	46	Hines & Love (28) (S-E)
9.5	0.0-13.0	-	-	-	-	-	-	-	24	Walsh (44) (S-E)
18.5±5.5	-	-	-	-	-	-	-	-	17	Chabner et al. (29) (S-E)
7.7	3.3-14.0	-	-	-	-	-	-	-	53	Anderson et al. (24) (S-M)
-	-	-	-	46.0	20.0-70.0	-	180	150-200	3	Fumita & Fujino (47) (W-F)
10.5±4.1	-	-	-	-	-	-	-	-	50	Lumeng et al. (45) (S-E)

N.M.-Not Measurable; S-Serum or Plasma; WB-Whole Blood; F-Fluorometric; E-Enzymatic; M-Microbiological.

Phenylhydrazone Colorimetric Method

The method of Wada and Snell (5) for the determination of PL and PLP is very suitable for the determination of these compounds in enzyme reaction mixtures. PL and PLP form hydrazones with a variety of aromatic hydrazines in acidified aqueous solution. Phenylhydrazine yields stable hydrazones with PL or PLP (Fig. 13). The product is of an intense yellow color with an absorption maximun at 410 nm. By decreasing the reaction temperature and increasing the acidity of the reaction mixture, the rate of color development as between PL and PLP could be increased to permit determination of PLP in the presence of a moderate excess of PL. Keto-acids like α-ketoglutaric and pyruvic acids do not interfere in the assay. Of the naturally occurring carbonyl compounds, only glyoxalate was found to interfere. However, when this method was applied to urine or tissue homogenates, the absorbancy at 410 nm was greater than can be accounted for by their PL contents.

5-Chloro 2,4-Disulfonyl Chloride-1-Aminobenzene Colorimetric Method

In this procedure preliminary separation of B-6 vitamers on an ion exchange resin columturn is combined with the formation of the colored diazo products (47). The isolated B-6 vitamers are coupled with diazotised 5-chloro 2,4-disulfonyl chloride-1-aminobenzene to produce characteristic orange products (Fig. 14). This method has been employed in the assay of B-6 vitamers in pharmaceutical products and some biological material. The sensitivity of the procedure is quite low (2-25 µg/ml) which limits its use in the assay of B-6 vitamers in blood or tissue homogenates.

Gas-liquid Chromatography

B-6 vitamers are not volatile enough because of the presence of polar groups in these compounds for their direct use in GLC separatory techniques. The preparation of suitable volatile derivatives thus becomes an important first step in the GLC analysis

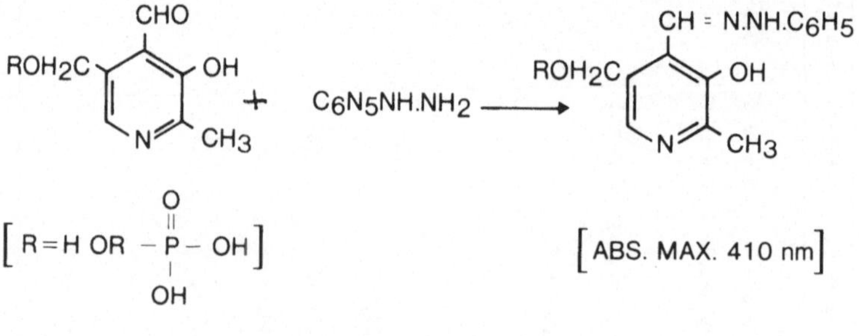

Fig. 13.   Phenylhydrazone of PL, PLP.

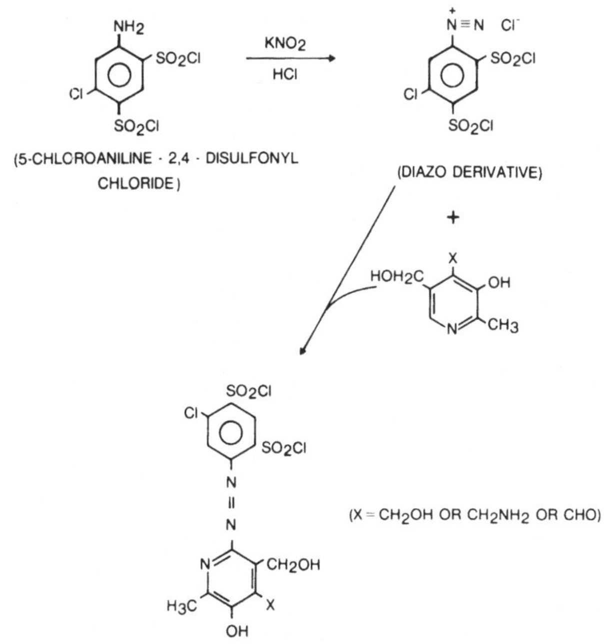

Fig. 14.   Diazo derivatives of PN, PM, and PL.

of these compounds. Studies on the chromatographic behavior of acetyl (48-50), benzyl (48), isopropylidene (48), trimethylsilyl (50,51), and trifluororacetyl (52) derivatives have been reported. Of these, acetylation has been considered to be satisfactory for the analysis of PN, PL, and PM.   The derivatization reactions are quantitative at ambient temperature.   Most of these methods use the more conventional flame ionization detector which has low sensitivity. These procedures are sensitive in the μg range and have been applied only to pure compounds like PN, PL, PM, and the lactone of 4PA or to pharmaceutical preparations.   The full potential of the GLC technique has not been realized for the separation of B-6 vitamers from biological material.   Preparation of suitable derivatives of the phosphorylated forms of PN, PL, and PM has not been reported so far.   Two attempts at increasing the sensitivity of these techniques are of significance in the context of their biological applicability. Imanari and Tamura (52) and Williams (53) have prepared the tri-fluoroacetyl derivatives of the nonphosphorylated B-6 vitamers as well as the lactone of 4PA.   The highly electronegative nature of these derivatives and the use of an electron capture detector have resulted in obtaining good resolution and response in the ng range. However, this method has been applied only to pure compounds.

Silylating or acetylating agents are single protecting group donors and they do not exploit the distinctive moieties of poly-functional compounds which could allow the use of more specific reagents involving proximal groups. Boronic acids react specifi-cally with 1,2 diols to form cyclic boronates. This method has been used for the chromatographic analysis of 4-hydroxy 3-methoxy-phenylethyleneglycol and 3,4-dihydroxy-phenylethyleneglycol in biological material (54,55). The presence of the 1,2 diol group in pyridoxine makes it amenable to such derivatization. The phenolic group of pyridoxine was methylated with diazomethane prior to boro-nation. The formation of the boronic ester (Fig. 15) is quantitative in yield. Conventional flame ionization detectors are adequate to detect up to 10 ng of PN. The response was linear from 10 to 100 ng per injection. As PM and PL can be quantitiatively converted to PN, this method could be used to determine all three B-6 vitamers. Application of this procedure to biological material is currently being investigated.

CONCLUSION

Determination of the vitamin B-6 content of biological material is complicated by the presence of the vitamers PN, PL, PM, and their phosphorylated forms. These compounds are decomposed by radiation in both the visible and ultraviolet range. Because of this, methods based on the native fluorescence of the B-6 vitamers are of limited value. Derivatization to form photostable compounds is a necessary prerequisite in their assay. The vitamers and their phosphates are separated by ion exchange column chromatography

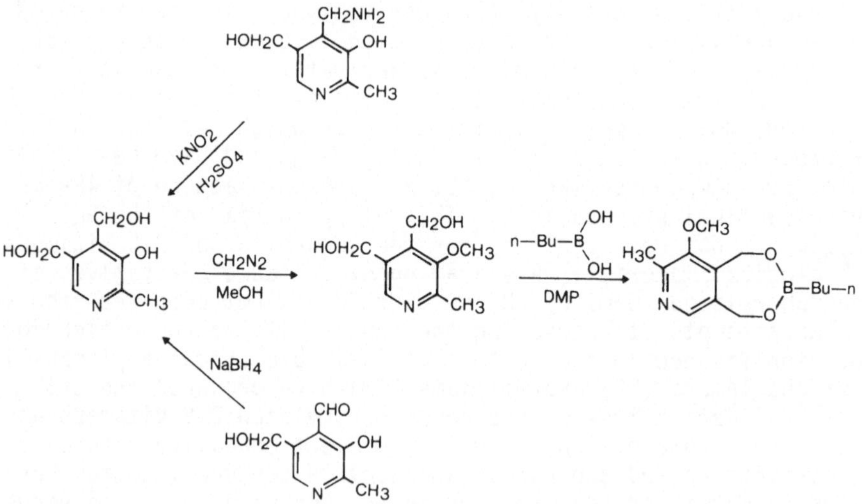

Fig. 15.   n-Butylboronic acid derivatives of PN, PM, and PL.

prior to derivatization. PL and PLP form stable cyanohydrins. PN, PM, and their phosphates can be converted quantitatively to PL or PLP before cyanohydrin formation. Thus, all the B-6 vitamers can be analyzed from a single sample of biological material. The potential of gas liquid chromatography for the assay of the B-6 vitamers has not been fully exploited.

LITERATURE CITED

1. Fujita, A., Matsuura, K. & Fujino, K. (1955) Fluorometric determination of vitamin B-6. Determination of pyridoxine. J. Vitaminol. 1, 267-274.
2. Fujita, A., Fujita, D. & Fumino, K. (1955) Flurometric determination of vitamin B-6. Determination of pyridoxamine. J. Vitaminol. 1, 275-278; Fluorometric determination of vitamin B-6. Fractional determination of pyridoxal and 4-pyridoxic acid. J. Vitaminol. 1, 279-289.
3. Coursin, D. B. & Brown, V. C. (1958) Measurement of compounds of vitamin B-6 group in blood. Proc. Soc. Expt. Biol. Med. 98, 315-318.
4. Bonavita, V. (1960) The reaction of pyridoxal 5'-phosphate with cyanide and its analytical use. Arch. Biochem. Biophys. 88, 366-372.
5. Wada, H. & Snell, E. E. (1961) The enzymatic oxidation of pyridoxine and pyridoxamine phosphates. J. Biol. Chem. 236, 2089-2095.
6. Toepfer, E. W., Polansky, M. M. & Hewston, E. M. (1961) Fluorometric determination of pyridoxamine by conversion to pyridoxal cyanide compound. Anal. Biochem. 2, 463-469.
7. Storvick, C. A., Benson, E. M., Edward, M. A. & Woodring, M. J. (1964) Chemical and microbiological determination of vitamin B-6. Methods in Biochem. Analysis 12, 183-276.
8. Contractor, S. F. & Shane, B. (1968) Estimation of vitamin B-6 compounds in human blood and urine. Clin. Chim. Acta 21, 71-77.
9. Loo, Y. H. & Badger, L. (1969) Spectrofluorometric assay of vitamin B-6 analogues in brain tissue. J. Neurochem. 16, 801-804.
10. Adams, E. (1969) Fluorometric determination of pyridoxal phosphate in enzymes. Anal. Biochem. 31, 118-122.
11. Tamura, Z. & Takanishi, S. (1970) Fluorometric determination of pyridoxal and pyridoxal 5'-phosphate in biological materials by the reaction with cyanide. In: Methods in Enzymology (McCormick, D. B. & Wright, L. D., eds.), vol. 18A, pp. 471-475, Academic Press, New York.
12. Takanishi, S. & Tamura, Z. (1970) Preliminary studies for fluorometric determination of pyridoxal and of its 5'-phosphate. J. Vitaminol. 16, 129-131.

13. Takanishi, S., Matrunaga, I. & Tamura, Z. (1970) Fluorometric
     determination of pyridoxal and its 5'-phosphate in biological
     materials. J. Vitaminol. 16, 132-136.
14. Durko, I., Yukhnovska, Y. V. & Ivanov, Ch. P. (1973) A new
     fluorometric method for the determination of vitamin B-6 in
     blood. Clin. Chim. Acta. 49, 407-414.
15. Shrivastava, S. K. & Beutler, E. (1973) A new fluorometric
     method for the determination of pyridoxal 5'-phasphate.
     Biochim. Biophys. Acta 304, 765-773.
16. Yasumoto, K. E., Tadera, K., Tsuji, H. & Mitsuda, H. (1975)
     Semi-automated system for analysis of vitamin B-6 complex by
     ion-exchange column chromatography. J. Nutr. Sci. Vitaminol.
     21, 117-127.
17. Chauhan, M. S. & Dakshinamurti, K. (1979) Fluorometric assay
     of pyridoxal. In: Methods in Enzymology (McCormick, D. B. &
     Wright, L. D., eds.), vol. 62D, pp. 405-407, Academic Press,
     New York.
18. Chauhan, M. S. & Dakshinamurti, K. (1979) Fluorometric assay
     of pyridoxal and pyridoxal 5'-phosphate. Anal. Biochem. 96,
     426-432.
19. Duggan, D. E., Bowman, R. L., Brodie, B. B. & Udenfriend, S.
     (1957) A spectrophotofluorometric study of compounds of
     biological interest. Arch. Biochem. & Biophys. 68, 1-14.
20. Toepfer, E. W. & Lehman, J. (1961) Procedure for chromato-
     graphic separation and microbiological assay of pyridoxine,
     pyridoxal and pyridoxamine in food extract. J. Assoc. Off.
     Agric. Chem. 44, 426-430.
21. Polansky, M. M., Murphy, E. W. & Toepfer, E. W. (1964)
     Components of vitamin B-6 in grains and cereal products. J.
     Assoc. Off. Agric. Chem. 47, 750-753.
22. Storvick, C. A. & Peters, J. M. (1964) Methods for the
     determination of vitamin B-6 in biological materials. Vit.
     & Horm. 22, 833-854.
23. Thiele, V. F. & Brin, M. (1966) Chromatographic separation
     and microbiological assay of vitamin B-6 in tissues from
     normal and vitamin B-6 depleted rats. J. Nutr. 90, 347-354.
24. Anderson, B. B., Peart, M. B. & Fulford-Jones, E. E. (1970)
     The measurement of serum pyridoxal by a microbiological assay
     using Lactobacillus casei. J. Clin. Pathol. 23, 232-242.
25. Haskell, B. E. & Snell, E. E. (1970) Microbiological
     determination of the vitamin B-6 group. In: Methods in
     Enzymology (McCormick, D. B. & Wright, L. D., eds.), vol. 18A,
     pp. 512-519, Academic Press, New York.
26. Brin, M. (1970) A simplified Toepfer-Lehman assay for the
     three vitamin B-6 vitamers. In: Methods in Enzymology
     (McCormick, D. B. & Wright, L. D., eds.), vol. 18A, pp. 519-
     523, Academic Press, New York

27. Dakshinamurti, K. & Stephens, M. C. (1969) Pryidoxine deficiency in the neonate rat. J. Neurochem. 16, 1515-1522.

28. Hines, J. D. & Love, D. S. (1969) Determination of serum and blood pyridoxal phosphate concentrations with purified rabbit skeletal muscle apophosphorylase b. J. Lab. Clin. Med. 73, 343-349.

29. Chabner, B. & Livingston, D. (1970) A simple enzymic assay for pyridoxal phosphate. Anal. Biochem. 34, 413-423.

30. Haskell, B. E. & Snell, E. E. (1972) An improved apotryptophanase assay for pyridoxal phosphate. Anal. Biochem. 45, 567-576.

31. Bhagavan, H. N., Koogler, J. M., Jr. & Coursin, D. B. (1974) Enzymatic micro-assay of pyridoxal-5'-phosphate using L-tyrosine apodecarboxylase and L-$(1-^{14}C)$ tyrosine. Internat. J. Vit. Nutr. Res. 46, 160-164.

32. Toepfer, E. W. & Polansky, M. M. (1964) Recent developments in the analysis for vitamin B-6 in foods. Vit. & Horm. 22, 825-832.

33. Ahrens, H. & Korytnyk, W. (1970) Thin-layer chromatography and thin-layer electrophoresis of vitamin B-6. In: Methods in Enzymology (McCormick, B. D. & Wright, L. D., eds.), vol. 18A, pp. 489-494, Academic Press, New York.

34. Columbini, C. E. & McCoy, E. E. (1970) Rapid thin-layer electrophoretic separation and estimation of all B-6 compounds and of some 5-hydroxyindoles. Anal. Biochem. 34, 451-458.

35. McCoy, E. E., Columbini, E. E. & Strynadka, K. (1979) High voltage electrophoresis and thin-layer chromatographic separation of vitamin B-6 compounds. In: Methods in Enzymology (McCormick, D. B. & Wright, L. D., eds.), vol. 62D, pp. 410-415, Academic Press, New York.

36. Heyl, D., Luz, E. & Harris, S. A. (1951) Phosphates of the vitamin B-6 group. IV. An oxidation product of codecarboxylase. J. Am. Chem. Soc. 73, 3437-3439.

37. Cordes, E. H. & Jencks, W. P. (1962) Semicarbazone formation from pyridoxal, pyridoxal phosphate and their Schiff bases. Biochemistry 1, 773-778.

38. Udenfriend, S. (1962) Vitamin B-6 Group. In: Fluorescence Assay in Biology and Medicine, pp. 253-263, Academic Press, New York.

39. Heyl, D. (1948) Phosphates of the vitamin B-6 group. II. 3-pyridoxal phosphoric acid. J. Am. Chem. Soc. 70, 3434-3436.

40. Fieser, L. F. & Fieser, M. (1967) In: Reagents for Organic Synthesis, pp. 456-478; 942-952. John Wiley & Sons, Inc., New York.

41. Metzler, D. E., Olivard, J. & Snell, E. E. (1959) Transamination of pyridoxamine and amino acids with glyoxylic acid. J. Am. Chem. Soc. 76, 644-648.

42. Chauhan, M. S. & Dakshinamurti, K. (1980) Fluorometric assay of vitamin B-6 vitamers in biological material. Clin. Chim. Acta. (In press).

43. Walsh, M. P. (1966) Determination of plasma pyridoxal phosphate with wheat germ glutamic-aspartic apotransaminase. Am. J. Clin. Path. 46, 282-285.

44. Lumeng, L., Cleary, R. E. & Li, T.-K. (1974) Effect of oral contraceptives on the plasma concentration of pyridoxal phosphate. Am. J. Clin. Nutr. 27, 326-333.

45. Hamfelt, A. & Wetterberg, L. (1969) Pyridoxal phosphate in acute intermittent porphyria. Ann. N.Y. Acad. Sci. 168, 361-364.

46. Fujita, A. & Fujino, K. (1954) Fractional determination of vitamin B-6 components and 4-pyridoxic acid in urine. J. Vitaminol. 1, 290-296.

47. Yasumoto, K., Tadera, K., Tsuji, H. & Mitsuda, H. (1975) Semi-automated system for analysis of vitamin B-6 complex by ion exchange column chromatography. J. Nutr. Sci. Vitaminol. 21, 117-127.

48. Korytnyk, W., Fricke, G. & Paul, B. (1966) Pyridoxine chemistry. XII. Gas chromatography of compounds in the vitamin B-6 group. Anal. Biochem. 17, 66-75.

49. Korytnyk, W. (1970) Gas chromatography of vitamin B-6. In: Methods in Enzymology (McCormick, D. B. & Wright, L. D., eds.), vol. 18A, pp. 500-504, Academic Press, New York.

50. Sheppard, A. J. & Prosser, A. R. (1970) Gas chromatography of vitamin B-6. In: Methods in Enzymology (McCormick, D. B. & Wright, L. D., eds.), vol. 18A, pp. 494-500, Academic Press, New York.

51. Sennello, L. T., Kummerow, F. A. & Argondelis, C. J. (1967) Synthesis and properties of trimethylsilyl derivatives of vitamin B-6. J. Heterocyclic. Chem. 4, 295-297.

52. Imanari, T. & Tamura, Z. (1967) Gas chromatography in vitamin B-6 group. Chem. Pharm. Bull. (Tokyo) 15, 896-898.

53. Williams, A. R. (1974) Vitamin B-6: Gas-liquid chromatography of pyridoxol, pyridoxal and pyridoxamine. J. Agric. Food Chem. 22, 107-109.

54. Anthony, O. M., Brooks, C. J. W., MacLean, I. & Sangster, I. (1969) Cyclic boronates as derivatives for gas chromatography. J. Chromatogr. Sci. 7, 623-631.

55. Biondi, P. A., Fedele, O., Motta, A. & Secchi, C. (1979) Determination of 3,4 dihydroxyphenylethyleneglycol in urine by gas chromatography with a flame ionization detector: a new rapid method. Clin. Chim. Acta 94, 155-161.

EXTRACTION AND QUANTITATION OF B-6 VITAMERS FROM ANIMAL TISSUES AND HUMAN PLASMA: A PRELIMINARY STUDY

Joseph T. Vanderslice, Catherine E. Maire and
Gary R. Beecher

Beltsville Human Nutrition Research Center
Human Nutrition
United States Department of Agriculture
Beltsville, MD   20705

Reports from recent conferences on vitamin B-6 metabolism indicate that it would be most useful to identify and quantitate all forms of vitamin B-6 in animal tissue and physiological fluids (1,2). Enzyme or microbiological assays by themselves do not yield information on the individual species, but chemical assays, particularly those involving high performance liquid chromatography (HPLC), do have this potential (3,4). The problem with chemical assays is that a suitable extraction procedure must be found which quantitatively extracts the compound(s) of interest from complex samples, prevents decomposition or metabolism during the extraction, and is compatible with the analytical HPLC systems.

Recently, an extraction procedure which satisfies these requirements has been developed and successfully applied to such complex foods as pork, beef, fish, dry milk, and cereals, as well as to human plasma (5-7). The use of a similar procedure in determining the concentrations of the B-6 vitamers in brain, liver, kidney, and muscle of rat to verify whether or not it would be suitable for metabolic investigations on animals is reported here, along with a brief review of the results for pork and human plasma.

MATERIALS AND METHODS

The complete procedure can be conveniently broken into major sections as shown in Fig. 1. Each procedure is discussed below.

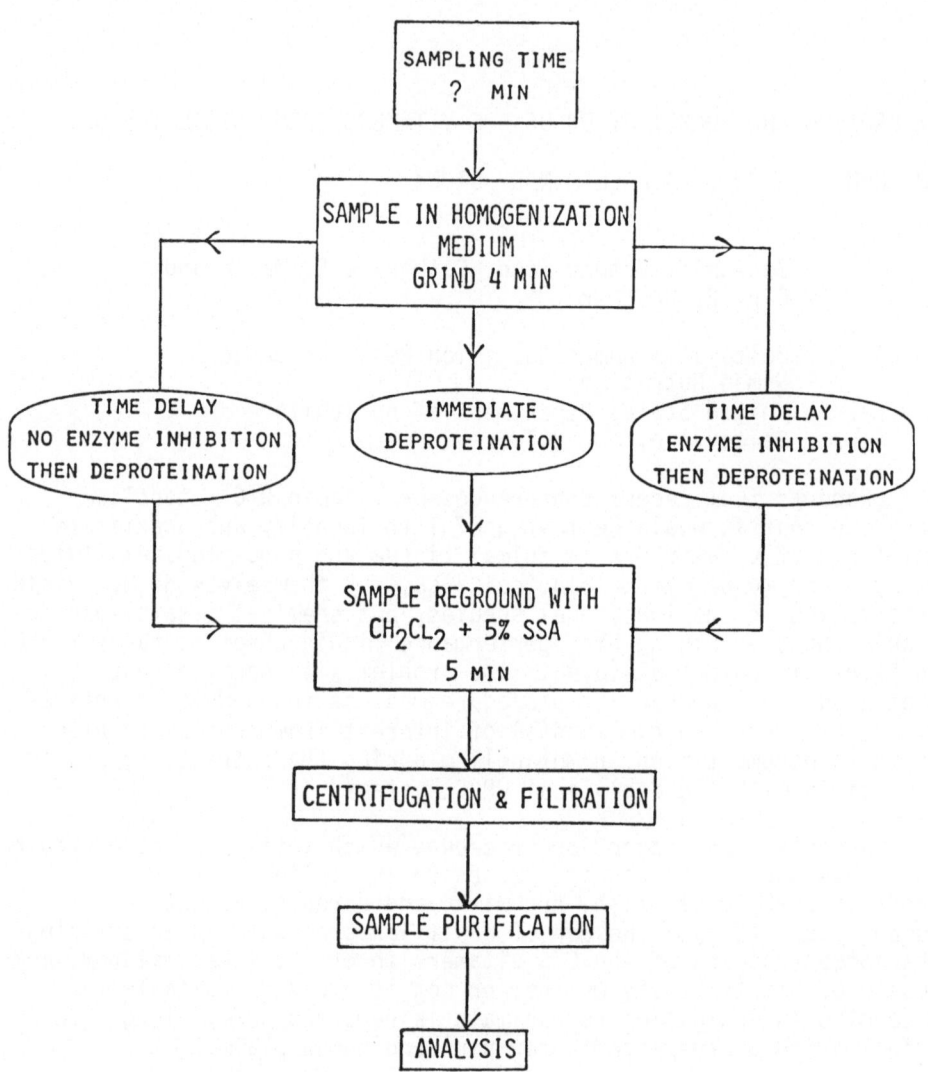

Fig. 1. Flow diagram of the sampling, homogenization, purification, and analysis system.

MATERIALS AND METHODS

Sampling

Rat tissues. Adult male Sprague-Dawley rats, obtained from the Charles River Breeding Laboratories, Wilmington, MA, and maintained on Purina Rat Chow, were used in this study. After decapitation during the feeding cycle, the organ or organs of interest were quickly removed and placed in various homogenization media (to be described). With the exception of muscle tissue (quadriceps group: vastus lateralis, v. intermedius, and v. medialis), all organs were in the medium within five minutes of decapitation. Muscle, which usually was removed with the other organs, reached the medium within 15 minutes. If more than one organ was removed, it was done in the order: liver, kidney, brain, and then muscle.

The vitamin B-6 content of rat liver was considered to be the one most sensitive to homogenization procedures and thus was investigated in more detail than the other organs. After removal of the liver, the large lobe was cut into sections (approximately 1 g) and after weighing, placed in the appropriate homogenization media for analysis. In some cases, one-half of the liver was frozen immediately in a Wollenberger Clamp (8), previously cooled to -50°, and kept for up to three days at -10° before thawing and subsequent analysis. Percent recovery was checked by adding known amounts of the different vitamers to one of duplicate samples.

The brain was usually divided, sagitally, into two portions for weighing and homogenization; to one sample was added a known amount of the six forms of the vitamin to determine percent recoveries. The two kidneys were each divided into two portions and half from each were taken to form a composite sample for weighing and homogenization.

Muscle tissue was first forced through a sieve (1 mm diameter holes) under pressure to remove a majority of the collagen which interferes with homogenization; the loss in mass amounted to approximately 10%. Tissues from the three muscles were thoroughly mixed before samples were taken for weighing and subsequent homogenization.

Raw pork loin. Fresh lean loin was ground in a Robot-Coup mixer for five minutes and immediately frozen. Normally, when the samples were to be analyzed, they were partially thawed, weighed, and placed in a homogenization medium (to be described). To test the effect of sample handling, some samples were frozen, thawed for 24 hours, refrozen, thawed, weighed, and then placed in the homogenization medium.

Human plasma. Blood was collected in a syringe containing 1 mg
sodium citrate dihydrate, 0.55 mg Na_2HPO_4 and 0.60 mg NaH_2PO_4 per
ml of sample. After centrifugation at 700 x g for 20 minutes at
4^0, the plasma was decanted and the extraction procedure begun.
Blood samples were donated by one of the male coauthors and were
taken: (1) while the subject was on his normal diet, (2) after the
diet was supplemented for four days with 100 mg PN per day and a
50 mg dose administered 2.5 hours before blood collection, and
(3) four days after supplementation ceased.

Extraction

The extraction procedure for animal tissue begins with homogenization of the sample in a liquid medium (5). Three types of
media were used. The simplest involves a 5% solution of sulfosalicylic acid (SSA) in water. This reagent denatures the protein in
the sample and releases the B-6 vitamers present. For solid samples,
10 ml of SSA solution were used for 1 g of sample. For plasma,
solid SSA was added to make the solution 5% in SSA.

The other two extraction procedures involve homogenization with
water or with water containing a phosphatase inhibitor. The samples
were ground for four minutes in the chosen medium, then allowed to
incubate for various amounts of time in that medium before solid SSA
was added to make a 5% (w/v) solution and deproteinate the sample.
During incubation, enzymes are released and become active until the
SSA is added. NaF (9) and Na_2HPO_4 at pH 7.5 (10,11) were used as
phosphatase inhibitors. These last two procedures were used
extensively with rat liver. Phosphatase inhibition and incubation
had no effort on muscle tissues, but did on liver, brain, and kidney.

The different homogenization procedures described in this section
were usually applied to liver with the resulting recommended procedure then being used for the final analysis on the other organs.
For all procedures, the final deproteinated solution was extracted
with an equal volume of methylene chloride for five minutes,
followed by centrifugation at 7,500 x g for 10 minutes at 4^0, and
removal and filtration of the water layer (5).

For plasma, 0.05 g of SSA were added per ml of plasma to make
a final concentration of 5% (w/v). The resulting solution was then
homogenized for three minutes before centrifugation at 700 x g for
20 minutes at 4^0, filtration, and purification.

Analytical Procedures

Sample purification. This step, described elsewhere in detail
(5), is used to remove SSA from the sample since SSA gradually changes
the characteristics of the final analytical column. Basically, the
purification system utilizes HPLC with fluorescence detection. The
anion exchange resin (Dowex AG 2-X8, 200-400 mesh, 10 cm x 6 mm)
completely binds SSA while permitting the vitamers to pass through.
Approximately 0.5 ml of sample was injected into a flowing stream
of 0.1 M HCl. As soon as the vitamers appeared at the detector,
the effluent was collected, normally 6-10 ml, for analysis and an
aliquot, usually 0.5 ml with a pH adjusted to 7.5, injected into
the analytical system. Approximately 15 samples can be injected
onto the purification column before it becomes saturated with SSA.
The column then can be either regenerated (5) or replaced.

Analysis. This procedure has been described elsewhere (4).
In essence, this HPLC system separates a given sample, usually 0.5
ml, into its vitamer components, measures the area of the eluted
peak, calculates the concentration of the given component on the
basis of a previous calibration and the known amount of internal
standard, 3-hydroxypyridine, added originally and finally, gives
a complete printout of all concentrations.

This system employs two columns, both packed with Bio-Rad A-25
resin; a Perkin-Elmer 650-40 fluorescence detector and a Shimadzu
C-R1A Chromatopac computing integrator. The first column is 24 cm
x 6 mm and is thermostated at 50° while the second is 24 cm x 3 mm
and is thermostated at 18°.

If only vitamer content is to be determined, a single buffer
(0.4 M NaCl, 0.01 M glycine, 0.005 M semicarbazide, adjusted to pH
10) is used. The flow rate is 1.25 ml/min. Following injection,
the buffer passes only through the first column for the initial
23.5 minutes during which time pyridoxamine phosphate (PMP),
pyridoxamine (PM), pyridoxine phosphate (PNP), and pyridoxine (PN)
are eluted. For the next 28 minutes, both columns are in line while
the pyridoxal phosphate (PLP) and 3-hydroxypyridine (HOP) peaks
appear. The second column is then switched out of line and at 63.4
minutes after injection, the pyridoxal (PL) peak appears. If pyridoxic acid (4PA) is to be detected, the original buffer is changed
to 0.4 M NaCl, 0.01 M glycine, pH 2.5, and the 4PA peak appears in
20 minutes. To detect PMP, PM, PNP, PN, and HOP, the excitation
and emission wavelengths are set at 310 and 380 nm, respectively.
PLP and PL are detected at 280 and 487 nm while 4PA is detected at
315 and 432 nm. A typical chromatogram for a sample of standards
is shown in Fig. 2.

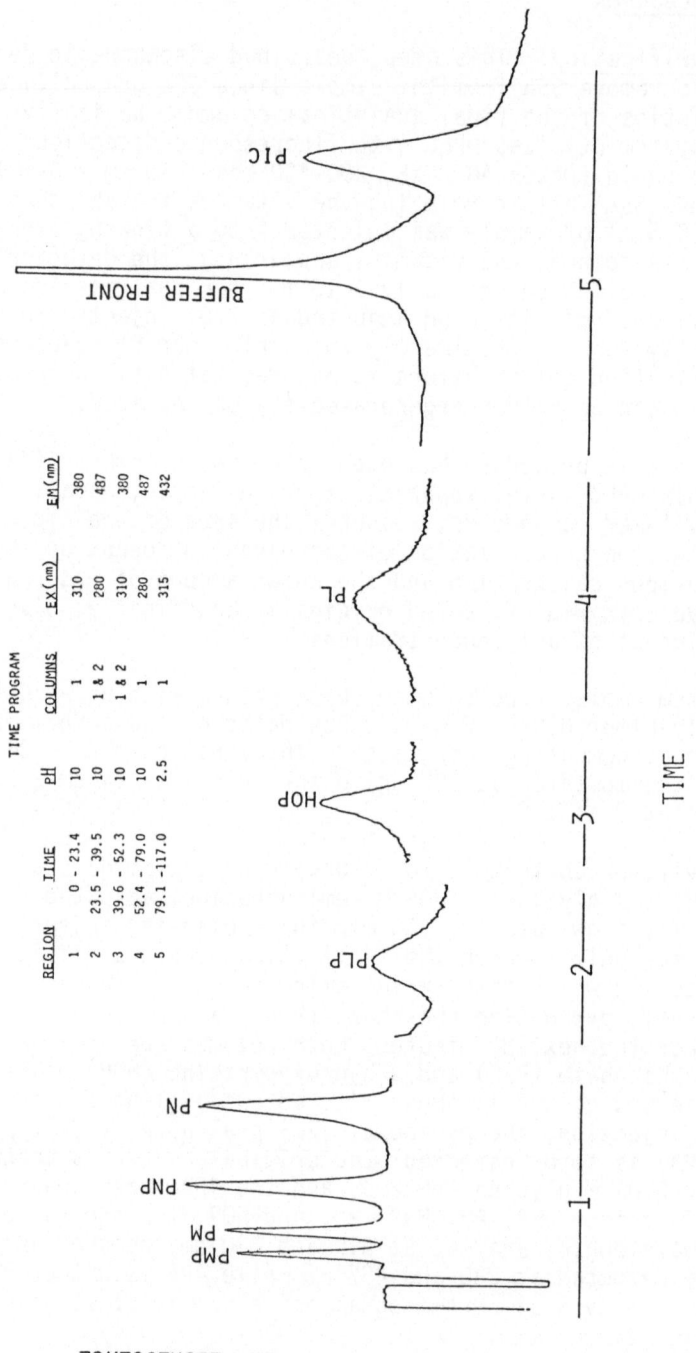

Fig. 2. Chromatogram of a solution of standards. The concentration of vitamers were approximately 4.7 ng/ml while the 4-pyridoxic acid (PIC) concentration was 0.6 ng/ml.

Reagents and supplies. Methylene chloride was of HPLC quality.
Most chemicals were obtained from Fisher Chemical Company and were
of analytical grade purity. However, sequanol grade sulfosalicylic
acid was obtained from Pierce Chemical Company, and 3-hydroxypyridine
came from Aldrich Chemical Company. With the exception of pyridoxine
phosphate, all pure forms of the vitamins were obtained from Sigma
Chemical Company. Pyridoxine phosphate was prepared by the method
of Peterson and Sober (12).

All aqueous solutions were prepared with water which was
distilled and then resin purified to at least 15 megohms resistance.
All glassware was detergent washed, rinsed thoroughly, then autoclaved at 121⁰ for 15 minutes in a Micro solution (International
Products Corporation, Trenton, NJ) and finally rinsed six times
in distilled water. All samples were ground in a Sorvall Omni Mixer
and the 50 ml containers were cleaned in the same manner as the
glassware.

RESULTS

Traces

Chromatographic traces obtained during analysis of the different
rat organs are shown in Figs. 3 and 4 with the vitamer peaks indicated by their appropriate abbreviations. All traces, independent
of the homogenization procedure, gave equally clean backgrounds.
Traces for spiked kidney and brain samples (i.e., samples to which
known amounts of vitamers were added) are shown in Fig. 5. Pork
samples gave equally clean backgrounds. Pyridoxic acid was not
determined for these sample but was for plasma. The plasma trace
is shown in Fig. 6. The absence of interfering compounds indicates
that the described extraction and cleanup procedures are worthy of
consideration.

Rat Tissue

The numerical results for the different rat organs are shown
in Tables 1-5. Chronologically, the sequence of experiments corresponds to the table numbering. Basically, we started with the procedure used for food where the sample was immediately deproteinated
with 5% SSA solution. Then, we concentrated on liver where we knew
the enzyme activity could be high. We homogenized the samples in
pure water or dilute solutions of phosphatase inhibitors and allowed
the resulting solutions to incubate for varying lengths of time
before deproteination. These results were compared with immediate
deproteination and subsequent incubation of samples for the same
lengths of time.

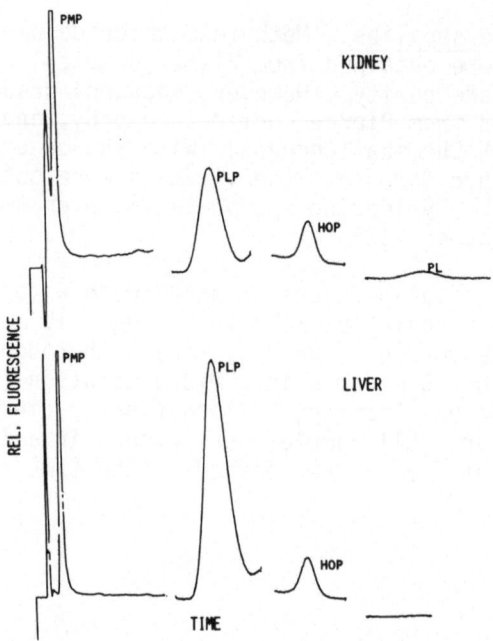

Fig. 3. Typical chromatographic traces from rat kidney and liver samples. Traces untouched except for deletion of instructions to integrator.

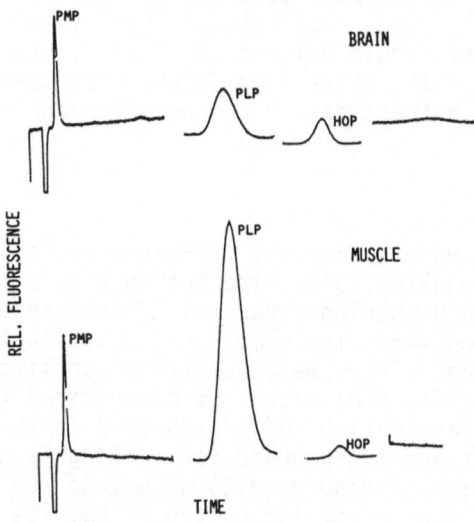

Fig. 4. Typical chromatograpnic traces from rat brain and muscle samples. Traces untouched except for deletion of instructions to integrator.

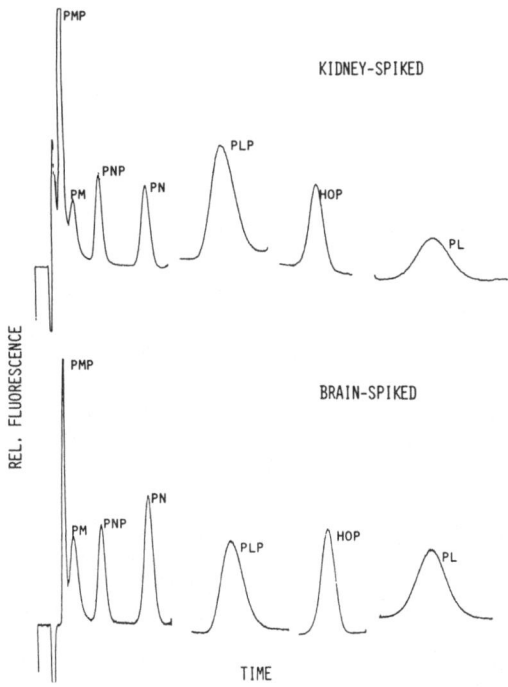

Fig. 5.   Typical chromatographic traces from spiked samples of rat
         kidney and brain.   Traces untouched except for deletion of
         integrator instructions.

    Duplicate runs were not generally considered, as the reproduc-
ibility has been better than 5%, which is confirmed by the recovery
studies on spiked samples. Also, spectral scans taken of the liver
vitamer peaks agreed with those obtained when pure standards were
run through the procedure.

    In Table 1, we present the results obtained when the samples
were immediately homogenized and deproteinated in a SSA solution
after removal from the animal. Results are presented for spiked
and unspiked samples. When the sample was spiked, it was added
after the SSA. We can conclude that recoveries for all vitamers
are close to 100% and that the principal forms of the vitamers in
all organs investigated are PMP and PLP, which is in agreement with
earlier observations (13). Under the conditions of these experiments
the only other forms, found in small amounts, were PN and PL in
liver and PL in kidney. (The lower limit of detection for the
overall method for forms other than PLP is 0.08 nmol/g, PLP is 0.4
nmol/g.)

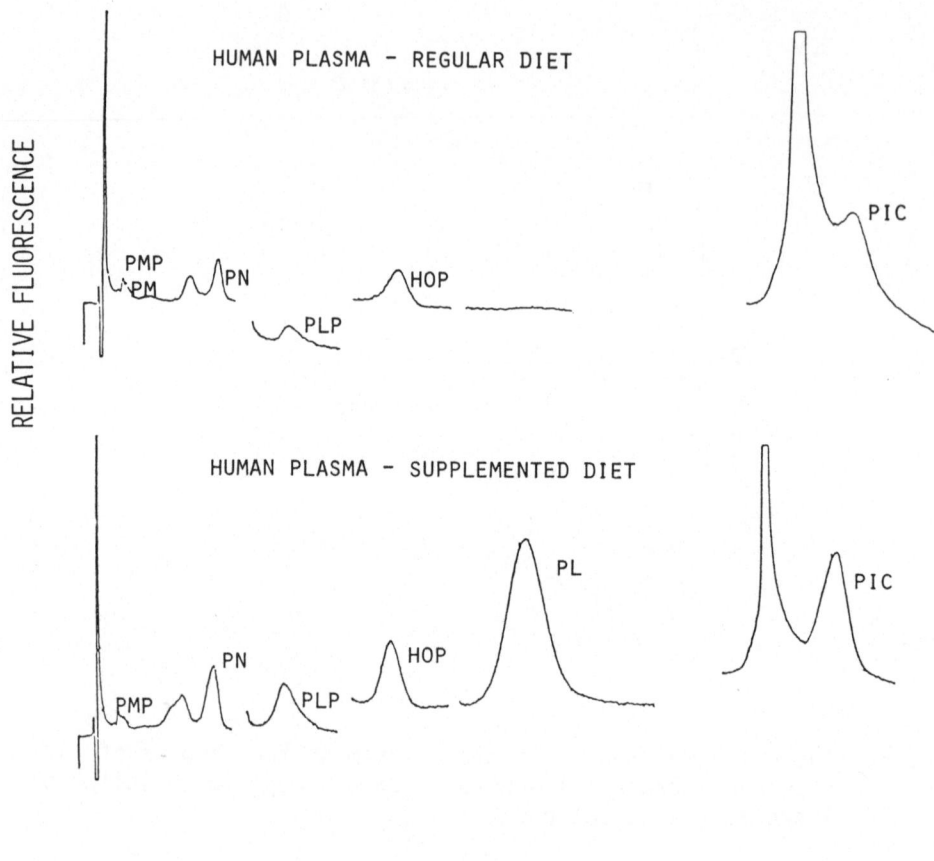

TIME

Fig. 6. Chromatographic traces for human plasma. See text for
         description of supplemental diet. Regular diet trace was
         taken four days after supplementation ceased.

        Table 2 shows the effect of allowing liver samples to incubate
in 5% SSA, H_2O or NaF for different lengths of time. As quickly as
was feasible after removal from the animal, the samples were homogenized in the media and allowed to incubate for times up to 3 hours.
Then, SSA was added to the H_2O and NaF homogenates to deproteinate
the sample as it was rehomogenized for 2 minutes. The results
indicate that the PLP values increase with incubation before
deproteination. The greatest increases occurred on incubation in
NaF. PMP values also increased in NaF media. The greatest increases
were found for cases where the homogenized sample was incubated in
a dilute solution of the enzyme inhibitor, NaF, for 10 minutes.

Table 1. B-6 Vitamer Recoveries – Immediate Deproteination[a]

Rat Mass	Tissue	Sampling Time	Code[b]	B-6 Vitamer Content (nmol/g) and % Recoveries						
g		min		PMP	PM	PNP	PN	PLP	PL	Totals
525	Brain	3	U	9.0	-	-	-	8.0	-	17.0
			S	20.9	21.5	11.9	19.9	16.0	18.4	108.7
			S+U	29.9	21.5	11.9	19.9	24.1	18.4	125.7
		3	A	28.2	21.8	11.6	21.7	21.9	19.1	124.3
			R	95	101	98	109	91	104	99
525	Muscle[c]	15	U	7.0	-	-	-	32.3	-	39.3
			S	5.7	5.9	3.2	5.4	4.4	5.0	29.6
			S+U	12.7	5.9	3.2	5.4	36.7	5.0	68.9
		15	A	12.9	6.5	3.4	5.0	35.3	4.6	68.2
			R	102	110	104	93	98	92	99
525	Liver	5[d]	U	30.3	-	-	0.9	34.8	4.1	70.1
			S	8.6	11.1	6.0	10.5	9.8	9.1	55.1
			S+U	38.9	11.1	6.0	11.4	44.6	13.2	125.2
		5[d]	A	37.2	11.0	5.9	10.8	41.5	13.6	120.0
			R	96	99	98	95	93	103	96

Table 1 (cont). B-6 Vitamer Recoveries - Immediate Deproteination[a]

Rat Mass	Tissue	Sampling Time	Code[b]	B-6 Vitamer Content (nmol/g) and % Recoveries						
				PMP	PM	PNP	PN	PLP	PL	Totals
g		min								
441	Kidney	2	U	28.8	-	-	-	11.9	0.9	41.5
			S	5.5	7.1	5.6	7.5	6.0	6.8	38.5
			S+U	34.3	7.1	5.6	7.5	17.9	7.7	80.0
		2	A	34.6	7.1	5.4	7.3	17.3	8.1	79.8
			R	101	100	96	97	97	105	100

[a]Sample homogenized in 5% SSA solution.
[b]U = unspiked sample analysis; S = amount of spike added; A = analysis of spiked samples;
R = % recovery.
[c]Collagen removed before weighing.
[d]Sample frozen 5 minutes after sacrifice; thawed after 24 hours and placed in homogenization
medium.

Table 2. Dependence of Vitamin B-6 Liver Values on Incubation Time and Enzyme Inhibitor, NaF

Rat Mass	Homogenization Medium	Sampling Time	Incubation Time	B-6 Vitamer Content[a]						
g		min	min	PMP	PM	PNP	PN	PLP	PL	Totals
				nmol/g						
441	5% SSA	5	0	20.3	–	–	–	31.5	–	51.8
	H₂O	5	180	19.4	–	–	0.8	35.8	5.8	61.8
	50 mM NaF	5	180	27.3	–	–	0.8	39.8	–	67.9
	5% SSA	2	b	26.5	–	–	0.9	23.1	4.7	55.2
710	5% SSA	1	10	21.6	–	–	–	40.1	–	61.7
	50 mM NaF	1	10	36.0	–	–	–	99.7	–	135.7
	5% SSA	1	30	24.5	–	–	–	40.2	–	64.7
	50 mM NaF	1	30	31.3	–	–	–	66.6	1.2	99.1
	5% SSA	1	180	24.0	–	–	0.8	37.6	–	62.4
	50 mM NaF	1	180	36.4	–	2.3	–	52.5	–	91.2
781	50 mM NaF	1	5	44.4	–	–	1.7	98.2	–	144.3
	50 mM NaF	1	10	49.4	–	–	–	105.1	–	154.4
	50 mM NaF	1	15	49.8	–	–	–	98.1	–	147.9

[a] Dashes indicate the compound was either below the limits of detection or absent.
[b] Sample frozen 72 hours before thawing and homogenization.

Longer and shorter times gave lower values of PLP. There is some
indication (seen by the appearance of PN and PL) that interconversions
between the vitamers are occurring and that the total amount of
vitamers are changing, as in the 10, 30, and 180 minute NaF samples,
presumably due to oxidase activity.

Table 3 shows the dependence of vitamin B-6 values on incubation
times but using Na_2HPO_4 instead of NaF. Again, an incubation of 10
minutes in a dilute solution of enzyme inhibitor gave maximum concentration values for PLP. These experiments also included sample
incubation in H_2O for different times. The total vitamin content
was greatest with inhibitor present and remained approximately
constant for 30 minutes. Interconversion from PLP to PMP appears
to be occurring. Without inhibitor present, the total vitamer
content was lower than with inhibitor and surprisingly remained
constant for 30 minutes. Dephosphorylations and interconversions
did occur to some extent, however, with PN and PL being the forms
produced.

In Table 4, we show the effect of enzyme activity on recovery
studies. Here, the homogenized samples were incubated for 10 minutes
before deproteination. The samples were spiked before, during, and
after deproteination. Unless deproteination is done before spiking,
total recovery is not achieved and there are conversions of PMP and
PLP into other forms as can be seen from the percent recoveries.
This is true even when the sample was spiked during deproteination
which indicates how rapid the enzymatic conversions were occurring.
Finally, note the relatively low vitamin B-6 values for the liver
sample that was frozen overnight. It is only 60% of the amount
obtained from the sample that was analyzed immediately after
excision from the animal.

In Table 5, we show the recovery results obtained with several
other tissues for incubation times of 10 minutes in 80 mM Na_2HPO_4.
In all cases, the recoveries are acceptable. Brain gives a total
recovery of only 94%, which is due to the low recoveries (90 and
91%) for PLP and PL.

In Table 6, we show a comparison of previously reported values
of PMP and PLP with results from the present study. For liver,
values from the present method agree reasonably well with those
obtained by others when the sample is immediately deproteinated.
When the sample cells are incubated for 10 minutes in an enzyme
inhibiting medium before deproteination, substantial increases in
PLP values are observed. A similar, but not as pronounced effect,
is seen in kidney, brain, and muscle.

Table 3. Dependence of Vitamin B-6 Liver Values on Incubation Times and Phosphatase Inhibitor, Sodium Phosphate[a]

Homogenization Medium	Incubation Time	B-6 Vitamer Content[b]						
		PMP	PM	PNP	PN	PLP	PL	Totals
	min	nmol/g						
80 mM Na$_2$HPO$_4$ pH 7.5	10	29.8	-	-	0.7	78.6	-	109.1
80 mM Na$_2$HPO$_4$ pH 7.5	20	34.2	-	-	-	68.9	-	103.1
80 mM Na$_2$HPO$_4$ pH 7.5	30	38.6	-	-	-	67.0	-	105.6
H$_2$O	10	33.4	-	-	0.7	70.2	-	104.2
H$_2$O	20	26.5	-	-	0.6	63.7	6.4	97.2
H$_2$O	30	29.1	-	-	1.3	61.3	8.7	100.4

[a] Rat Mass = 623 g; all samples removed within 1 minute of decapitation.
[b] Dashes indicate the compound was below the limits of detection.

Table 4. B-6 Vitamer Recoveries from Liver; Dependence on Enzyme Activity[a]

Rat Mass	Time of Spiking	Code[b]	B-6 Vitamer Content (nmol/g) and % Recoveries						
			PMP	PM	PNP	PN	PLP	PL	Totals
g									
623	10 minutes before deproteination	U	29.8	-	-	0.7	78.6	-	109.1
		S	18.3	14.8	8.8	16.2	14.3	14.3	86.7
		S+U	48.1	14.8	8.8	16.9	92.9	14.3	195.8
		A	44.1	21.7	9.8	19.9	72.4	15.4	183.3
		R	92	147	111	118	78	108	94
798	Simultaneous addition with SSA	U	35.7	-	-	-	101.3	-	137.0
		S	9.5	7.1	3.7	10.5	11.3	4.6	46.7
		S+U	45.3	7.1	3.7	10.5	112.6	4.6	183.7
		A	40.6	14.0	6.0	16.3	92.6	5.9	175.4
		R	90	197	162	155	82	128	95
798	3 minutes after deproteination	U[c]	23.3	-	-	0.6	54.6	4.0	82.5
		S	11.3	8.4	4.4	12.5	13.5	5.5	55.6
		S+U	34.6	8.4	4.4	13.1	68.7	9.5	138.1
		A[c]	33.5	8.7	4.5	13.2	68.5	9.2	137.6
		R	97	104	102	101	101	97	100

[a] Homogenization medium = 80 mM Na_2HPO_4 at pH 7.5; incubation time = 10 minutes prior to deproteination with SSA. All samples removed within 1 minute of decapitation.
[b] U = unspiked sample analysis; S = amount of spike added; A = analysis of spiked sample; R = % recovery.
[c] Sample frozen overnight; thawed and homogenized.

Table 5. B-6 Vitamer Recoveries from Rat Tissues; Incubation in Phosphate Buffer[a]

Tissue	Sampling Time	Code[b]	PMP	PM	PNP	PN	PLP	PL	Totals
	min								
Kidney	1	U	25.1	-	-	-	16.9	0.3	42.3
		S	15.7	14.4	7.7	21.3	18.2	12.2	89.5
		S+U	40.8	14.4	7.7	21.3	35.1	12.5	131.8
	1	A	46.1	14.2	7.7	20.5	37.2	12.0	137.7
		R	113	99	100	96	106	96	104
Brain	1	U	8.4	-	-	-	8.7	-	17.1
		S	31.2	28.6	15.3	42.4	36.2	24.2	177.9
		S+U	39.6	28.6	15.3	42.4	44.9	24.2	195.0
	1	A	37.3	29.4	13.9	40.2	40.3	22.0	183.1
		R	94	103	91	95	90	91	94
Muscle[c]	15	U	5.1	-	-	-	26.0	-	31.1
		S	11.7	10.8	5.7	16.0	13.6	9.1	66.9
		S+U	16.8	10.8	5.7	16.0	39.6	9.1	98.0
	15	A	15.3	10.4	5.3	14.6	42.7	7.8	96.1
		R	91	96	92	91	108	86	98

[a] Incubation for 10 minutes in 80 mM Na_2HPO_4, pH 7.5. Rat Mass = 470 g.
[b] U = unspiked sample analysis; S = amount of spike added; A = analysis of spiked sample; R = % recovery.
[c] Collagen removed before weighing.

Table 6. Ratios of PLP/PMP Concentrations in Different Tissues[a]

Tissue	Rat Mass	PMP	PLP	PLP/PMP	Sample Treatment
	g	nmol/g	nmol/g		
Liver	-	32.0	30.8	0.96	Lumeng and Li values (9)
	~175	28.5	22.0	1.30	Thiele and Brin values (14)[b]
	441	20.3	31.5	1.55	Immediate deproteination
	525	30.3	34.8	1.15	Sample frozen overnight; thawed; immediate deproteination
	441	26.5	23.1	0.87	Sample frozen 72 hours; thawed, immediate deproteination
	710	36.0	99.7	2.77	Sample incubated 10 minutes in NaF before deproteination
	781	49.4	105.1	2.12	Sample incubated 10 minutes in NaF before deproteination
	623	29.8	78.6	2.64	Sample incubated 10 minutes in Na_2HPO_4 before deproteination
	798	35.7	101.3	2.84	Sample incubated 10 minutes in Na_2HPO_4 before deproteination

Table 6 (cont). Ratios of PLP/PMP Concentrations in Different Tissues[a]

Tissues	Rat Mass	PMP	PLP	PLP/PMP	Sample Treatment
	g	nmol/g	nmol/g		
Kidney	~175	24.1	13.7	0.57	Thiele and Brin values (14)[b]
	441	28.8	11.9	0.41	Immediate deproteination
	470	25.1	16.9	0.67	Incubated in Na_2HPO_4 for 10 minutes before deproteination
Brain	–	9.8	5.7	0.58	Lumeng and Li values (9)
	~175	11.7	7.7	0.66	Thiele and Brin values (14)[b]
	525	9.0	8.0	0.89	Immediate deproteination
	470	8.4	8.7	1.04	Incubated in Na_2HPO_4 for 10 minutes before deproteination

Table 6 (cont). Ratios of PLP/PMP Concentrations in Different Tissues[a]

Tissue	Rat Mass	PMP	PLP	PLP/PMP	Sample Treatment
	g	nmol/g	nmol/g		
Muscle	–	4.6	21.8	4.74	Lumeng and Li values (9)
	~175	7.3	18.5	2.53	Thiele and Brin values (14)[b]
	525	7.0	32.3	4.61	Immediate deproteination[c]
	470	5.1	26.0	5.10	Incubated in Na_2HPO_4 for 10 minutes before deproteination[c]

[a] Mature male Charles River rats used in this study during the feeding cycle. Weanling male rats used by Thiele and Brin. All rats raised on regular laboratory food.
[b] Reported nmol/g values of PM and PL assumed to be PMP and PLP.
[c] Collagen removed before weighing.

Finally, at the suggestion of T.-K. Li, we performed a joint experiment with R. D. Reynolds. Extracted and purified samples from rat liver (prepared as described in this paper) were analyzed for PLP for incubation times of 0 and 10 minutes by two different methods. Reynolds used a tyrosine decarboxylase enzymatic procedure (15) while we used the present method. The results are shown in Table 7. Increases of PLP were observed with incubation by both groups although the observed increases with the enzymatic method were not as great. NaF also appears to suppress the enzymatic reaction as evidenced by the overall decrease in observed PLP values for samples 5 and 6.

Raw Pork Loin

Table 8 shows results obtained with raw pork. The results for pork loin handled in the two different ways described previously are compared to those of Polansky and Toepfer (8) who obtained lower values for total vitamin B-6 primarily due to lower values of PLP. Until analyses are performed on identical samples, no conclusions can be drawn. Note, however, the decrease by 10% of total vitamin B-6 for the sample that was thawed and refrozen.

Human Plasma

Finally, in Table 9, results are given from a preliminary investigation on the vitamin B-6 content of human plasma. Here the subject was on a regular diet, on a supplemented diet for 4 days, and off the supplemented diet for 4 days when analyses were made. It is interesting to note the high values of PN obtained when compared to other investigators even though the concentration of the other vitamers are in reasonable agreement. (Another subject tested also exhibited high PN values.) As a check, the eluting PN peak was scanned during a run and the fluorescent spectrum was compared to that obtained with a PN standard. The spectra were identical. For plasma, the lower limits of detection were 9 pmol/ml for all vitamers except for pyridoxal phosphate with a lower limit of 14 pmol/ml. Pyridoxic acid has a lower limit of less than 1 pmol/ml.

CONCLUSIONS

This preliminary study suggests that the vitamin B-6 extraction and analytical procedure previously described for food and plasma samples can be successfully and accurately applied to animal tissue. The method should be of considerable value for nutritional studies on both animals and humans and may lead to significant findings in metabolic work as individual vitamer content and interconversions can be followed directly.

Table 7. Comparison of HPLC and Enzymatic Methods for
          PLP in Incubated and Non-incubated Samples of
          Rat Liver[a]

Sample[b]	HPLC	Enzymatic	Incubation Time	Inhibitor
	nmol/g	nmol/g	min	
1	46.8	46.2	0	PO_4
2	72.5	59.5	10	PO_4
3	46.4	42.3	0	PO_4
4	70.0	56.3	10	PO_4
5	44.7	35.1	0	F
6	68.0	41.0	10	F

[a]All samples taken from same liver, rat mass = 477 g.
[b]Lower numbered samples treated first.

Table 8. B-6 Vitamer Content of Raw Pork Loin

Sample	PMP	PM	PNP	PN	PLP	PL	Total
				nmol/g			
Pork Loin (raw)[a]	4.3	–	0.4	1.2	31.2	–	37.1
Pork Loin (raw)[b]	2.2	1.0	–	1.2	28.9	0.3	33.6
Pork Loin (raw)[c]	–	5.5	–	3.4	–	16.4	24.9

[a]Sample frozen, thawed, then analyzed.
[b]Sample frozen, thawed 24 hours, refrozen, thawed, then analyzed.
[c]Data of Polansky and Toepfer (16).

    Initial treatment of samples affects the numerical results.
While we do not claim to have arrived at the optimal conditions for
the different tissues, it is clear that the overall procedures do
yield reliable results. Handling of food samples must be considered
when identifying the individual vitamer forms present. Future
refinements must account for active enzymes in the sample as it is
being homogenized.

Table 9. B-6 Vitamer Content of Human Plasma[a]

PMP	PM	PNP	PN	PLP	PL	Total	4PA	Source
				pmol/ml				
24	12	-	216	77	-	329	n.d.	regular diet
35	-	-	358	376	1996	2765	914	supplement--4 days
35	-	-	242	159	-	436	448	4 days after discontinuation of supplement
5	6.2	-	18.6	76.9	17.4	124.1	n.d.	Lumeng and Li (17)
80.8	46	-	-	54.6	7.7	189.1	174	whole blood, Shane (18)
-	-	-	-	21-33[b]	-	-	-	Wachstein et al. (19)
-	-	-	-	20-68[b]	-	-	-	Hamfelt (20)

[a] Sample collected into syringes containing 1 mg sodium citrate dihydrate, 0.55 mg Na_2HPO_4 0.60 mg NaH_2PO_4 per ml blood.
[b] Analyzed for PLP only.

The speed with which these analyses can be performed may be the reason why large concentrations of PLP are obtained. Enzyme activity can be stopped whenever desired and the sample can be ready for final analysis in a total of 30 minutes from collection if necessary.

This analytical system was originally designed to analyze food samples where sample size is not usually a problem. Obvious improvements can be made in miniaturizing the system as well as increasing the operating pressure. Such refinements ought to reduce the necessary sample size and substantially reduce the analysis times.

ACKNOWLEDGMENT

The authors wish to thank Dr. R. D. Reynolds of the Beltsville Human Nutrition Research Center, U.S. Department of Agriculture, Beltsville, MD, for his participation in the cooperative study on rat liver.

This work was supported in part by an Interagency Reimbursable Agreement No. 2YO1-HB 60041-05 from the National Heart, Lung and Blood Institute, NIH.

LITERATURE CITED

1. National Research Council (1978) Human vitamin B-6 requirements. Nat. Acad. Sci., Washington, DC.
2. Tryfiates, G. P., ed. (1980) Vitamin B-6 metabolism and role in growth. Food and Nutrition Press, Inc., Westport, CT.
3. Vanderslice, J. T., Stewart, K. K. & Yarmas, M. M. (1979) Liquid chromatographic separation and quantification of B-6 vitamers and their metabolite, pyridoxic acid. J. Chromatogr. 176, 280-285.
4. Vanderslice, J. T. & Maire, C. E. (1980) Liquid chromatographic separation and quantification of B-6 vitamers at plasma concentration levels. J. Chromatogr. 196, 176-179.
5. Vanderslice, J. T., Maire, C. E., Doherty, R. F. & Beecher, G. R. (1980) Sulfosalicylic acid as an extraction agent for vitamin B-6 in food. J. Agric. Food Chem. (In press).
6. Vanderslice, J. T., Maire, C. E. & Beecher, G. R. (1980) B-6 vitamer analysis in human plasma by HPLC: a preliminary study. Am. J. Clin. Nutr. (In press).
7. Vanderslice, J. T., Maire, C. E. & Yakupkovic, J. E. (1980) Vitamin B-6 in ready-to-eat cereals: analysis by high performance liquid chromatography. J. Food Sci. (In press).
8. Hess, B. & Brand, K. (1963) Cell and tissue disintegration. In: Methods of Enzymatic Analysis (Bergmeyer, H. V., ed.), 2nd edition, pp. 396-409, Academic Press, New York.

9. Nordstrom, J. L., Rodwell, V. W. & Mitschelen, J. J. (1977) Interconversion of active and inactive forms of rat liver hydroxmethylglutaryl-CoA reductase. J. Biol. Chem. 252, 8924-8934.

10. Anderson, B. B. (1980) Red-cell metabolism of vitamin B-6. In: Vitamin B-6 Metabolism and Role in Growth (Tryfiates, G. P., ed.), pp. 53-84, Food and Nutrition Press, Inc., Westport, CT.

11. Lumeng, L. & Li, T.-K. (1980) Mammalian vitamin B-6 metabolism: regulatory role of protein-binding and the hydrolysis of pyridoxal 5'-phosphate in storage and transport. In: Vitamin B-6 Metabolism and Role in Growth (Tryfiates, G. P., ed.), pp. 27-51, Food and Nutrition Press, Westport, CT.

12. Peterson, E. A. & Sober, H. A. (1954) Preparation of crystalline phosphorylated derivatives of vitamin B-6. J. Am. Chem. Soc. 76, 169-175.

13. Bain, J. A. & Williams, H. L. (1960) Concentrations of B-6 vitamers in tissues and tissue fluids. In: Inhibitions in the Nervous System and Gammaaminobutyric Acid (Baxter, C. F., Harreveld, A. V., Wiersma, C. A. G., Adley, W. R. & Killam, K. F., eds.), pp. 275-281, Pergamon Press, New York.

14. Thiele, V. F. & Brin, M. (1966) Chromatographic separation and microbiological assay of vitamin B-6 in tissues from normal and vitamin B-6-depleted rats. J. Nutr. 90, 347-353.

15. Sloger, M. S., Scholfield, L. G. & Reynolds, R. D. (1978) Loss of in vitro inactivation of rat liver tyrosine aminotransferase with dietary vitamin B-6 restriction. J. Nutr. 108, 1355-1360.

16. Polansky, M. M. & Toepfer, E. W. (1969) Vitamin B-6 components in some meats, fish, dairy products and commercial infant formulas. J. Agric. Food Chem. 17, 1394-1397.

17. Lumeng, L. & Li, T.-K. (1978) Plasma content of B-6 vitamers and its relationship to hepatic vitamin B-6 metabolism. Fed. Proc. 37, 588.

18. Shane, B. (1978) Vitamin B-6 and blood. In: Human Vitamin B-6 Requirements, pp. 111-128, Nat. Acad. Sci., Washington, DC. National Research Council, Washington, DC.

19. Wachstein, M., Kellner, J. D. & Ortiz, J. M. (1960) Pyridoxal phosphate in plasma and leukocytes in patients with leukemia and other diseases. Proc. Soc. Exp. Biol. Med. 105, 563-566.

20. Hamfelt, A. (1962) A method of determining pyridoxal phosphate in blood by decarboxylation of L-tyrosine-[14]C(U). Clin. Chim. Acta 7, 746-748.

DETERMINATION OF VITAMIN B-6 COMPOUNDS BY SEMIAUTOMATED CONTINUOUS-FLOW AND CHROMATOGRAPHIC METHODS

Jesse F. Gregory III and James R. Kirk

Food Science and Human Nutrition Department
University of Florida
Gainesville, FL   32611

The development of instrumental methods for the quantitative analysis of the various vitamin B-6 compounds has been the subject of extensive research. The need for alternative analytical methods stems largely from the limitations of many of the conventional procedures and the requirement for accurate, rapid, and simple methods for food analysis, research, and nutritional assessment purposes. Microbiological methods for the biologically active B-6 vitamers are often limited by the cumbersome nature of the analysis, poor precision, and potential variation in growth response. Enzymatic procedures for the vitamin B-6 coenzymes (pyridoxal 5'-phosphate, PLP and pyridoxamine 5'-phosphate, PMP), while extremely sensitive, are not well suited for multiple routine analyses and may be subject to certain interferences. Likewise, conventional methods for the determination of 4-pyridoxic acid (4PA), the primary excretory form of vitamin B-6, have not been widely employed because of their lengthy nature.

At the present time, no universally applicable instrumental method has been devised for the determination of all vitamin B-6 compounds in foods and other biological materials. Great progress has been made, however, in the development of analytical methods for certain vitamin B-6 compounds in specific materials. This review will deal with instrumental techniques for vitamin B-6 compounds which employ continuous-flow semiautomated methods, gas-liquid chromatography (GLC), and high-performance liquid chromatography (HPLC). These techniques will be discussed in terms of their practical suitability and potential applicability to food and other biological analyses.

149

SEMIAUTOMATED CONTINUOUS-FLOW METHODOLOGY

A variety of chemical methods for the determination of vitamin B-6 have been based on the conversion of the B-6 vitamers to a common derivative, followed by fluorometric quantitation. The fluorophores employed in these methods include 4PA lactone and 4-pyridoxic acid 5'-phosphate (1-18), pyridoxal (PL) semicarbazone and pyridoxal 5'-phosphate semicarbazone (19,20), and recently methyl-N-4'-pyridoxylanthranilate and its 5'-phosphate (21). Several colorimetric methods have been devised although they are not sufficiently sensitive for biological analysis.

Most of the chemical methods are suitable for at least partial automation, the result of which would ordinarily be increased precision and rate of analysis. The 4PA lactone procedure is the only chemical method for vitamin B-6 to be partially automated to date, having been adapted to semiautomated continuous-flow analysis using a Technicon AutoAnalyzer II system (17). The quantitation of the 4PA lactone fluorophore is performed at a rate of 40 to 60 samples per hour using the continuous-flow system to provide pH adjustment, air segmentation, mixing, and fluorometric measurement. In spite of the high rate of continuous-flow fluorometry, the rate limiting nature of the sample extraction, preparative chromatography, and chemical derivatization procedures prevent this method from filling the need for a rapid instrumental procedure for vitamin B-6 analysis.

Further limitations of the 4PA lactone procedure became apparent when its results were compared with those of other analytical techniques and literature values for vitamin B-6 in selected foods and model systems (Table 1). Observed vitamin B-6 values were significantly greater when determined by the 4PA lactone method than by Saccharomyces uvarum, rat bioassay, reverse phase HPLC, or literature values bases on S. uvarum analysis (17,22,23). These results indicate that the semiautomated 4PA lactone method, in its present form, would probably yield results which seriously overestimate the vitamin B-6 content of many foods and biological materials.

Limited studies have been conducted in an effort to determine the presence of or identity of interfering fluorophores (22). The fluorescence emission spectra of extracts from various processed model cereal systems, prepared for the semiautomated assay, were found to be qualitatively identical to the emission spectrum of 4PA lactone prepared from pure B-6 vitamers. These results suggest that the interfering compound(s) may be structurally similar to PL or 4PA and, upon reaction with cyanide, produces a fluorophore with spectral emission characteristics identical to 4PA lactone.

Table 1. Comparison of Total Vitamin B-6 in Selected Model Cereal Systems and Foods as Determined by 4-pyridoxic Acid Lactone, Saccharomyces uvarum, HPLC, and Rat Bioassay Methods

Sample	Assay Procedure			
	4PA Lactone	S. uvarum	Rat Bioassay[a]	HPLC
	μg vitamin B-6/g sample			
Model Cereal System Control[b]				
No fortification	19.0	1.1	–	1.0
PN fortification	34.5	19.6	–	18.7
PM fortification	35.2	9.7	–	19.8
PLP fortification	25.3	13.6	–	14.4
Roasted (180°, 25 min)[b]				
No fortification	5.2	1.0	0.1	–
PN fortification	14.4	9.3	5.4	–
PM fortification	10.5	6.2	4.1	–
PLP fortification	11.0	5.1	6.4	–
Stored (0.6 a_w, 128 days, 37°)[c]				
No fortification	13.5	0.5	-0.7	0.5
PN fortification	24.0	11.9	11.6	12.8
PM fortification	16.3	6.3	6.9	7.5
PLP fortification	13.4	2.9	2.7	4.2

Table 1 (cont).   Comparison of Total Vitamin B-6 in Selected Model Cereal Systems and Foods as Determined by 4-pyridoxic Acid Lactone, Saccharomyces uvarum, HPLC, and Rat Bioassay Methods

Sample	Assay Procedure			
	4PA Lactone	S. uvarum	Rat Bioassay[a]	HPLC
	μg vitamin B-6/g sample			
Cornflakes	33.7[d]	15[e]	—	—
Infant formula (powdered)	13.4[d]	1.4[f]	—	—
Cured ham	13.5[d]	3.2[f]	—	—

[a] Rat bioassay values are means of data derived from rat growth, feed efficiency, erythrocyte aspartate aminotransferase activity, and PLP stimulation in vitro.
[b] Mean standard error approximately 1.9 μg/g.
[c] Reference 22.   HPLC data unpublished.
[d] Reference 23.
[e] Reference 17.
[e] Label claim 25% USRDA/oz.
[f] Previously published data, not same sample.   Reference 24.

The semiautomated 4PA lactone method has been found to be fully reliable for the determination of vitamin B-6 in mixtures of simple composition. The results to date indicate that modification and detailed reexamination of this procedure are required before the semiautomated 4PA lactone method is employed for food or biological analysis or nutritional assessment.

GAS-LIQUID CHROMATOGRAPHY

Although gas-liquid chromatography has shown promise for the separation and quantitation of vitamin B-6 compounds, this technique has received little application to the analysis of food or other biological materials. Derivatization is essential for GLC analysis because of the low volatility of the vitamin B-6 compounds. Numerous derivatization methods have been reported for quantitation of the free base B-6 vitamers and several vitamin B-6 analogues. These methods include the formation of acetyl, heptafluorobutyryl, trifluoroacetyl, trimethylsilyl, 3-0-benzyl, and isopropylidene derivatives. GLC separations have been performed using stationary liquid phases such as methyl silicone (with or without added neopentyl glycol succinate) or methyl phenyl silicone. Detailed discussion of GLC methodology for vitamin B-6 compounds is available in the publications by Williams (25), Sheppard and Prosser (27), and Korytnyk (26).

The only report of GLC for the determination of vitamin B-6 in biological materials is an abstract by Haskell (28) which involved animal tissue PLP analysis. Further research is needed before GLC methodology can be adapted to the analysis of vitamin B-6 compounds in food and other biological materials. The major disadvantages of GLC for the determination of B-6 vitamers are the sensitivity of many of the derivatization methods to water or alcohols in the sample extract and the need to remove nonvolatile materials. The reported chromatographic efficiency and sensitivity of several of the methods employing β-ionization or electron capture detection indicate that such applications may be feasible if adequate extract cleanup methods were employed.

HIGH-PERFORMANCE LIQUID CHROMATOGRAPHY

Recent advances in column and instrument technology have permitted the development of methods for the quantitative analysis of many biological compounds by HPLC. Many researchers have recently reported HPLC separations involving vitamin B-6 compounds and several applications for the HPLC determination of B-6 vitamers in foods and other biological materials. The principal chromatographic modes for the HPLC separation of vitamin B-6 compounds, ion exchange and reverse phase, will be discussed here.

Ion Exchange HPLC

The ionogenic nature of the vitamin B-6 compounds makes them well suited for separation by ion exchange chromatography, which is the basis of many preparative methods. Although Tiselius (29) has demonstrated that a sulfonated cation exchange resin (Dowex AG 50W-X8) can be employed for the preparative separation of PM, PL, PN, PLP, PMP, PNP, and 4PA, HPLC applications using similar resins have only involved the nonphosphorylated forms of vitamin B-6. Callmer and Davies (30) first applied cation exchange HPLC for the analysis of PN in multivitamin preparations. The HPLC separation of PL, PN, and PM was first achieved by Williams and Cole (31) and Yasumoto et al. (32), both of whom employed Aminex A-5 cation exchange resins (Bio-Rad Laboratories). High resolution and efficiency were achieved in these separations when the B-6 vitamers were eluted with either a continuous linear gradient (31) or a step gradient (32). Poorer separation was obtained with isocratic elution (31). Yasumoto et al. (32) developed a post-column derivatization method which permitted the chromogenic labeling of the eluted B-6 vitamers with the diazide of 5-chloroaniline 2,4-disulfonyl chloride to enhance the specificity of the assay. This procedure was successfully applied to the analysis of pharmaceutical products, yeast, cereal-grains, and liver. Although the chromogenic labeling method provided the first viable HPLC technique for the determination of B-6 vitamers in biological materials, it has not been widely employed because of the complex instrumentation, slow elution (ca 120 min/sample), and lack of sensitivity.

Other attempts to apply cation exchange HPLC to food and other biological analysis have met with variable success. Wong (33) reported an isocratic cation exchange separation similar to that of Williams and Cole (31). In spite of the use of a sensitive 210 nm absorption detector, the naturally occurring B-6 vitamers in several fruits and vegetables could not be quantified by this procedure. Thompson (34) reported that cation exchange resins (Aminex A-5 or preferably Aminex A-9, each from Bio-Rad Laboratories) were suitable for the isocratic HPLC determination of PN in fortified infant formulas using fluorometric detection. Gradient elution permitted the separation and fluorometric quantitation of the naturally occurring B-6 vitamers in milk, although quantitative data were not presented.

Anion exchange HPLC was employed by Hill et al. (25) in a study which showed that several water soluble vitamins, including PN, could be separated using a μBondapak NH$_2$ column (Waters Associates). The anionic nature of the B-6 vitamers in alkaline media has been recently utilized for an anion exchange HPLC separation of PM, PN, PL, PLP, PMP, PNP, and 4PA. Vanderslice et al. (36) employed an Aminex A-25 anion exchange resin (Bio-Rad Laboratories) to achieve the HPLC separation, which permitted the simultaneous analysis of these seven vitamin B-6 compounds. This procedure would appear to be ideal for the determination of the complete distribution of vitamin B-6 in foods or other biological materials; however, the only reported application to date has been the analysis of breakfast cereals (37). The disadvantages of the Aminex A-25 anion exchange procedure include a slow elution (ca 75 min) for the B-6 vitamers, relatively low chromatographic efficiency, incomplete resolution of PMP, PM, and PNP, and the need for dual refrigerated fluoro- meters for the detection system. The reported detection limits of the method (ca 10 ng for each vitamer) are only slightly higher than those achieved using the reverse phase fluorometric methods (23,38,39). This sensitivity would be satisfactory for natural vitamin B-6 levels in many foods and biological materials, although it would be insufficient for plasma PLP analysis. Several recent modifications (37) have improved the separation and provided sensi- tivity which is suitable for most biological analysis. Wider appli- cation of this procedure is dependent upon the development of suitable extraction and extract cleanup methods.

Anion exchange HPLC methods have also been applied to in vitro studies of vitamin B-6 enzymology. Korytnyk et al. (40) and Gregory (41) used this technique to examine the phosphorylation of B-6 vitamers and structural analogues by PL kinase. These separa- tions involved isocratic HPLC of kinase reaction mixtures using Bondapak AX/Corasil (40) and μBondapak NH_2 (41) columns (each from Waters Associates). Although ultraviolet absorption detection was suitable for each application, the use of absorption and fluorescence detectors in series (41) greatly facilitated the simultaneous quantitation of substrates and products.

Recently, ion exchange HPLC has been employed in a novel approach to PLP analysis. This method is based on the quantitation of a tyrosine apodecarboxylase procedure using HPLC (42). L-3,4- dihydroxylphenylalanine (L-DOPA) was employed as the substrate for the PLP-dependent decarboxylase reaction. Cation exchange HPLC with electrochemical detection was used to quantify the dopamine formed, thus providing an extremely sensitive indirect assay for PLP. A similar apoenzyme-based PLP assay could conceivably be performed using a recently developed HPLC assay for tryptophanase (43). Although this method was not specifically designed for PLP analysis, the sensitive fluorometric detection of the reaction product indole and the efficient reverse phase separation may provide another viable alternative to conventional enzymatic assay methods. As with other apoenzyme assay procedures for PLP, however, these methods would be subject to interference by materials which could inhibit the recon- stitution of the holoenzyme or alter the rate of the enzyme-catalyzed reaction (44).

Reverse Phase HPLC

Reverse phase chromatography is based on the use of polar
mobile phases and columns packed with nonpolar stationary phase
materials (e.g., octadecylsilica). Much of the original work
concerning the separation of the B-6 vitamers by reverse phase HPLC
involved "ion pair" chromatography; i.e., HPLC using hydroorganic
mobile phases containing ionic surfactants. Several procedures
for the separation of PM, PN, and PL have been based on the use of
ion-pairing agents such as alkyl sulfonates, camphor sulfonate,
sodium dodecyl sulfate, and dioctyl sulfosuccinate, in methanol-
water-acetic acid mobile phases (45-47). These methods have not
been applied to the analysis of biological materials, although ion
pair HPLC methods have been reported for the determination of PN
in pharmaceutical multivitamin preparations (46,48).

Detailed studies by Horvath and associates have demonstrated
that reverse phase HPLC is very well suited for the separation of
weak acids, weak bases, and zwitterions in the absence of ion pairing
agents (49,50). The retention and separation of these compounds
are the result of reversible hydrophobic or "solvophobic" association with the nonpolar stationary phase. Retention is a function
of the ionization and hydrocarbonaceous surface area of the sample
components and the mobile phase pH, ionic strength, temperature,
and organic modifier content.

Shortly after the initial reports concerning solvophobic HPLC
of ionogenic compounds (49,50), we found that the free base B-6
vitamers (PM, PL, and PN), PLP, and 4PA could be separated with
high chromatographic efficiency using a μBondapak C_{18} column (Waters
Associates) and a 0.033 M potassium phosphate (pH 2.2) mobile phase.
Under these acidic conditions, the pyridine ring nitrogen of the
B-6 compounds is protonated, resulting in relatively short retention
times and high efficiency. Elevation of the mobile phase pH induces
increased retention and a loss of resolution and efficiency as the
phenolic hydroxyl group ionizes (pK_a 3.5 to 5.0). This pH-dependent
alteration in retention time provides a convenient technique for
studies of the acid-base behavior of B-6 vitamers and analogues.

We have subsequently examined a variety of commercial reverse
phase columns for their suitability in the HPLC analysis of the free
base B-6 vitamers, PLP, and several derivatives (ϵ-pyridoxyllysine,
4'-deoxypyridoxine, PL- and PLP-semicarbazone, and PL- and PLP-oxime);
those columns tested including Ultrasphere IP, LiChrosorb RP-8, and
Spherisorb ODS from Altex Scientific, Partisil 10 ODS-3 from Whatman,
Inc., and μBondapak C_{18} from Waters Associates. Each of these columns
was found to provide the separation of PM, PN, PL, and certain of
the other vitamin B-6 compounds when the acidic phosphate mobile
phase was employed. The chromatographic efficiency of certain columns
(e.g., Ultrasphere IP) has been observed to increase significantly

when 1.0 M ammonium sulfate was added to the mobile phase, as
described by Horvath et al. (49,50). Of the columns listed, the
Ultrasphere IP (5 μm octadecylsilica) ordinarily provides the
greatest resolution and efficiency for vitamin B-6 separations;
however, we have also used the LiChrosorb RP-8, Partisil 10 ODS-3,
and μBondapak C_{18} columns with satisfactory results in many cases.
The phosphorylated B-6 vitamers can also be separated under these
conditions, with retention times very similar to their respective
free base forms. Certain columns can provide partial or complete
separation of PLP from PL under optimal conditions. Typical
separations are shown in Fig. 1.

        This reverse phase method and all others developed in our
laboratory were performed using Waters Associates ALC/GPC 204 and/
or Altex Scientific Model 312 liquid chromatographs. Other comparable instruments would undoubtedly suffice. Fluorometric detection
was performed using an American Instrument Company FluoroMonitor
in all cases.

        The first research application of the solvophobic separation
technique was an examination of vitamin B-6 stability during the
storage of dehydrated model cereal systems (23). In this study,
the phosphorylated B-6 vitamers were determined as their respective
free base forms following acid phosphatase treatment of acetate
buffer extracts. The trichloroacetic acid used to deproteinize the
extracts was found to enhance the retention and resolution of the
B-6 vitamers. While both ultraviolet (280 nm) absorption and
fluorescence (American Instrument Company 295 nm interference
excitation filter; Turner Associates 405 or Corning 7-51 emission
filter; and General Electric Germicidal lamp, Model C4T41) detection
methods provided adequate sensitivity, fluorometric monitoring
greatly enhanced the specificity of the procedure (Fig. 2).
ε-Pyridoxyllysine in protein hydrolysates was determined using the
same method (23).

        The application of this direct assay method to the determination
of vitamin B-6 in other materials has met with varied success. The
HPLC procedure was recently tested for the determination of PN in
fortified cereal products (Fig. 3) and found to be superior to the
S. uvarum method with respect to accuracy and precision (51). The
direct fluorometric HPLC analysis of milk (52) and liver (Gregory,
unpublished) extracts was only partially successful because of
incomplete resolution from interfering compounds. Recently, Lim et
al. (53) reported a very similar separation of PM, PL, and PN and
proposed its application to milk analysis. This method employed a
Spherisorb ODS column, 0.033 M phosphate mobile phase (1.0% acetonitrile, pH 2.2), and 280 nm absorption detection. Although several
peaks from the milk extract chromatogram corresponded to the
retention times of B-6 vitamers, their identity was not confirmed

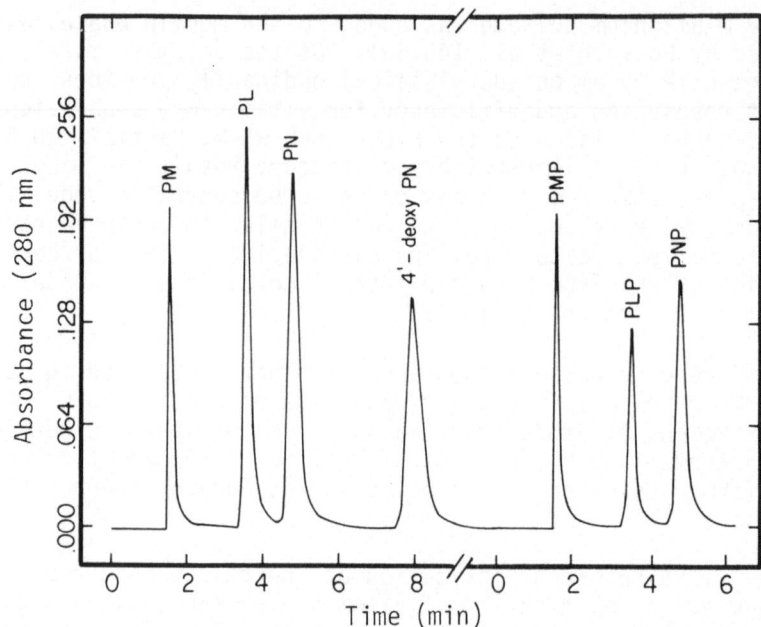

Fig. 1. Typical separation of vitamin B-6 compounds using reverse
         phase HPLC. Column = Partisil 10 ODS-3; mobile phase =
         0.033 M potassium phosphate, pH 2.2; flow rate = 2.0 ml/
         min; detection = 280 nm absorption; injection volume =
         50 µl; temperature = ambient; inlet pressure = 1100 psi.
         Vitamin B-6 solutions were prepared in the mobile phase
         buffer at 100 µg/ml for each vitamer.

by spectral means. The observed differences between standard and
sample peak widths for PL and PN strongly suggest inadequate resolution and detection specificity. Another fluorometric reverse
phase procedure, employing a pH 5.5 buffer mobile phase and a Toyo
Soda Gel LS-160 column, was reported for the determination of the
B-6 vitamers in blood following phosphatase treatment (54). This
procedure was suitable for pharmacokinetic studies of experimental
vitamin B-6 supplementation; however, the stated detection limits
indicate that the sensitivity is inadequate for the assay of normal
physiological levels of vitamin B-6 in blood.

    A significant advance in vitamin B-6 methodology was the
adaptation of reverse phase HPLC to the determination of 4PA in
urine (38). In this procedure urine samples (4 ml) are prepared
for analysis by adding 1 ml distilled water or 1 ml of distilled
water containing 10 µg 4PA, followed by the addition of 1 ml 40%
(w/v) trichloroacetic acid to precipitate proteins. Samples are

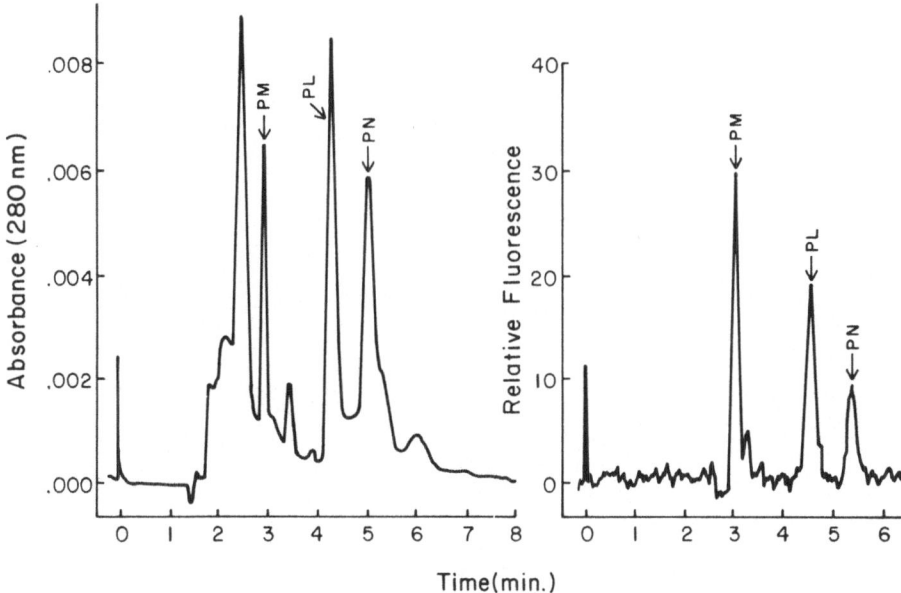

Fig. 2.   Reverse phase HPLC chromatograms from the determination
of vitamin B-6 in a stored dehydrated model system
simulating breakfast cereals (storage at 37°C, 97 days,
0.6 water activity). Model system samples were spiked
prior to analysis to provide 0.75 μg of each free base
vitamer per ml final injection solution. Left chromatogram, 280 nm absorption detection; right chromatogram,
fluorometric detection.   Column = μBondapak C_{18}; mobile
phase = 0.033 M potassium phosphate, pH 2.2; flow rate =
2.0 ml/min; inlet pressure = 1800 psi; temperature =
ambient. (Reprinted from ref. 23, p. 1804. Copyright
(1978) Institute of Food Technologists.)

then centrifuged for 15 minutes at 1000 x g. The HPLC analysis is
performed using a μBondapak C_{18} or comparable reverse phase column,
with a mobile phase of 0.033 M potassium phosphate, pH 2.2,
containing 5.0% (v/v) methanol. Fluorometric detection (American
Instrument Company FluoroMonitor; Corning 7-60 nm excitation filter;
Wratten 47B emission filter; General Electric Blacklight Model
F4T4-BL) was shown to be specific for 4PA and was sufficiently
sensitive for the detection of physiological concentrations of 4PA
(i.e., >10 ng 4PA/ml urine). The minimal sample preparation, no
cleanup, and short elution time (ca 5.4 min) are distinct advantages
and permit the analysis of large numbers of samples (Fig. 4). A
statistical comparison of the results of this method with those of
previous 4PA procedures has not yet been performed, but spectro-
photofluorometric examination of 4PA peaks from samples and standards
strongly supports the validity of the HPLC method.

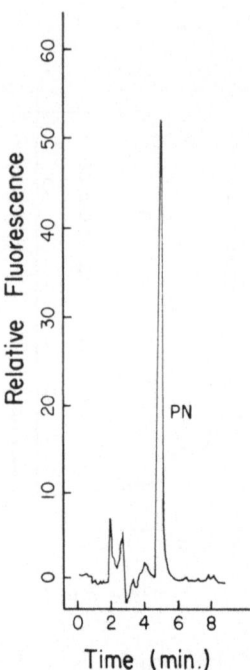

Fig. 3.   Reverse phase HPLC chromatogram from the determination of
          vitamin B-6 in a ready-to-eat breakfast cereal (Fruity
          Pebbles).   Column = μBondapak C_{18}; mobile phase = 0.033 M
          potassium phosphate, pH 2.2; flow rate = 2.0 ml/min;
          inlet pressure = 1300 psi; injection volume = 50 μl;
          temperature = ambient; fluorometric detection.   (Reprinted
          from ref. 51, p. 488.   Copyright (1980) American Chemical
          Society.)

     Another recent application of reverse phase HPLC to the quanti-
tation of vitamin B-6 in biological samples was the development of
an assay procedure for PL and PLP in animal tissues (39).   This
method was based on the treatment of neutralized perchloric acid
tissue extracts with semicarbazide to form semicarbazone derivatives
of PL and PLP.   Two ml portions of 33% tissue homogenate (in 0.1 M
potassium phosphate, pH 7.0) are prepared for analysis by adding
1 ml distilled water or 1 ml distilled water containing 10 μg PLP,
followed by protein precipitation with 2 ml 3 N perchloric acid and
centrifugation.   The supernatants are removed and the pellets
resuspended in 2 ml 1 N perchloric acid and recentrifuged.   Both
supernatants from samples are combined and the perchloric acid is
precipitated by neutralization with KOH.   The formation of the
semicarbazone derivatives of PL and PLP is performed by treating
2 ml aliquots of the extracts with 0.5 ml 0.2 M semicarbazide in

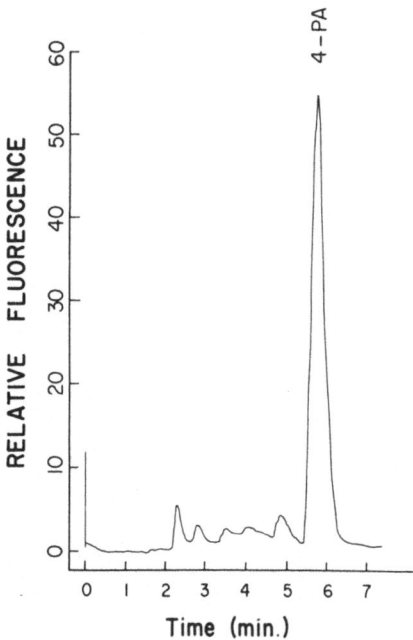

Fig. 4.   Reverse phase HPLC chromatogram from the determination of
4-pyridoxic acid in human urine. Urine sample contained
4.8 μg 4-pyridoxic acid per ml. Column = μBondapak C_{18};
mobile phase = 0.033 M potassium phosphate, 5.0% (v/v)
methanol, pH 2.2; flow rate = 2.0 ml/min; injection
volume = 50 μl; inlet pressure = 1800 psi; temperature =
ambient; fluorometric detection. (Reprinted from ref. 38,
p. 880. Copyright (1979) American Society for Clinical
Nutrition.)

a capped tube at 100°. Following cooling and the addition of 0.5 ml
0.2 M H_3PO_4, the samples are analyzed by HPLC. Chromatographic
separation and quantitation are performed using a Lichrosorb RP-8
column (Altex Scientific) or equivalent, a 0.033 M potassium phosphate mobile phase (pH 2.2) containing 2.5% acetonitrile, and a
fluorometric detector (American Instrument Company FluoroMonitor;
Corning 7-51 excitation filter; Wratten 8 emission filter; General
Electric Blacklight, Model F4T4-BL). Derivatization was employed
to enhance the fluorescence and increase the retention of PL and
PLP, thereby permitting their resolution from interfering compounds
and increasing the sensitivity of the procedure (Fig. 5). Approxi-
mate recovery values for PLP added to tissue homogenates were 75%
for liver, 80 to 85% for muscle, and 95 to 100% for brain, with
typical coefficients of variation of about 5%. This method has
been used to quantitate rat bioassays; typical dose-response data

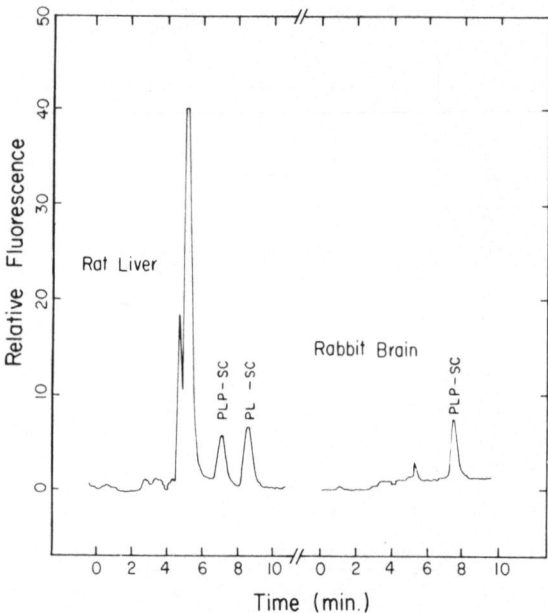

Fig. 5.   Reverse phase HPLC chromatograms from the determination
          of PLP and PL in rat liver and rabbit brain as their
          respective semicarbazone derivatives (PLP-SC and PL-SC).
          Column = LiChrosorb RP-8; mobile phase = 0.033 M potassium
          phosphate, 2.5% (v/v) acetonitrile, pH 2.2; flow rate =
          1.3 ml/min; inlet pressure = 600 psi; temperature =
          ambient; injection volume = 50 µl; fluorometric detection.
          Rat liver contained 3.6 µg PLP/g and 3.4 µg PL/g; rabbit
          brain contained 1.4 µg PLP/g. (Reprinted from ref. 39,
          p. 376. Copyright (1980) Academic Press, Inc.)

for dietary PN and liver PLP concentration are shown in Table 2.
The semicarbazone procedure is a favorable alternative to the
enzymatic methods for tissue PLP because of its technical simplicity,
specificity, and the fact that it is a direct physicochemical analysis. Attempts have been made to adapt this HPLC method to the
determination of plasma and erythrocyte PLP concentration. Peaks
corresponding to PLP-semicarbazone have been detected in these
samples; however, a 10- to 20-fold increase in sensitivity is
required for optimum routine quantitation. (Note: The reported
sensitivity of several commercial fluorometric detectors would
probably be sufficient for the analysis of blood fractions by this
method, although other detectors have not yet been evaluated.)

Table 2. Dose-response Data Relating Rat
          Liver PLP and Dietary PN Concen-
          tration[a]

PN Added to Basal Diet	Liver PLP
μg/g	μg/g wet weight
0.00	2.9 + 0.2
0.25	3.4 + 0.3
0.50	5.1 + 0.3
1.00	5.9 + 0.2
2.50	10.1 + 0.4

[a]Liver PLP determined by the HPLC semicarbazone method (39). PLP data = X̄
+ SEM (6 to 7 rats per group). Data
from control rats employed in quantification of bioassays in references 52
and 55.

        The semicarbazone method (39) has been modified to permit the
determination of total vitamin B-6 in animal tissues (56). Tissue
extracts are treated with sodium glyoxylate (6) to convert PMP and
PM to PLP and PL, respectively. Specifically, 2 ml aliquots of the
neutralized extracts are mixed with 0.2 ml 1.0 M KH_2PO_4 and 0.05 ml
0.5 M sodium glyoxylate or 0.05 ml water in a capped tube, then
held in a boiling water bath for 15 minutes. Subsequent HPLC
analysis using the semicarbazide derivatization technique is then
performed (Fig. 6). The tissue concentration of PLP, PL, PMP, and
PM can be routinely calculated from the semicarbazone peak heights
obtained from extracts prepared with and without glyoxylate treatment. Typical data are presented in Table 3. Further studies have
shown that PNP plus PLP and PN plus PL can be determined by the
semicarbazone method by initial treatment of the tissue extract with
manganese dioxide (56). As previous studies have shown PNP and PN
to be minor components of the vitamin B-6 pool in animal tissues
(24,57-61), an accurate assessment of "total" vitamin B-6 in tissues
can be readily obtained by the glyoxylate-semicarbazide adaptation
of the reverse phase HPLC method.

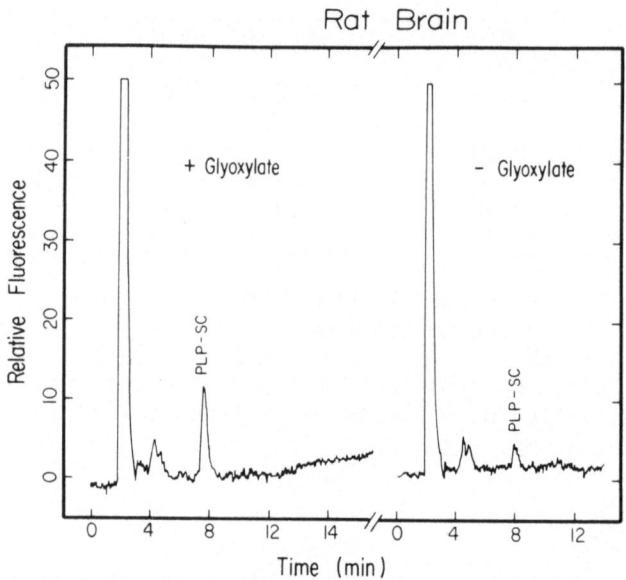

Fig. 6. Reverse phase HPLC chromatograms from the determination
of total vitamin B-6 in rat brain by the semicarbazone
method. Column = Ultrasphere IP; mobile phase = 0.033 M
potassium phosphate, 2.5% (v/v) acetonitrile, pH 2.2;
flow rate = 2.0 ml/min; inlet pressure = 2500 psi;
injection volume = 100 µl; temperature = ambient;
fluorometric detection. The chromatogram on the left is
from a glyoxylate-treated extract, thus the PLP-semicarbazone peak represents the sum of brain PLP and PMP.
The chromatogram on the right is from an extract prepared
without glyoxylate treatment, thus the PLP-semicarbazone
peak represents brain PLP only. The concentrations of
PLP and PMP in the brain sample were 0.57 and 1.34 µg/g,
respectively; PL and PM were not detectable. The retention
time of PL-semicarbazone was 14.6 minutes under these
conditions.

Table 3. B-6 Vitamer Content of Selected Animal
Tissues Determined by the Semicarbazone
HPLC Method[a]

B-6 Vitamer	Bovine Liver	Rat Brain	Ground Beef
	µg/g	µg/g	µg/g
PLP	0.39 + 0.02[b]	0.57 + 0.06	0.56 + 0.16
PL	ND[c]	ND	ND
PMP	0.31 + 0.10	1.34 + 0.13	1.16 + 0.28
PM	1.26 + 0.09	ND	ND

[a]Calculations were based on PLP- and PL-semicarbazone
peak heights of perchlorate extracts prepared with
and without glyoxylate treatment.
[b]$\overline{X}$ + SD (N = 3-4).
[c]ND = not detected.

Research is underway to adapt the direct analysis and/or
semicarbazone HPLC methods to the determination of vitamin B-6 in
processed animal products, vegetables, and fruits. It is unlikely
that HPLC methodology will totally replace the conventional microbiological and enzymatic methods for the determination of the B-6
vitamers. Sample extraction and extract purification appear to be
major problems in the development of universally applicable chrpo-
matographic methods of analysis. It is anticipated, however, that
HPLC methods will be extended to permit the rapid, precise, and
accurate determination of vitamin B-6 in a wide variety of foods
and other biological materials.

ACKNOWLEDGEMENT

The research of the authors was supported in part by a grant
from the Nutrition Foundation and USDA/SEA Grant No.
5901-0410-9-0305-0.

LITERATURE CITED

1. Fujita, A., Masuura, K. & Fujino, K. (1955) Fluorometric
    determination of vitamin B-6. I. Determination of pyridoxine.
    J. Vitaminol. 1, 267-271.
2. Fujita, A., Fujita, D. & Fujino, K. (1955) Fluorometric
    determination of vitamin B-6. II. Determination of pyri-
    doxamine. J. Vitaminol. 1, 272-278.

3. Fujita, A., Fujita, D. & Fujino, K. (1955) Fluorometric
    determination of vitamin B-6. III. Fractional determination
    of pyridoxal and 4-pyridoxic acid. J. Vitaminol. 1, 279-289.
4. Bonavita, V. (1960) The reaction of pyridoxal 5-phosphate
    with cyanide and its analytical use. Arch. Biochem. Biophys.
    88, 366-372.
5. Hennessy, D. J., Steinberg, A. M., Wilson, G. S. & Keaveney,
    W. P. (1960) Fluorometric determination of added pyridoxine
    in enriched white flour and in bread baked from it. J. Assoc.
    Off. Agric. Chem. 43, 765-768.
6. Toepfer, E. W., Polansky, M. M. & Hewston, E. M. (1961)
    Fluorometric determination of pyridoxamine by conversion to
    pyridoxal cyanide compound. Anal. Biochem. 2, 463-469.
7. Polansky, M. M., Camarra, R. T. & Toepfer, E. W. (1964) Pyri-
    doxine determined fluorometrically as pyridoxal cyanide compound.
    J. Assoc. Off. Agric. Chem. 47, 827-828.
8. Contractor, S. F. & Shane, B. (1968) Estimation of vitamin
    B-6 compounds in human blood and urine. Clin. Chim. Acta 21,
    71-77.
9. Ohishi, N. & Fukui, S. (1968) Further study on the reaction
    products of pyridoxal and pyridoxal 5'-phosphate with cyanide.
    Arch. Biochem. Biophys. 128, 606-610.
10. Loo, Y. H. & Badger, L. (1969) Spectrofluorometric assay of
    vitamin B-6 analogues in brain tissue. J . Neurochem. 16,
    801-804.
11. Takanashi, S., Matsunaga, I. & Tamura, Z. (1970) Fluorometric
    determination of pyridoxal and its 5'-phosphate in biological
    materials. J. Vitaminol. 16, 132-136.
12. Tamura, Z. & Takanashi, S. (1970) Fluorometric determination
    of pyridoxal and pyridoxal 5'-phosphate in biological materials
    by the reaction with cyanide. In: Methods in Enzymology,
    (McCormick, D. B. & Wright, L. D., eds.), vol. 18A, pp. 471-
    475, Academic Press, New York.
13. Columbini, C. E. & McCoy, E. E. (1970) Rapid thin-layer
    electrophoretic separation and estimation of all vitamin B-6
    compounds and of some 5-hydroxyindoles. Anal. Biochem. 34,
    451-458.
14. Masukawa, K., Nakama, A., Monaka, H., Kondo, T. & Okumura, K.
    (1971) Differential determination of pyridoxal, pyridoxamine,
    pyridoxal 5'-phosphate, and pyridoxamine 5'-phosphate in
    biological materials. Vitamins 44, 168-175.
15. Fiedlerova, V. & Davidek, J. (1974) Fluorometric determination
    of pyridoxal in dried milk. Z. Lebensm. Unters.-Forsch. 155,
    277-281.
16. Chin, Y.-P. (1975) Chromatographic separation and fluorometric
    determination of pyridoxal, pyridoxamine, and pyridoxine in
    food system. M.S. Thesis, pp. 1-79, Michigan State University,
    East Lansing.

17. Gregory, J. F. & Kirk, J. R. (1977) Improved chromatographic
     separation and fluorometric determination of vitamin B-6 com-
     pounds in foods. J. Food Sci. 42, 1073-1076.
18. Adams, E. (1979) Fluorometric determination of pyridoxal
     phosphate in enzymes. In: Methods in Enzymology, (McCormick,
     D. B. & Wright, L. D., eds.), vol. 62, pp. 407-410, Academic
     Press, New York.
19. Srivastava, S. K. & Beutler, E. (1973) A new fluorometric
     method for the determination of pyridoxal 5'-phosphate.
     Biochim. Biophys. Acta 304, 765-773.
20. Spector, R. (1978) Vitamin B-6 transport in the central
     nervous system: in vivo studies. J. Neurochem. 30, 881-887.
21. Chauhan, M. S. & Dakshinamurti, K. (1979) Fluorometric assay
     of pyridoxal. In: Methods in Enzymology, (McCormick, D. B. &
     Wright, L. D., eds.), vol. 62, pp. 405-407, Academic Press,
     New York.
22. Gregory, J. F. & Kirk, J. R. (1978) Assessment of roasting
     effects on vitamin B-6 stability and bioavailability in dehy-
     drated food systems. J. Food Sci. 43, 1585-1589.
23. Gregory, J. F. & Kirk, J. R. (1978) Assessment of storage
     effects on vitamin B-6 stability and bioavailability in dehy-
     drated food systems. J. Food Sci. 43, 1801-1815.
24. Polansky, M. M. & Toepfer, E. W. (1969) Vitamin B-6 compo-
     nents in some meats, fish, dairy products, and commercial
     infant formulas. J. Agric. Food Chem. 17, 1394-1397.
25. Williams, A. K. (1974) Vitamin B-6: gas-liquid chromatog-
     raphy of pyridoxol, pyridoxal, and pyridoxamine. J. Agric.
     Food Chem. 22, 107-109.
26. Korytnyk, W. (1970) Gas chromatography of vitamin B-6. In:
     Methods in Enzymology, (McCormick, D. B. & Wright, L. D., eds.),
     vol. 18A, pp. 500-504, Academic Press, New York.
27. Sheppard, A. J. & Prosser, A. R. (1970) Gas chromatography
     of vitamin B-6. In: Methods in Enzymology, (McCormick, D. B.
     & Wright, L. D., eds.), vol 18A, pp. 494-500, Academic Press,
     New York.
28. Haskell, B. E. (1968) Gas liquid chromatographic analysis
     of pyridoxal phosphate. Fed. Proc. 27, 554 (abstract).
29. Tiselius, H.-G. (1972) A chromatographic separation of the
     different forms of vitamin B-6. Clin. Chim. Acta 40, 319-324.
30. Callmer, K. & Davies, L. (1974) Separation and determination
     of vitamin B-1, B-2, B-6, and nicotinamide in commercial
     vitamin preparations using high performance cation-exchange
     chromatography. Chromatographia 7, 644-650.
31. Williams, A. K. & Cole, P. D. (1975) Vitamin B-6: ion
     exchange chromatography of pyridoxal, pyridoxol, and pyridox-
     amine. J. Agric. Food Chem. 23, 915-916.

32. Yasumoto, K., Tadera, K., Tsuji, H. & Mitsuda, H. (1975) Semi-automated system for analysis of vitamin B-6 complex by ion-exchange column chromatography. J. Nutr. Sci. Vitaminol. 21, 117-127.

33. Wong, F. F. (1978) Analyses of vitamin B-6 in extractives of food materials by high-performance liquid chromatography. J. Agric. Food Chem. 26, 1444-1446.

34. Thompson, J. N. (1978) Analysis of vitamins in foods using high performance liquid chromatography. In: Symposium Proceedings: Application of High Pressure Liquid Chromatographic Methods for Determination of Fat Soluble Vitamins A, D, E, and K in Foods and Pharmaceuticals, pp. 62-83. Presented by Association of Vitamin Chemists in conjunction with Waters Associates.

35. Hill, R. B. H., Shaw, C. G. & Day, W. R. (1977) Analysis of water soluble vitamins by high pressure liquid chromatography. J. Chromatogr. Sci. 15, 262-266.

36. Vanderslice, J. T., Stewart, K. K. & Yarmas, M. M. (1979) Liquid chromatographic separation and quantification of B-6 vitamers and their metabolite, pyridoxic acid. J. Chromatogr. 176, 280-285.

37. Vanderslice, J. T., Maire, C. E. & Yakupkovic, J. (1980) High performance liquid chromatographic analysis of vitamin B-6 in ready-to-eat breakfast cereals. Paper #201, presented at the 40th annual meeting of the Institute of Food Technologists, New Orleans.

38. Gregory, J. F. & Kirk, J. R. (1979) Determination of urinary 4-pyridoxic acid using high performance liquid chromatography. Am. J. Clin. Nutr. 32, 879-883.

39. Gregory, J. F. (1980) Determination of pyridoxal 5'-phosphate as the semicarbazone derivative using high-performance liquid chromatography. Anal. Biochem. 102, 374-379.

40. Korytnyk, W., Hakala, M. T., Potti, P. G. G., Angelino, N. & Chang, S. C. (1976) On the inhibitory activity of 4-vinyl analogues of pyridoxal: enzyme and cell culture studies. Biochemistry 15, 5458-5466.

41. Gregory, J. F. (1980) Effects of ε-pyridoxyllysine and related compounds on liver and brain pyridoxal kinase and liver pyridoxamine (pyridoxine) 5'-phosphate oxidase. J. Biol. Chem. 255, 2355-2359.

42. Allenmark, S., Hjelm, E. & Larsson-Cohn, U. (1978) New method for quantitative analysis of pyridoxal-5'-phosphate in biological material. J. Chromatogr. 146, 485-489.

43. Krstulovic, A. M. & Matzura, C. (1979) Rapid assay for tryptophanase using reversed-phase high-performance liquid chromatography. J. Chromatogr. 176, 217-224.

44. Suelter, C. H., Wang, J. & Snell, E. E. (1976) Application
     of a direct spectrophotometric assay employing a chromogenic
     substrate for tryptophanase to the determination of pyridoxal
     and pyridoxamine 5'-phosphates. Anal. Biochem. 76, 221-232.
45. Waters Associates, Inc. (1976) Liquid Chromatography School
     Manual, pp. LS23-LS28, Waters Associates, Inc., Milford, MA.
46. Wittmer, D. P. & Haney, W. G. (1976) Water-soluble vitamins.
     In: GLC and HPLC Analysis of Therapeutic Agents (Tsuji, K. &
     Morozowitch, W., eds.), Ch. 29, Dekker, New York.
47. Williams, A. K. (1979) High-performance chromatography of
     vitamin B-6. In: Methods in Enzymology (McCormick, D. B. &
     Wright, L. D., eds.), vol. 62, pp. 415-422, Academic Press,
     New York.
48. Kirchmeier, R. L. & Upton, R. P. (1978) Simultaneous deter-
     mination of niacin, niacinamide, pyridoxine, thiamine, and
     riboflavin in multivitamin blends by ion-pair high-pressure
     liquid chromatography. J. Pharmaceut. Sci. 67, 1444-1446.
49. Horvath, C., Melander, W. & Molnar, I. (1976) Solvophobic
     interactions in liquid chromatography with nonpolar stationary
     phases. J. Chromatogr. 125, 129-156.
50. Horvath, C., Melander, W. & Molnar, I. (1977) Liquid chroma-
     tography of ionogenic substances with nonpolar stationary
     phases. Anal. Chem. 49, 142-154.
51. Gregory, J. F. (1980) Comparison of high performance liquid
     chromatographic and Saccharomyces uvarum methods for the
     determination of vitamin B-6 in fortified breakfast cereals.
     J. Agric. Food Chem. 28, 486-489.
52. Gregory, J. F. (1980) Bioavailability of vitamin B-6 in
     nonfat dry milk and a fortified rice breakfast cereal product.
     J. Food Sci. 45, 84-86.
53. Lim, K. L., Young, R. W. & Driskell, J. A. (1980) Separation
     of vitamin B-6 components by high-performance liquid chroma-
     tography. J. Chromatogr. 188, 285-288.
54. Yoshida, T., Yunoki, N., Nakazima, Y., Kaito, T. & Anmo, T.
     (1978) Simultaneous determination of the vitamin B-6 group
     in blood by high-performance liquid chromatography (HPLC).
     J. Pharmaceut. Soc. Japan 98, 1319-1326.
55. Gregory, J. F. (1980) Effects of ε-pyridoxyllysine bound to
     dietary protein on the vitamin B-6 status of rats. J. Nutr.
     110, 995-1005.
56. Gregory, J. F., Manley, D. & Kirk, J. R. (1980) Determination
     of total vitamin B-6 in animal tissues by reverse phase liquid
     chromatography. J. Agric. Food Chem. (submitted for publication).
57. Brin, M. & Thiele, V. F. (1967) Relationships between vitamin
     B-6 vitamer content and the activities of two transaminase
     enzymes in rat tissues at varying intake levels of vitamin B-6.
     J. Nutr. 93, 213-221.

58. Johansson, S., Lindstedt, S. & Tiselius, H.-G. (1968) Metab-
     olism of ($^3H_8$) pyridoxine in mice. Biochemistry 7, 2327-2332.
59. Johansson, S., Lindstedt, S. & Tiselius, H.-G. (1974) Metab-
     olic interconversions of different forms of vitamin B-6. J.
     Biol. Chem. 249, 6040-6046.
60. Thiele, V. F. & Brin, M. (1966) Chromatographic separation
     and microbiologic assay of vitamin B-6 in tissues from normal
     and vitamin B-6-depleted rats. J. Nutr. 90, 347-353.
61. Thiele, V. F. & Brin, M. (1968) Availability of vitamin B-6
     vitamers fed orally to Long-Evans rats as determined by tissue
     transaminase activity and vitamin B-6 assay. J. Nutr. 94,
     237-242.

METHODOLOGY FOR DETERMINATION OF BLOOD AMINOTRANSFERASES

J. H. Skala, P. P. Waring, M. F. Lyons, M. G. Rusnak
and J. S. Alletto

Division of Research Support
Letterman Army Institute of Research
Presidio of San Francisco, CA   94129

Nutritional interest in the blood aminotransferases is concerned with the in vitro functional evaluation of the relative degree of saturation of total endogenous apoenzyme with vitamin B-6 vitamers, principally pyridoxal-5'-phosphate (PLP). The transamination reactions catalysed by aspartate and alanine aminotransferases (AST and ALT) are outlined in Fig. 1. Both enzymes facilitate the transfer of the amino group from the respective amino acid to 2-oxoglutarate forming L-glutamate and the keto acid corresponding to the original amino acid. Both enzymes are believed to be a mixture (as measured directly by current techniques) of two or more isomers requiring different B-6 vitamers to form the active holoenzyme. A significant portion of the total activity responds to PLP. The ratio of the increase in the endogenous enzyme activity resulting from exogenous adjunct of PLP to the original endogenous activity is used by some as an indicator of vitamin B-6 status. The ratio is usually assigned one of three coefficient designations: activity, saturation, or stimulation.

Alanine Aminotransferase (ALT)

$$\text{L-Alanine + 2-Oxoglutarate} \underset{}{\overset{\text{ALT}}{\rightleftharpoons}} \text{Pyruvate + L-Glutamate}$$

Aspartate Aminotransferase (AST)

$$\text{L-Aspartate + 2-Oxoglutarate} \underset{}{\overset{\text{AST}}{\rightleftharpoons}} \text{Oxalacetate + L-Glutamate}$$

Fig. 1.   Reactions catalyzed by alanine and aspartate aminotransferase (ALT and AST).

The endogenous activity of the specimen is usually called the unsaturated or unstimulated activity (designated with U in this paper). Likewise, the activity amplified by exogenous PLP is usually called the saturated or stimulated activity (designated with S in this paper). Emphasis in the following discussion will center on efforts in recent years to optimize procedures to establish U and S activity levels in various specimens with somewhat less emphasis on the interpretation of the calculated coefficients.

The principle steps in the contemporary evolution of routine methodology for AST and ALT are shown in Tables 1 and 2. Tonhazy et al. (1) introduced a colorimetric procedure for AST in tissues which involved converting the oxalacetate formed via the trans-amination reaction to pyruvate with aniline citrate. The pyruvate-dinitrophenylhydrazone is formed, extracted with toluene, and color is developed with strong alkali. Cabaud et al. (2) adapted the method to serum. Reitman and Frankel (3) refined the procedure and extended the technique to the determination of serum ALT. Marsh et al. (4) used the procedure in whole blood hemolysates, but criticized the lack of sensitivity. The procedure has been labeled non-specific because the 2,4-dinitrophenylhydrazine reacts with keto acids other than pyruvic acid (5).

Karmen et al. (6) introduced the coupled enzyme spectrophoto-metric procedure for AST in serum in the appendix to their 1955 paper. Fig. 2 outlines the principles of the reaction in which the basic transaminase reaction is coupled with the reaction catalyzed by malic dehydrogenase (MDH) in which oxidation of reduced nicotine-adenine-dinucleotide ($NADH_2$ or NADH) is measured as a decrease in absorbance at 340 nm (the indicator reaction). The chief weakness of the Karmen procedure lies in the fact that it was conducted at room temperature.

The coupled enzyme procedure was subsequently refined as out-lined in Table 1, beginning in 1960 with the procedures by Henry et al. (7). These workers increased the L-asparate concentration and performed the analysis at 32°. The Committee on Enzymes of the Scandinavian Society for Clinical Chemistry and Clinical Physiology (SSCC & CP (8)) in 1974, presented their recommendations for serum AST determination employing a pH 7.7 Tris buffer, increased concentration of L-aspartate and 2-oxoglutarate and a reaction temperature of 37°. Beutler (9) and Beutler et al. (10) presented a method for erythrocyte AST in a 1:20 hemolysate at 37° with a markedly reduced concentration of L-aspartic acid in the final reaction mixture. The method incorporated PLP (in lieu of water) for the saturated value at a final reaction concentration of 0.02 mM.

Table 1. Recent Evolution of Methods for Aspartate Aminotransferase

Method	Characteristics				
		Buffer		mM Final Reaction Mixture		
		Type	pH	Buffer	L-Aspartate	2-Oxoglutarate
Colorimetric Tonhazy et al. (1)	Oxalacetate produced by enzyme reaction, converted to pyruvate with aniline citrate, and 2,4 dinitrophenyl-hydrazone of pyruvate determined					
Reitman et al. (3)	Refined Tonhazy procedure and extended it to ALT					
Coupled Enzyme						
Karmen et al. (6)		phosphate	7.4	33	33	6.6
Henry et al. (7)		phosphate	7.4	43	125	6.7
SSCC & CP (8)		Tris	7.7	20	200	12.0
Beutler (9,10)		Tris	8.0	100	10	10.0
Bergmeyer et al. (11) and IFCC (12)		Tris	7.8	80	240	12.0

Table 2.   Recent Evolution of Methods for Alanine Aminotransferase

Method	Characteristics				
		Buffer		mM Final Reaction Mixture	
		Type	pH	Buffer	L-Alanine	2-Oxoglutarate
Colorimetric Reitman et al. (3)	Refined Tonhazy procedure and extended it to ALT					
Coupled Enzyme						
Wroblewski et al. (20)		phosphate	7.4	33	33	6.6
Henry et al. (7)		phosphate	7.4	43	167	6.7
SSCC & CP (8)		Tris	7.4	20	400	12.0
IFCC (13)		Tris	7.8	80	400	12.0
Bergmeyer et al. (11)		Tris	7.5	100	500	15.0

REACTION PRINCIPLES
Aspartate Aminotransferase (AST) Determination

L-Aspartate + 2-Oxoglutarate $\xrightarrow{\text{AST}}$ Oxalacetate + L-Glutamate

Oxalacetate + $NADH_2$ $\xrightarrow{\text{MDH}}$ L-Malate + NAD

Pyruvate + $NADH_2$ $\xrightarrow{\text{LDH}}$ L-Lactate + NAD

Fig. 2.   Reaction principles involved in the determination of
aspartate aminotransferase by the coupled enzyme technique.

Finally, Bergmeyer et al. (11) published a comprehensive study
outlining optimized methods for both AST and ALT which, doubtless,
contributed to the corresponding recommendations for serum AST of
the Expert Panel on Enzymes (of which Bergmeyer was a member) of the
International Federation of Clinical Chemistry (IFCC (12). The
recommendations for serum AST call for pH 7.8 Tris buffer, increased
L-aspartic acid, and a reaction temperature of 30°. It was also
recommended that PLP at a final reaction concentration of 0.10 mM
be incorporated as a standard reaction component. This has been
received with mixed reaction by domestic diagnostic kit manufacturers;
those who do not incorporate the PLP usually defer to the lack of
data for interpreting the elevated saturated values. The reaction
mixture includes lactic dehydrogenase (LDH--see Fig. 2) for the
reduction of endogenous pyruvate and diminution of competing NADH
oxidation interference. The reagents (except 2-oxoglutarate) are
incubated for 10 minutes to allow saturation of the specimen apoenzyme with PLP and permit the LDH clearing reaction to occur. The
reaction is then initiated by the addition of 2-oxoglutarate and
monitored for a period of 5 minutes.

Methodology for ALT (Table 2) evolved in much the same manner
and almost concomitantly with that for AST. The same general
pattern existed shifting from the colorimetric to the coupled enzyme
procedure which is outlined in Fig. 3. The evolution of the coupled
enzyme procedure involved optimization through changes from phosphate
to Tris buffer, increases in concentration for the buffer and substrates, and utilization of controlled temperatures.

REACTION PRINCIPLES
Alanine Aminotransferase (ALT) Determination

L-Alanine + 2-Oxoglutarate $\xrightarrow{\text{ALT}}$ Pyruvate + L-Glutamate

Pyruvate + NADH $\xrightarrow{\text{LDH}}$ L-Lactate + NAD

Fig. 3.   Reaction principles involved in the determination of
alanine aminotransferase by the coupled enzyme technique.

Most emphasis on optimization presented here has been expressed by clinical chemists primarily interested in improved serum methodology for diagnostic applications. Nutritional scientists have generally adapted these or earlier procedures to specimens pertinent to their studies. Our situation has been much the same. This paper will report two automated systems using chemistries adapted to a variety of specimens from the optimized serum procedures; a general consideration of both nuances and principle problem areas in these determinations will be given.

MATERIALS AND METHODS

Centrifugal Analyzer Procedures

The centrifugal analyzer used is a Gemsaec (research configuration) manufactured by Electro-Nucleonics, Inc., Fairfield, NJ. Among the more important features pertinent to this type of analytical application are the facts that it has a diffraction grating monochromator coupled with interference filters, programmable reading interval capability, and electronic temperature control with internal calibration. The principle disadvantage of this type of equipment is that the reaction (end-point or kinetic) must be observed through the sample matrix.

The working reagent and final reaction concentrations for the determination of AST U and S, and ALT U and S are shown in Tables 3 and 4, respectively. During the determination of the unsaturated (U) activities, the aqueous PLP is replaced by distilled water so that the volume relationships are maintained. These concentrations (with the exception of NADH and PLP) are the same ratio, but are approximately half the concentration recommended by the IFCC (12). PLP is incorporated at the IFCC concentration and NADH at approximately 75% of the recommendation. These adjustments were required to scale down to the optimal ratio between activity and substrate requirements imposed by this automated system.

The reagents and sample are automatically loaded into the teflon distribution disc (good heat sink). The analysis is initiated by the sample in this procedure, so a single buffered reagent is used which includes the usual substrates for all the reactions plus 2-oxoglutarate. For the unsaturated (U) activities, the loader is programmed to deliver 10 μl sample followed by 140 μl of flush (aqueous 0.1% Triton X-100) into Well B of the disc, and 300 μl of the working reagent into Well C. For the saturated (S) activities, 50 μl of the aqueous working PLP is delivered into Well B (we use a Reagent Dispenser with 50 μl cartridge, Micromedic Systems, Inc., Horsham, PA). The disc is then placed on the loader programmed to deliver 10 μl of sample, followed by 90 μl of flush (aqueous 0.16%

Table 3. Reagent Concentrations for Automated Analysis of AST

Reagent	Concentrations				Units
	Continuous Flow		Centrifugal Analyzer		
	Working Reagent	Final Reaction	Working Reagent	Final Reaction	
Tris (hydroxymethyl-aminomethane)	104	82	65	43	mM
L-Aspartate	505	200	188	126	mM
NADH	0.12	0.12	0.21	0.14	mM
LDH	-	-	1210	800	U/l
MDH	610	610	1210	800	U/l
2-Oxoglutarate	80	12	9.4	6.3	mM
pH	7.8	7.8	7.8	7.8	-
PLP	0.66	0.10	0.15	0.10	mM
Volume fraction of sample	0.25	(0.025-0.04)	-	0.022	-

Table 4.   Reagent Concentrations for Centrifugal
           Analysis of ALT

Reagent	Concentrations		Units
	Working Reagent	Final Reaction	
Tris (hydroxymethyl-aminomethane)	65	43	mM
L-Alanine	315	210	mM
NADH	0.21	0.14	mM
LDH	1550	1030	U/1
2-Oxoglutarate	9.4	6.3	mM
pH	7.4	7.4	-
PLP	0.15	0.10	mM
Volume fraction of sample	-	0.022	-

of Triton X-100) into Well B where it mixes with the PLP, and 300
µl of working reagent into Well C. When determinging AST stimulation,
the disc is wrapped in plastic wrap and incubated at 30° for 10
minutes to maximize saturation. ALT stimulation did not show evidence of further beneficial effect due to incubation, but rather a
more erratic reading to reading variability. Consequently, we have
performed this analysis immediately after loading.

The samples analyzed have been either hemolysates of whole blood
or erythrocytes, serum, and plasma. We have generally used as anti-
coagulants EDTA or heparin. We have discovered that we can achieve
maximum response from human cells through incorporation of Triton
X-100 as a dispersant at 0.1% concentration in saline as the diluent
after cell disruption by freezing. The dilution of whole blood is
1 + 17 with the saline plus Triton. The twice-washed (saline)
erythrocytes are processed in graduated tubes so that they can be
diluted to the equivalent volume of whole blood and then further
diluted (1 + 17), eliminating the need for involving hematocrit
consideration when expressed as erythrocyte activity (IU) per liter
of whole blood. The stability of rat hemoglobin appears to be quite
low; consequently, it precipitates extensively after being frozen in
aqueous solution. This occurs without loss of enzyme activity and
results in reduction of the matrix effect and use of much lower
dilutions. This phenomenon has not been observed in human whole
blood or erythrocytes, nor in rat whole blood. The usual preparation
involves adding 1.0 ml of distilled water to the twice-washed erythrocytes from 0.5 ml of EDTA blood and freezing. Further dilution
with an equal volume of saline plus Triton is made after thawing and
before analysis.

Table 5. Centrifugal Analyzer

Parameter List

EASTU,S; WASTU,S; PASTU,S
EALTU,S; WALTU,S; PALTU,S
IU
30°
U = S10/F140/R300
S = S10/PLP50/F90/R300
IR = 120 (varies)
RI = 60
NR = 8
SC = 1.0
KT = 7235 (x Dil. Factor)
TF = 1.0
TC = 2
SA = 0.6

The pertinent operating parameters of the centrifugal analyzer program for determining AST and ALT U and S in a variety of samples are shown in Table 5. The initial reading (IR) can be varied to compensate for unusually long lag phases (rare) or unusually long nonlinear initial response (more common). The reading interval (R) is normally 60 seconds. The total number of readings (NR) can be as low as 6 and still encompass a 5-minute observation period, but we usually take 8 observations (7 minutes) to ensure coverage of the zero-order kinetic portion of the reaction. The test constant (KT) is determined using the fomula:

$$KT = \frac{1000 \text{ (assay volume)}}{\text{(sample volume) (6.22)}}$$

where 6.22 is the molar absorptivity of $NADH_2$ $(cm^2/\mu mol)$. The KT is the critical multiplier in calculating the International Unit (IU) which is defined as that amount of enzyme which converts 1 μmol of 2-oxoglutarate to 1 μmol of L-glutamate per minute per liter of sample with the concurrent oxidation of 1 μmol of $NADH_2$. A dilution factor can also be included in the value for KT.

The analysis time with the parameters set as they are in Table 5 is 9 minutes; an additional 1 to 2 minutes is required for data output (hard copy). Recent models of this equipment incorporate faster computers and line printers. It would not be improbable to analyze 6 discs per hour with 13 unknowns plus 2 quality controls per disc for a throughput of 78 per hour.

Continuous Flow Procedure

The continuous flow analyzer used is an Autoanalyzer II, manufactured by Technicon Instruments Corp., Tarrytown, NY. This system incorporates in line dialysis which, though limited, minimizes matrix effects. The response of the system must be calibrated with a known chemistry standard. It is intended primarily for end-point chemistry, although additional data points may be collected by incorporating additional analysis channels with time delays; but the cost effectiveness of performance is greatly diminished beyond a two-channel, two-point kinetic measurement.

The working reagent and final reaction concentrations for the determination of AST U and S are shown in Table 3. These are the concentrations recommended. The Tris buffer contains 10 ml Triton X-405 per liter. Individual reagent preparations in buffer were made with the exception of aqueous PLP. The flow diagram in Fig. 4 shows the integration of the reactants into the system. The unsaturated (U) activity is obtained by substituting water for the PLP input (see Fig. 4). The indicator reaction takes place on the recipient side of the dialyzer. The analysis is 2-oxoglutarate-initiated as suggested by IFCC (13).

The system is calibrated with known standards. In the case of the controlled rat depletion/repletion study described later, this was accomplished with aliquots of 5 erythrocyte pools from vitamin B-6-deficient and sufficient rats. These specimens were repetitively analyzed by the centrifugal analyzer procedure prior to use, so that a confidence interval could be established. One set of quality controls was analyzed with each tray of specimens ($N = 5 + 35 = 40$).

The improved continuous flow procedure has, thus far, been applied only in the rat depletion/repletion study. Rat hemolysates, prepared as described in the centrifugal analysis procedure, are thawed and vortexed; 1.8 ml of Tris buffer is added to 0.2 ml of the aqueous hemolysate in a sample cup and the dilution mixed well. Controls are treated in an identical manner. The system can be operated at 50 samples per hour. A procedure for ALT has not been finalized for the continuous flow analyzer.

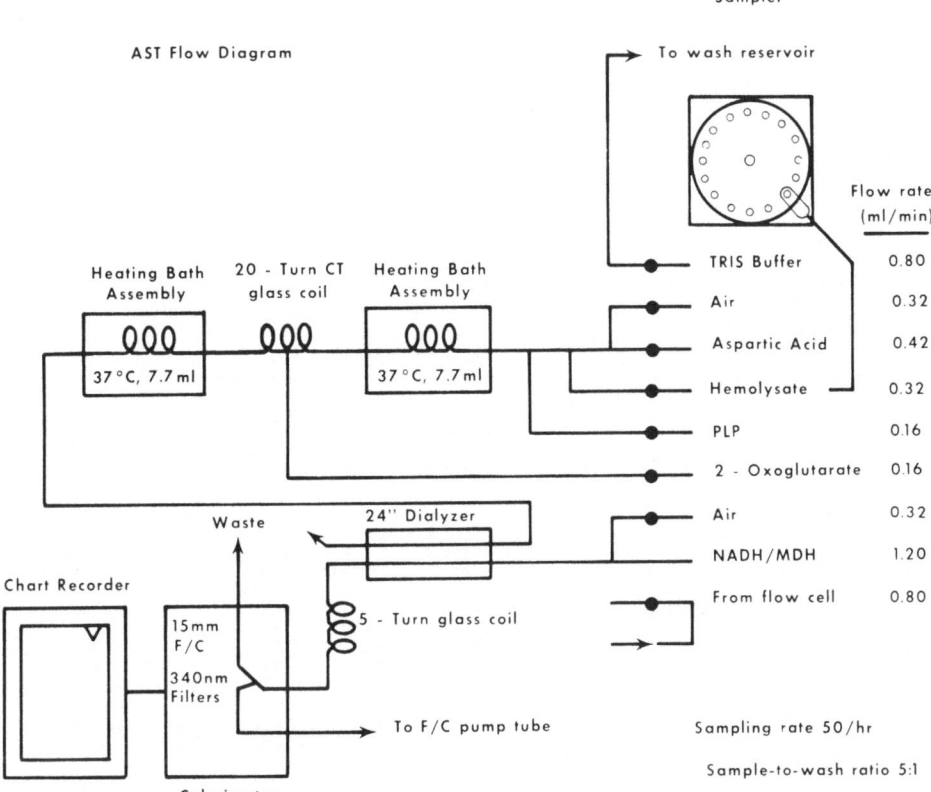

Fig. 4.   Manifold flow diagram for continous flow determination
of aspartate aminotransferase in hemolysates.

RESULTS AND DISCUSSION

Performance of the Centrifugal Analysis Procedure

The output format for the centrifugal analysis of rat erythrocyte ALT U and ALT S are shown in Figs. 5 and 6, respectively.
The analysis was performed on a 1 + 3 dilution of the hypotonic
hemolysate. The results (IU) shown need multiplication by (1 +
hematocrit/100) to compensate for the preliminary dilution. Examination of the data points printed in the lower portion of each
format reveals the starting absorbance range of the assay and the
reproducibility of minute-by-minute readings within specimens by
analysis. A generally recognized fault with the determination of
ALT in erythrocytes is the difficulty in reading the relatively
low activity of this enzyme through the sample matrix, so that it

```
                              GEMSAEC RUN
          TEST HEADER:  GOT              WORKSHEET:  A15FEB
DET:       EALTU        IR:    120     AD:     4      HI:    20.0000
DATE:     5 JUN 80      RI:     60     CD:     1      LO:     5.0000
RUN:      5             NR:      8     TC:     2      SA:     0.6000
TEMP:     30' C         KT:   28940    TF:    1.0     DI:     1

              RAD FOOD MALES 15 FEB 80

   CUV ABS/MIN    LAB #'S    IU    ******* FLAGS ***************
                                   RANGE         OPERATIONAL
    2 -0.0027     124162    77.9   HI    DECR              /    8
    3 -0.0043     496235   124.7   HI    DECR              /    8
    4 -0.0041        434   117.4   HI    DECR              /    8
    5 -0.0035        441   100.5   HI    DECR              /    8
    6 -0.0039        452   112.1   HI    DECR              /    8
    7 -0.0035        464   102.3   HI    DECR              /    8
    8 -0.0043        475   124.8   HI    DECR              /    8
    9 -0.0041        505   118.3   HI    DECR              /    8
   10 -0.0041        506   119.8   HI    DECR              7    8
   11 -0.0036        515   103.0   HI    DECR              7    8
   12 -0.0040        531   116.9   HI    DECR              7    8
   13 -0.0033        546    95.2   HI    DECR              7    8
   14 -0.0043        573   123.7   HI    DECR              /    8
   15 -0.0038        589   108.6   HI    DECR              7    8
   16 -0.0117     496234   338.5   HI    DECR              7    8

  MDP                    DETERMINATION: EALTU            RUN:      5
  POINT    ABS+DELTA ABS     ABS+DELTA ABS     ABS+DELTA ABS     ABS+DELTA ABS
                 1                  2                 3                 4
    1                        1.0215  0.0000   0.9829  0.0000   1.0502  0.0000
    2                        1.0186 -0.0029   0.9780 -0.0049   1.0458 -0.0044
    3                        1.0162 -0.0024   0.9742 -0.0038   1.0421 -0.0037
    4                        1.0137 -0.0024   0.9692 -0.0051   1.0376 -0.0044
    5                        1.0104 -0.0033   0.9649 -0.0043   1.0336 -0.0041
    6                        1.0078 -0.0026   0.9610 -0.0039   1.0296 -0.0039
    7                        1.0056 -0.0022   0.9569 -0.0041   1.0259 -0.0037
    8                        1.0025 -0.0031   0.9526 -0.0043   1.0216 -0.0043
                 5                  6                 7                 8
    1    1.0367  0.0000       1.0540  0.0000   1.0382  0.0000   1.0330  0.0000
    2    1.0329 -0.0038       1.0494 -0.0046   1.0341 -0.0042   1.0284 -0.0046
    3    1.0303 -0.0026       1.0464 -0.0031   1.0309 -0.0031   1.0245 -0.0039
    4    1.0263 -0.0040       1.0422 -0.0042   1.0274 -0.0036   1.0197 -0.0048
    5    1.0227 -0.0036       1.0381 -0.0041   1.0236 -0.0038   1.0153 -0.0044
    6    1.0194 -0.0033       1.0344 -0.0037   1.0206 -0.0030   1.0113 -0.0040
    7    1.0162 -0.0032       1.0306 -0.0037   1.0169 -0.0036   1.0074 -0.0039
    8    1.0122 -0.0041       1.0267 -0.0039   1.0131 -0.0039   1.0025 -0.0049
                 9                 10                11                12
    1    1.0405  0.0000       1.0421  0.0000   1.0377  0.0000   1.0308  0.0000
    2    1.0361 -0.0044       1.0375 -0.0046   1.0334 -0.0043   1.0262 -0.0046
    3    1.0323 -0.0038       1.0339 -0.0036   1.0304 -0.0030   1.0227 -0.0036
    4    1.0281 -0.0043       1.0301 -0.0038   1.0264 -0.0041   1.0185 -0.0042
    5    1.0235 -0.0046       1.0252 -0.0048   1.0227 -0.0037   1.0142 -0.0043
    6    1.0201 -0.0034       1.0213 -0.0039   1.0194 -0.0033   1.0104 -0.0038
    7    1.0161 -0.0039       1.0172 -0.0041   1.0162 -0.0032   1.0066 -0.0038
    8    1.0116 -0.0045       1.0129 -0.0043   1.0126 -0.0036   1.0023 -0.0043
                13                 14                15                16
    1    1.0282  0.0000       1.0366  0.0000   1.0886  0.0000   0.9689  0.0000
    2    1.0246 -0.0036       1.0319 -0.0046   1.0847 -0.0039   0.9568 -0.0121
    3    1.0217 -0.0028       1.0281 -0.0039   1.0812 -0.0036   0.9456 -0.0113
    4    1.0182 -0.0036       1.0240 -0.0041   1.0773 -0.0039   0.9338 -0.0117
    5    1.0144 -0.0038       1.0189 -0.0051   1.0734 -0.0039   0.9217 -0.0121
    6    1.0117 -0.0026       1.0150 -0.0039   1.0702 -0.0031   0.9102 -0.0115
    7    1.0086 -0.0031       1.0112 -0.0038   1.0662 -0.0040   0.8988 -0.0114
    8    1.0049 -0.0037       1.0064 -0.0049   1.0621 -0.0042   0.8868 -0.0120
```

Fig. 5.   Data output from centrifugal analyzer for determination
          of unsaturated alanine aminotransferase in erythrocyte
          hemolysates.

```
                             GEMSAEC RUN
         TEST HEADER:  GOT              WORKSHEET:  A15FEB
 DET:      EALTS       IR:    120    AD:    4      HJ:    20.0000
 DATE:    5 JUN 80     RI:    60     CD:    1      LO:     5.0000
 RUN:     13           NR:    8      TC:    2      SA:     0.6000
 TEMP:    30' C        KT:  28940    TF:   1.0     DI:     1

                   RAD FOOD MALES 15 FEB 80

 CUV ABS/MIN    LAB #'S    IU   ******* FLAGS ***************
                               RANGE         OPERATIONAL
  2 -0.0028    124162     82.1  HI   DECR                7   8
  3 -0.0044    496235    127.9  HI   DECR                /   8
  4 -0.0046       434    132.4  HI   DECR                7   8
  5 -0.0041       441    118.9  HI   DECR                /   8
  6 -0.0041       452    118.8  HI   DECR                /   8
  7 -0.0037       464    107.2  HI   DECR                /   8
  8 -0.0048       475    137.6  HI   DECR                7   8
  9 -0.0043       505    124.4  HI   DECR                7   8
 10 -0.0044       506    127.6  HI   DECR                7   8
 11 -0.0037       515    106.7  HI   DECR                7   8
 12 -0.0043       531    124.7  HI   DECR                7   8
 13 -0.0034       546     97.9  HI   DECR                /   8
 14 -0.0045       573    129.5  HI   DECR                /   8
 15 -0.0043       589    123.9  HI   DECR                7   8
 16 -0.0119    496234    344.4  HI   DECR                7   8
```

```
 MDP                     DETERMINATION: EALTS          RUN:     13
 POINT    ABS+DELTA ABS      ABS+DELTA ABS      ABS+DELTA ABS     ABS+DELTA ABS
              1                  2                  3                  4
  1                        1.0261  0.0000     0.9825  0.0000     1.1869  0.0000
  2                        1.0229 -0.0033     0.9783 -0.0042     1.1824 -0.0045
  3                        1.0199 -0.0030     0.9732 -0.0051     1.1779 -0.0046
  4                        1.0172 -0.0026     0.9684 -0.0048     1.1727 -0.0052
  5                        1.0152 -0.0021     0.9654 -0.0030     1.1701 -0.0026
  6                        1.0117 -0.0035     0.9605 -0.0049     1.1642 -0.0059
  7                        1.0086 -0.0031     0.9557 -0.0047     1.1591 -0.0051
  8                        1.0061 -0.0024     0.9514 -0.0043     1.1549 -0.0043
              5                  6                  7                  8
  1    1.1742  0.0000     1.1951  0.0000     1.1757  0.0000     1.1735  0.0000
  2    1.1700 -0.0043     1.1901 -0.0049     1.1717 -0.0039     1.1679 -0.0056
  3    1.1661 -0.0039     1.1861 -0.0040     1.1685 -0.0032     1.1633 -0.0046
  4    1.1617 -0.0043     1.1819 -0.0043     1.1641 -0.0044     1.1584 -0.0049
  5    1.1589 -0.0028     1.1794 -0.0025     1.1621 -0.0020     1.1545 -0.0039
  6    1.1544 -0.0046     1.1742 -0.0051     1.1574 -0.0046     1.1493 -0.0052
  7    1.1493 -0.0051     1.1696 -0.0046     1.1531 -0.0044     1.1442 -0.0051
  8    1.1451 -0.0042     1.1659 -0.0037     1.1496 -0.0034     1.1399 -0.0043
              9                 10                 11                 12
  1    1.1875  0.0000     1.1836  0.0000     1.1799  0.0000     1.1734  0.0000
  2    1.1830 -0.0045     1.1787 -0.0049     1.1756 -0.0043     1.1689 -0.0045
  3    1.1784 -0.0046     1.1744 -0.0044     1.1724 -0.0032     1.1644 -0.0045
  4    1.1737 -0.0047     1.1693 -0.0051     1.1685 -0.0039     1.1595 -0.0049
  5    1.1709 -0.0028     1.1667 -0.0026     1.1662 -0.0023     1.1566 -0.0029
  6    1.1665 -0.0044     1.1616 -0.0051     1.1620 -0.0042     1.1520 -0.0046
  7    1.1609 -0.0056     1.1564 -0.0051     1.1572 -0.0047     1.1472 -0.0048
  8    1.1572 -0.0037     1.1525 -0.0039     1.1536 -0.0037     1.1428 -0.0044
             13                 14                 15                 16
  1    1.1722  0.0000     1.1781  0.0000     1.2369  0.0000     0.9686  0.0000
  2    1.1683 -0.0039     1.1729 -0.0051     1.2318 -0.0051     0.9562 -0.0124
  3    1.1651 -0.0032     1.1686 -0.0043     1.2279 -0.0039     0.9444 -0.0118
  4    1.1612 -0.0039     1.1642 -0.0044     1.2235 -0.0044     0.9324 -0.0121
  5    1.1593 -0.0019     1.1606 -0.0036     1.2207 -0.0027     0.9209 -0.0115
  6    1.1552 -0.0041     1.1559 -0.0047     1.2157 -0.0050     0.9091 -0.0118
  7    1.1512 -0.0041     1.1507 -0.0051     1.2106 -0.0052     0.8967 -0.0123
  8    1.1483 -0.0029     1.1462 -0.0046     1.2064 -0.0042     0.8850 -0.0117
```

Fig. 6.   Data output from centrifugal analyzer for determination
          of saturated alanine aminotransferase in erythrocyte
          hemolysates.

must be done in dilute solution with a low signal to noise ratio.
This caused a problem evident in Fig. 6 in the determination of ALT
S where MDP point 5 is uniformly low across all cuvettes, 2-15,
where the absorbance change is low. This would normally be noted
and the run repeated.

Various aspects of the reproducibility of the centrifugal analyzer
procedures are presented in Tables 6-8. The within-day precision of
repeated analysis for plasma AST U and S, ALT U and S in an abnormal
aqueous matrix standard, and AST and ALT U in a normal range human
lyophilized serum pool are shown in Table 6. These are used as
quality controls on the chemistries involved in these studies. The
statistics were derived from 11 individual determinations on each
control, each day, on 6 different days. Also shown in Table 6 is
the within-day precision of repeated analysis of AST U in two erythrocyte pooled controls, control (normal) and deficient, which were
analyzed 15 times each daily on 2 days. The day-to-day precision
of repeated AST U and S and ALT U and S analyses on the plasma
controls is shown in Table 7. These data were derived from statis-
ical analysis of results obtained on 6 days, 11 times each day. The
day-to-day precision of repeated AST U and S, and ALT U and S
analyses of the erythrocyte controls are presented in Table 8.
These statistics were derived from analysis of the controls on 10
days for AST (duplicate aliquots each day) and 4 days for ALT
(duplicate aliquots each day).

Performance of the Continuous Flow Procedure

The analogue performance characteristics of the continuous
flow system for AST are shown in Figs. 7 and 8. Fig. 7 reveals the
linearity of system response for AST U and S throughout the full
output range produced by various dilutions of the same (deficient)
rat pool. Fig. 8 shows the peak height and separation in AST U
determination of the 5 pooled erythrocyte controls run at a rate of
50 samples per hour (upper), and the same rate with a buffer cup
between controls (effective rate = 25 samples per hour). It can be
seen that there is very little peak carryover and the peak height
response is the same.

The within-day and day-to-day precision of repeated AST U
analyses by the continuous flow procedure are shown in Table 9.
These data are expressed as the mean (of the 5 pooled controls)
response in IU value assigned by the centrifugal analyzer procedure
per chart unit of peak height. The within-day statistics were
derived from analysis of 20 each of the 5 controls on the same day.
The between-day precision was established by analyzing 5 each of
the 5 controls on each of 6 days.

Table 6. Within Day Precision by Centrifugal Analyzer

Analysis/Sample	Mean Activity	Standard Deviation	Coefficient of Variation
	IU/L (30°)	±	%
AST, Plasma[a]			
Normal, U[b]	19.1	1.0	5.4
Abnormal, U[c]	42.0	1.6	3.8
Abnormal, S	68.6	1.8	2.6
ALT, Plasma[a]			
Normal, U	21.5	1.1	5.2
Abnormal, U	86.5	2.6	3.0
Abnormal, S	92.6	3.4	3.6
AST, Erythrocytes[d]			
Control, U	722	8	1.1
Deficient, U	300	6	2.1

[a]N = 11 observations per day each of 6 days, each group.
[b]Lyophilized human pool.
[c]Aqueous fabricated control.
[d]N = 15 observations per day each of 2 days, each group;
rat erythrocyte pools, activity expressed as IU of
erythrocyte activity per liter of whole blood.

Application and Correlation of Methods

Results of the application of the centrifugal analyzer procedures in analysis of specimens from rats in depleted, control, and
repleted (two levels PN) groups sampled at deficiency and 1, 2, and
4 weeks after repletion are shown in Tables 10-13. There were 12
male and 12 female rats in each group. The plasma ALT and AST U
activities are shown in Table 10. It can be noted that there is
distinction between the groups at deficiency, but both aminotransferase activities are quickly restored. The whole blood AST U and
S (Table 11), and the erythrocyte AST U and S (Table 12) show a
tendency for the activity of the two repletion groups to be restored
somewhat more slowly, at least through the second week of repletion.
Whole blood values appear to be inordinately larger than the
corresponding erthrocyte values. They should be higher due to the
inclusion of the plasma contribution, but the differential is even
larger, possibly because the whole blood aliquots were analyzed
within 2 days of collection, while the erythrocyte determinations

Table 7. Day-to-day Precision--Plasma AST and ALT by
          Centrifugal Analyzer

Analysis/Sample	Mean Activity	Standard Deviation	Coefficient of Variation
	IU/L (30°)	±	%
AST[a]			
Normal, U[b]	19.0	0.5	2.4
Abnormal, U[c]	42.0	1.4	3.3
Abnormal, S	68.6	1.6	2.3
ALT			
Normal, U	21.5	1.0	4.5
Abnormal, U	86.5	3.6	4.1
Abnormal, S	92.6	3.4	3.7

[a]N = 6 days, 11 observations per day, each group.
[b]Lyophilized human pool.
[c]Aqueous fabricated control.

Table 8. Day-to-day Precision--Erythrocyte AST and ALT
          by Centrifugal Analyzer

Analysis/Sample	Mean Activity[a]	Standard Deviation	Coefficient of Variation
	IU/L (30°)	±	%
AST[b]			
Control, U	727	17	2.4
Control, S	817	17	4.1
Deficient, U	300	18	6.0
Deficient, S	531	26	4.8
ALT[c]			
Control, U	130	6	4.5
Control, S	140	3	2.1
Deficient, U	40	4	8.9
Deficient, S	49	2	4.5

[a]Activity expressed as IU of erythrocyte activity per
   liter of whole blood; rat erythrocyte pools.
[b]N = 10 days, 2 observations per day, each group.
[c]N = 4 days, 2 observations per day, each group.

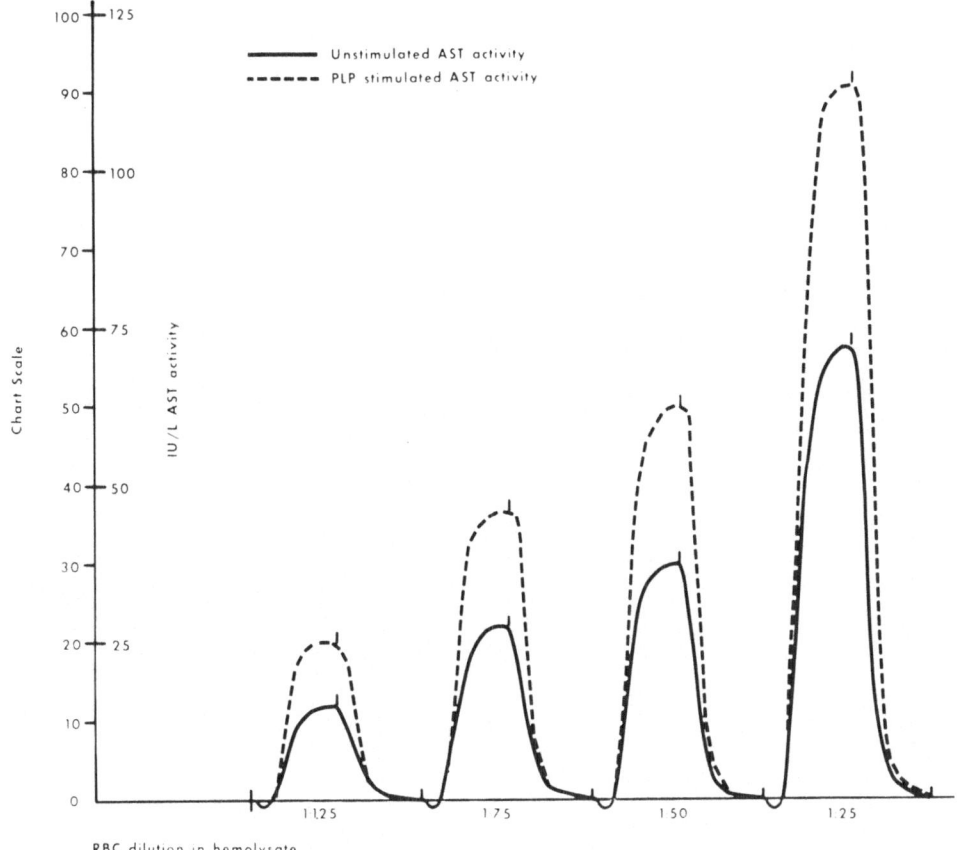

Fig. 7. Response of continuous flow determination of unsaturated
         and saturated aspartate aminotransferase in various
         dilutions of a vitamin B-6 deficient rat hemolysate.

were performed on duplicate hemolysates which had been stored beyond
the known limits of stability. The erythrocyte ALT U activity
(Table 13) of the suboptimal repletion group remained lower through
4 weeks of repletion while the activity of the higher repletion
group was restored earlier.

     The continuous flow procedure for AST was used to analyze the
same specimens in the rat study. The paired data from the depletion
and first week repletion samplings were subjected to linear regression analysis. The regression data are shown in Figs. 9-11 for
AST U, S, and the activity coefficient, respectively. The correlations are highly significant. While a strong relationship between

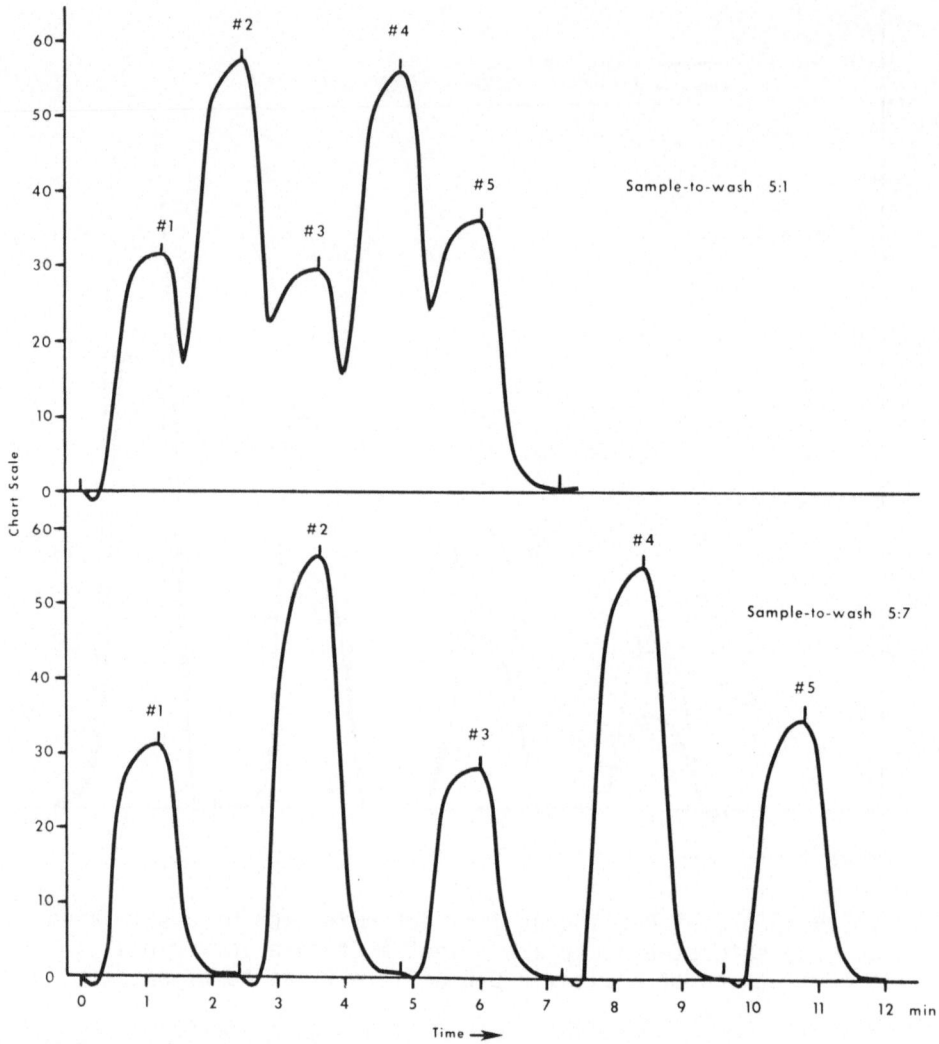

Fig. 8.   Continuous flow determination of unsaturated aspartate
          aminotransferase in five rat erythrocyte controls at two
          sample:wash ratios, 5:1 and 5:7.

methods might be expected because one calibrates the other, it is
not necessarily a correct corollary. The interesting fact is that
the response is so similar, even though one technique is serum-
initiated at 30° and the other is 2-oxoglutarate-initiated at 37°.

Table 9.   Precision of Continuous Flow Analyzer
Determination of AST in Erythrocytes

Precision Type	Mean Response[a]	Standard Deviation	Coefficient of Variation
	IU/L/Chart Unit	±	%
Within day[b]	11.5	0.5	4.2
Day-to-day[c]	13.2	0.7	6.2

[a] IU/L activity observed per recorder chart unit under the peaks.
[b] N = 20 each of 5 different rat erythrocyte pools.
[c] N = 5 each of 5 different rat erythrocyte pools on each of 6 days.

General Considerations

Specimen and reagent handling are routinely carried out in subdued, indirect room light. This is particularly critical when handling aqueous PLP. Reagents are stored in brown or foil-covered glassware.

Spectrophotometric characteristics for application in amino-transferase determinations by the coupled enzyme technique require narrow band-width (<10 nm) wavelength accuracy with 2 nm, and absorbance readout capability to 0.001 unit. To use IFCC recommended reagent strengths and sample volume fractions, instrument reading range capability of 3.0 absorbance units would be required. The system should allow for constant monitoring of the reaction (recorder) or monitoring at regular intervals (13). Temperature should be accurately determined and maintained (IFCC (14) ± 0.05°) during the observation period, both within days and between days, and during any incubations. In our earlier attempts to establish reference values for the erythrocyte quality controls used in the controlled rat study, we employed a spectrophotometer system with a jacketed cuvette assembly controlled by an external recirculating bath at 30°. Values obtained were consistently lower by 8-10% than activities obtained with the centrifugal analyzer. It was (finally) ascertained that when the cuvette cell cover was removed to add the 2-oxoglutarate (4 aliquots) the temperature dropped 1 degree plus a fraction and did not recover for the period of observation. The temperature factors usually given for enzyme reaction corrections change 6-7% per degree around 30°, and would account for the observed discrepancy. The recommendation for continuous or frequent

Table 10. Plasma Aminotransferases (Unsaturated IU/L) in Depleted/Repleted Rats[a]

Period	ALT			AST		
	Control Group	Repletion Group		Control Group	Repletion Group	
		2.5 mg PN per kg feed	12 mg PN per kg feed		2.5 mg PN per kg feed	12 mg PN per kg feed
Deficiency	20 ± 5	4 ± 1		44 ± 8	16 ± 3	
1 week repletion	20 ± 5	17 ± 4	27 ± 6	44 ± 12	38 ± 7	43 ± 8
2 weeks repletion	22 ± 5	18 ± 4	25 ± 5	46 ± 13	44 ± 10	50 ± 14
4 weeks repletion	21 ± 5	18 ± 4	23 ± 6	46 ± 12	46 ± 14	49 ± 16

[a] N = 12 female and 12 male rats per group.

Table 11. Whole Blood AST (IU/L) in Depleted/Repleted Rats[a]

Period	Unsaturated			Saturated		
	Control Group	Repletion Group		Control Group	Repletion Group	
		2.5 mg PN per kg feed	12 mg PN per kg feed		2.5 mg PN per kg feed	12 mg PN per kg feed
Deficiency	845 ± 113	306 ± 41		1003 ± 113	653 ± 68	
1 week repletion	823 ± 153	628 ± 120	764 ± 107	965 ± 153	839 ± 74	918 ± 102
2 weeks repletion	941 ± 124	891 ± 130	1001 ± 119	1070 ± 160	1104 ± 183	1151 ± 134
4 weeks repletion	945 ± 142	934 ± 154	980 ± 153	1107 ± 151	1134 ± 182	1123 ± 161

[a] N = 12 female and 12 male rats per group.

Table 12. Erythrocyte AST (IU/L Whole Blood) in Depleted/Repleted Rats[a]

Period	Unsaturated			Saturated		
	Control Group	Repletion Group		Control Group	Repletion Group	
		2.5 mg PN per kg feed	12 mg PN per kg feed		2.5 mg PN per kg feed	12 mg PN per kg feed
Deficiency	798 $\pm$ 99	252 $\pm$ 34		876 $\pm$ 108	506 $\pm$ 55	
1 week repletion	772 $\pm$ 106	439 $\pm$ 75	618 $\pm$ 114	860 $\pm$ 120	662 $\pm$ 103	724 $\pm$ 127
2 weeks repletion	839 $\pm$ 115	764 $\pm$ 146	892 $\pm$ 135	951 $\pm$ 121	956 $\pm$ 168	1022 $\pm$ 158
4 weeks repletion	853 $\pm$ 153	831 $\pm$ 142	920 $\pm$ 150	933 $\pm$ 159	990 $\pm$ 162	1030 $\pm$ 161

[a] N = 12 female and 12 male rats per group.

Table 13.   Erythrocyte ALT (IU/L Whole Blood) in
            Depleted/Repleted Rats[a]

	Unsaturated		
Period	Control Group	Repletion Group	
		2.5 mg PN per kg feed	12 mg PN per kg feed
Deficiency	139 ± 20	35 ± 3	
1 week repletion	145 ± 30	48 ± 5	70 ± 11
2 weeks repletion	155 ± 18	64 ± 14	122 ± 17
4 weeks repletion	169 ± 31	97 ± 13	155 ± 22

[a]N = 12 female and 12 male rats per group.

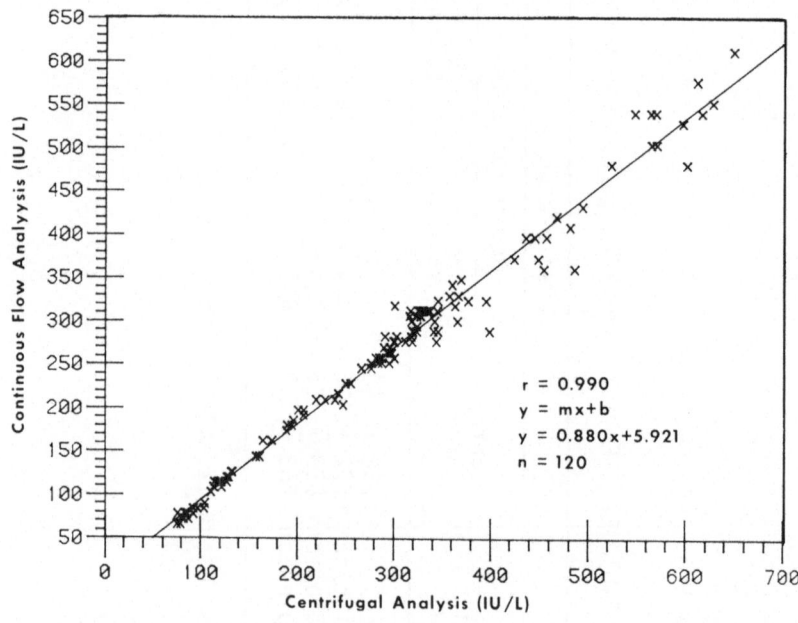

Fig. 9. Correlation between measurements of unstimulated AST
        activity in rat hemolysates using continuous flow analysis
        or centrifugal analysis.

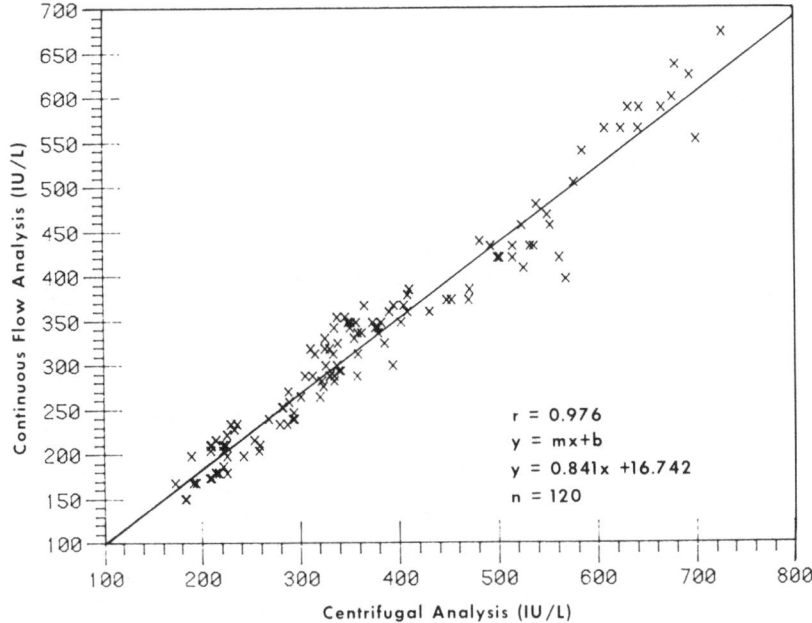

Fig. 10.   Correlation between measurements of PLP stimulated AST
           activity in rat hemolysates using continuous flow analysis
           or centrifugal analysis.

fixed interval monitoring of the reaction is to ensure that observations are taken in the zero-order region. An example is shown in
Table 14 of the effect of arbitrary preselection of reading interval,
particularly on the saturated value which could subsequently affect
the calculated coefficient. The Δ Abs. values are the mean of 3
aliquots. It can be readily discerned that a 2-point assay can
lead to this variation. This phenomenon which we have casually
observed in greater degree in specimens from more mature human
subjects and rat models may arise from the endogenous chemistry of
the matrix, as suggested by Rodgerson and Osberg (15). This
prompted Lustig and Redman (16) to recommend omission of the LDH
clearing reaction in the AST reaction scheme and incorporation of
sodium oxamate, a competitive inhibitor of LDH. This may eliminate
part of this initial rapid oxidation, but it would still be advis-
able to monitor the entire observation period because of the fact
that the maximum carry-over oxidation may occur coincident with the
incorporation of PLP as indicated in Table 14, which would imply
other enzyme involvement.

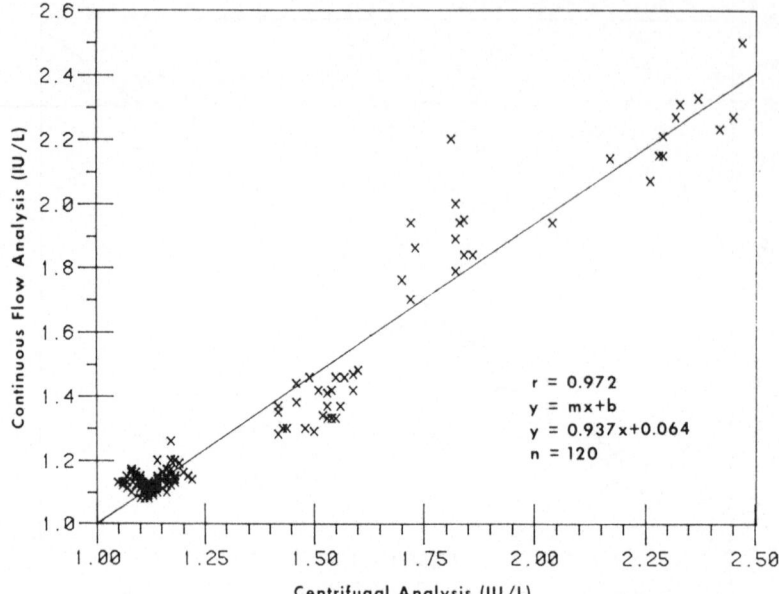

Fig. 11.   Regression of AST activity coefficients derived by
continuous flow analysis on coefficients derived from
centrifugal analysis.

The reaction component contribution and the potential effect
of reagent contaminants to the overall AST reagent response is
shown in Table 15. The response factors are the mean of 6 repli-
cations on each of 2 days. Various combinations of the AST reagent
components were made according to IFCC concentrations as shown, and
their reactivity when loaded with an erythrocyte specimen or water
was observed. The observation period was for 10 minutes after
mixing in the disc of the centrifugal analyzer. It is apparent that
there was little AST activity stimulated by endogenous 2-oxoglutarate
in the specimen or reagents. It is also apparent that in the presence
of 2-oxoglutarate, there was negligible blank activity (water),
except in the presence of PLP. The label on the MDH used in this
evaluation indicated an AST contaminant level of 0.02%, which was
apparently much greater in the presence of PLP. This emphasizes
the importance of monitoring purity of individual reagents if
preparing them from individually procured components.

Specimen storage stability can be of paramount interest. While
we conducted certain storage studies, they were directed at the
anticipated limits of analysis delay and, inadvertently, to actual
delays experienced. The studies reported in Tables 16-18 are not
finite for the reason they were not designed to extend beyond the

Table 14.   Reading Interval Selection--Erythrocyte
AST Values, Age 50 Male Subject

Reaction Interval (min)	Δ Abs. Unsaturated	IU/L (30°)	Δ Abs. Saturated	IU/L (30°)
0	-		-	
1	-0.0082		-0.0151	
2	-0.0068		-0.0124	
3	-0.0072		-0.0127	
4	-0.0080		-0.0130	
5	-0.0080	976	-0.0127	1540
6	-0.0073		-0.0109	(AC=1.58)[a]
7	-0.0084		-0.0122	
8	-0.0071		-0.0110	
9	-0.0076		-0.0118	
10	-0.0078	966	-0.0113	1440
11	-0.0080		-0.0115	(AC=1.49)[a]
12	-0.0080		-0.0119	
13	-0.0071		-0.0102	
14	-0.0071		-0.0113	
15	-0.0081		-0.0113	
16	-0.0079		-0.0111	
17	-0.0077		-0.0119	
18	-0.0083		-0.0113	

[a]AC = Activation coefficient.

limits shown. As shown in Table 16, ALT and AST activities were
recoverable in plasma stored up to 14 days at -70°. Results are
means of triplicate aliquots. Demetriou et al. (17) reported that
serum ALT was stable for 1 week at refrigeration temperatures, 2
days at room temperature, and that freezing was not recommended;
serum AST was reported to be stable for at least 2 weeks at refrigerator temperatures. As shown in Table 17, ALT U and S activities
were recoverable at 60 days of storage at -70°, although the ALT
U activity of the erythrocyte pool tended to drop off. As shown
in Table 18, the erythrocyte AST of 4 control pools was recoverable
through 60 days of -70° storage and, in this case, after 76 days.

Reagents are generally stable (with the exception of NADH and
PLP) if kept refrigerated and there is no evidence of microbiological
growth. NADH should be made up daily for maximum extension of
response. PLP was made fresh weekly. For these reasons, it is
best to make these reagents up separately for incorporation in the
overall reaction mixture.

Table 15.   Response Due to Components of the AST Reagent System[a]

Sample	NADH + Aspartic Acid				NADH + Aspartic Acid + 2-Oxoglutarate			
	Bkg	+MDH	+LDH	+MDH, LDH	Bkg	+MDH	+LDH	+MDH, LDH
				$-\Delta$ Abs. x 10^4				
Unsaturated								
Erythrocyte	2	18	2	2	626	650	645	677
Water	3	2	1	3	1	16	14	26
Saturated								
Erythrocyte	2	2	4	4	681	825	690	828
Water	0	4	2	14	3	133	19	144

[a]N = 6 observations per day, each reagent treatment, on 2 days.

Table 16.   Short-term Stability of Plasma AST
            and ALT at -70°

Analysis of Plasma Pool[a]	Initial IU/L (30°)	Recovery of Initial Value	
		3 Days	14 Days
	$\bar{x} \pm SD$	%	%
AST	38.8 + 0.4	100	99
ALT	27.5 + 0.2	102	105

[a]N = 3 replicate aliquots per examination.

Table 17.   ALT Storage Stability at -70°

Sample[a]	Initial IU/L (30°)	% Recovery of Initial Value After 60 Days
	$\bar{x} \pm SD$	$\bar{x} \pm SD$
Unsaturated		
Whole Blood Pool	156 + 9	101 + 6
Erythrocyte Pool	113 + 3	92 + 3
Saturated		
Whole Blood Pool	188 + 9	103 + 5
Erythrocyte Pool	152 + 5	110 + 3

[a]N = 3 replicate aliquots per examination.

Table 18.   Erythrocyte AST Storage Stability at -70°

Sample[a]	Initial IU/L (30°)	% Recovery of Initial Value After	
		60 Days	76 Days
	x̄ ± SD	x̄ ± SD	x̄ ± SD
Unsaturated			
A	735 ± 26	102 ± 1	100 ± 1
B	181 ± 10	108 ± 2	109 ± 4
C	690 ± 11	104 ± 2	106 ± 2
D	273 ± 10	111 ± 1	109 ± 3
Saturated			
A	814 ± 7	108 ± 1	104 ± 1
B	409 ± 3	111 ± 1	105 ± 3
C	774 ± 4	107 ± 5	107 ± 5
D	496 ± 2	115 ± 2	107 ± 3

[a]N = 3 replicate aliquots per examination.

Selected principle chemistries were adapted to the centrifugal analyzer in a manner which did not compromise their effectuality; the only one which was scaled down proportionally was the IFCC procedure we adapted. The results are shown in Table 19; the values are not the activities in IU, but rather the mean response (-Δ Abs/min x 10^4) produced by the chemistries in two normal and two deficient erythrocyte pools analyzed in triplicate by each method. It can be seen that the IFCC (12) procedure and that of Henry et al. (7) for AST U and S did not differ, whereas the IFCC (13) recommendation for ALT yielded much higher values than did the Henry et al. (7) procedure, particularly with regard to the saturated value. The Beutler (9,10) procedure was compared with the IFCC (12) centrifugal analyzer adaptation at 37° as recommended, yet we only obtained 77% of the U activity and 72% of the S activity. Not shown in Table 19 is a recently completed comparison of the IFCC (13) recommendation for serum ALT determination with the Bergmeyer et al. (11) procedure. The Bergmeyer reagents did elicit a slightly greater (8%) response from the erythrocyte controls with a somewhat cleaner reading-to-reading reaction.

Selection of proper reference standards for quality control can cause some apprehension. Lyophilized serum pools, aqueous matrix standards, and frozen erythrocyte pools have been used here. Evans[1]

---

[1]Personal communication to Dr. H. E. Sauberlich.

Table 19. Relative Response of Selected Chemistries Adapted to the Centrifugal Analyses for Four Erythrocyte Controls ($\overline{X} \pm$ SD)[a]

Analysis	IFCC(12) 30^0	Henry et al.(7) 30^0	IFCC(13) 30^0	IFCC(12) 37^0	Beutler(9,10) 37^0
			$-\Delta$ Abs/min x 10^4		
AST, U	150 + 3.6	151 + 3.5	-	214 + 2.5	165 + 4.8
AST, S	208 + 2.4	202 + 4.6	-	283 + 5.0	203 + 9.3
ALT, U	-	20 + 3.3	33 + 3.3	-	-
ALT, S	-	19 + 5.9	41 + 9.5	-	-

[a]N = 6 replicates on each of 2 days, each method.

has suggested and produced a freeze-dried erythrocyte pool for control purposes. This may provide the long-term quality control
coverage that is needed for study-to-study precision.

Comprehensive summaries of the effects of drugs (18) and
disease (19) on the aminotransferases and other clinical tests have
been published. These are important to consider in survey or
uncontrolled studies because of the heavy impact on serum and plasma
levels. Less is known about the effect on erythrocyte levels; a
potential effect may arise from chronic exposures. In general,
drugs and disease which affect the liver and the heart will cause
alterations in circulating aminotransferases.

In conclusion, we believe that the coupled enzyme procedure
for AST, based on IFCC recommendations, provides good precision when
applied to hemolysates or serum. The ALT recommendation, while
optimized and workable, when applied to hemolysates and monitored
with instrumentation such as the centrifugal analyzer, must be
performed at an undesirably low signal to noise ratio. The solution
may be found in an improved continuous flow procedure, or in a
process for reducing the hemoglobin background which is non-
destructive to enzyme activity. Extended storage stability study
is needed, not so much for sample retention as for quality control
stability for study-to-study precision. In this regard, the
possibility of using a freeze-dried erythrocyte pool has strong
potential. In addition to quality control application, it is
apparent that good instrumentation and a rigid protocol for per-
forming the analysis are necessary for acceptable precision.

LITERATURE CITED

1. Tonhazy, N. E., White, N. G. & Umbreit, W. W. (1950) A rapid
    method for the estimation of the glutamic-aspartic transami-
    nase in tissues and its application to radiation sickness.
    Arch. Biochem. 28, 36-42.
2. Cabaud, P., Leeper, R. & Wroblewski, F. (1956) Colorimetric
    measurement of serum glutamic oxaloacetic transaminase. Am.
    J. Clin. Path. 26, 1101-1105.
3. Reitman, S. & Frankel, S. (1957) Colorimetric method for
    the determination of serum glutamic-oxaloacetic and glutamic-
    pyruvic transaminases. Am. J. Clin. Path. 28, 56-63.
4. Marsh, E. M., Greenberg, L. D. & Rinehart, J. F. (1955) The
    relationship between pyridoxine ingestion and transaminase
    activity. I. Blood hemolysates. J. Nutr. 56, 115-127.
5. Henley, K. S. & Pollard, H. M. (1955) A new method for the
    determination of glutamic oxalacetic and glutamic pyruvic
    transaminase in plasma. J. Lab. Clin. Med. 46, 785-789.

6. Karmen, A., Wroblewski, F. & LaDue, J. S. (1955) Transaminase
    activity in human blood. J. Clin. Invest. 34, 126-133.
7. Henry, R. J., Chiamori, N., Golub, O. J. & Berkman, S. (1960)
    Revised spectrophotometric methods for the determination of
    glutamic-oxalacetic transaminase, glutamic-pyruvic transaminase
    and lactic acid dehydrogenase. Am. J. Clin. Path. 34, 381-398.
8. Scandinavian Society for Clinical Chemistry and Clinical
    Physiology, Committee on Enzymes, R. Keiding, Chairman (1974)
    Recommended methods for the determination of four enzymes in
    blood. Scand. J. Clin. Lab. Invest. 32, 291-306.
9. Beutler, E. (1975) Red Cell Metabolism. Grune & Stratton,
    New York.
10. Beutler, E., Blume, K. G., Kaplan, J. C., Lohr, G. W., Ramot,
    B. & Valentine, W. N. (1977) International Committee for
    Standardization in Hematology: Recommended methods for red-
    cell enzyme analysis. Brit. J. Hematol. 35, 331-340.
11. Bergmeyer, H. U., Scheibe, P. & Wahlefeld, A. W. (1978)
    Optimization of methods for aspartate aminotransferase and
    alanine aminotransferase. Clin. Chem. 24, 58-73.
12. International Federation of Clinical Chemistry (1978)
    Provisional recommendations on IFCC methods for the measure-
    ment of catalytic concentrations of enzymes. Part 3. Revised
    IFCC method for aspartate aminotransferase. Clin. Chem. 24,
    720-721.
13. International Federation of Clinical Chemistry (1977) Provi-
    sional recommendations on IFCC methods for the measurement of
    catalytic concentrations of enzymes. Part 2. IFCC method
    for aspartate aminotransferase. Clin. Chem. 23, 887-899.
14. International Federation of Clinical Chemistry (1976) Pro-
    visional recommendation (1974) on IFCC methods for the measure-
    ment of catalytic concentration of enzymes. Clin. Chem. 22,
    384-391.
15. Rodgerson, D. O. & Osberg, I. M. (1974) Sources of error in
    spectrophotometric measurement of aspartate aminotransferase
    and alanine aminotransferase activities in serum. Clin. Chem.
    20, 43-50.
16. Lustig, V. & Redman, L. W. (1980) Improved serum-initiated
    aspartate aminotransferase assay by inhibition of lactic
    dehydrogenase with oxamate. Clin. Chem. 26, 831-834.
17. Demetriou, J. A., Drewes, P. A. & Gin, J. B. (1974) Enzymes.
    In: Clinical Chemistry, Principles and Technics (Henry, R. J.,
    Cannon, P. C. & Winkelman, J. W., eds.), second ed., pp. 882,
    888, Harper & Row, Hagerstown, MD.
18. Young, D. S., Pestaner, L. C. & Gibberman, V. (1975) Effects
    of drugs on clinical laboratory tests. Clin. Chem. 21, 1D-
    432D.

19. Friedman, R. B., Anderson, R. E., Entine, S. M. & Hirshberg,
     S. B. (1980) Effects of disease on clinical laboratory tests.
     Clin. Chem. 26, 1D-476D.
20. Wroblewski, F. & LaDue, J. S. (1956) Serum glutamic pyruvic
     transaminase in cardiac and hepatic disease. Proc. Soc. Exp.
     Biol. Med. 91, 569-571.

VITAMIN B-6 STATUS ASSESSMENT: PAST AND PRESENT

H. E. Sauberlich

Letterman Army Institute of Research and
USDA-SEA Western Nutrition Research Center
Presidio of San Francisco, CA 94129

OCCURRENCE OF VITAMIN B-6 DEFICIENCY IN THE HUMAN

In 1934, György established the existence of vitamin B-6 (1,2). Following the synthesis of vitamin B-6 in 1939 by Harris and Folkers (3), Gyorgy suggested that "In accordance with the chemical nature of vitamin B-6, which is a pyridine derivative containing several methoxyl groups, the term 'pyridoxine' appears appropriate" (4). György recognized that vitamin B-6 deficiency in the rat produced lesions of the extremities that resembled those observed in human acrodynia rather than of pellagra.

In 1939, Spies et al. (5) was treating undernourished subjects with niacin, thiamin, and riboflavin. Some of the subjects failed to respond to these vitamins and developed symptoms that included extreme nervousness, insomnia, weakness, irritability, abdominal pains, and difficulty in walking. When crystalline vitamin B-6 became available in 1939, Spies et al. (5) injected some of the subjects who failed to respond to previous treatment, with 50 mg of vitamin B-6. Dramatic relief was observed within 24 hours. In some of the patients, a load of pyridoxine was administered and the amount lost in the urine determined (6). Only a small amount was found to be present which was interpreted to mean the subjects were depleted of vitamin B-6. Smith and Martin (7) also observed that pyridoxine was effective in healing cheilosis which did not respond to riboflavin.

Table 1 lists significant reports on the occurrence of vitamin
B-6 deficiency in the human. Convincing evidence of the essentiality
of vitamin B-6 in human nutrition was provided in 1951-1953 when a
syndrome of hyperirritability and convulsive seizures occurred in
young infants maintained on an autoclaved commercial liquid formula
low in vitamin B-6 (8-10). The seizures and abnormal electroencephalograms were corrected with the administration of pyridoxine (9).
The abnormal urinary excretion of xanthurenic acid was also corrected
by the administration of vitamin B-6. It is interesting to note
that the central nervous system symptoms in these patients were
aggravated by the addition of protein to the diet but were diminished
with a carbohydrate diet (9). In 1957, Bessey et al. (11) described
a similar syndrome in infants who were breast fed as their source
of nourishment. These infants had a microcytic hypochromic anemia
in addition to convulsive seizures and an elevated excretion of
xanthurenic acid following a DL-tryptophan test load. They observed
that small therapeutic doses of vitamin B-6 corrected the convulsive
seizures but larger quantities were required to reverse the abnormal
excretion of xanthurenic acid.

In 1954, Hunt et al. (12) reported on an entirely different
type of vitamin B-6 related condition. They observed an infant
that required levels of pyridoxine that far exceeded normal nutritional requirements. Subsequently, additional pyridoxine-dependent
infants with convulsive seizures have been described (13).

An adult with sideroblastic anemia was studied by Harris and
associates (14). The patient required a daily intake of 50 mg of
pyridoxine to prevent the observed anemia and abnormal tryptophan
metabolism. Electroencephalograms were normal at all times. This
and subsequent reports (15,16) have established a role for vitamin
B-6 in human erythropoiesis. Other types of vitamin B-6 dependen-
cies have since been identified (17). In some cases, excessive
loss of vitamin B-6 occurred in the urine while others may have
had an abnormal metabolism of sulfur amino acids. Cystathioninuria
patients excrete excess cystathionine which can be enhanced with
methionine loads (17). Large supplements of pyridoxine generally
correct the abnormal excretion of cystathionine. Similarly,
patients with xanthurenic aciduria respond to large doses of vitamin
B-6. Following a tryptophan load test, these patients excrete
abnormal amounts of kynurenine, 3-hydroxykynurenine, and xanthurenic
acid (18). Although vitamin B-6 dependency syndromes are relatively
rare, they have provided signs and symptoms of a vitamin B-6 deficiency as well as guides to procedures to assess a vitamin B-6
status.

Table 1. Vitamin B-6 Deficiency in the Human: Historical Development

Author	Date	Subjects	Means of Assessment
Spies et al. (5)	1939	Pellagrin injected with 50 mg pyridoxine	Relief of clinical signs and symptoms
Spies et al. (6)	1940	Patients with a suspected vitamin B-6 deficiency	Vitamin B-6 load, measurement of loss in urine
Smith & Martin (7)	1940	Clinical patients	Healed cheilosis that failed to respond to riboflavin
Malony & Parmelee (8)	1954	Infants on commercial milk formula	Reversal of convulsive seizures and irritability
Coursin (9)	1954	Infants on commercial milk formula	Reversal of seizures and abnormal EEG, xanthurenic acid excretion
Hunt et al. (12)	1954	Infants on commercial milk formula	Reversal of convulsive seizures, tryptophan load
Bessey et al. (11)	1957	Infants on commercial milk formula	Anemia, tryptophan load, convulsive seizures
Waldinger & Berg (13)	1963	Pyridoxine-dependent infants	Convulsive seizures

Table 1 (cont). Vitamin B-6 Deficiency in the Human: Historial Development

Author	Date	Subjects	Means of Assessment
Harris, et al. (14)	1956	Anemia patients	Sideroblastic anemia responds to vitamin B-6, tryptophan load
Hines & Harris (15)	1964	Anemia patients	Response of anemia to vitamin B-6
Mudd (16)	1971	Anemia patients	Anemia response to vitamin B-6
Frimpter et al. (17)	1969	Vitamin B-6 dependency	Abnormal urinary metabolites, tryptophan or methionine load
Spannuth et al. (19)	1977	Uremic patients	Plasma PLP and EGOT
Walsh et al. (20)	1966	Alcoholics	Tryptophan load, plasma PLP
Li (21)	1978	Alcoholics	Plasma PLP
Rose (22) (23)	1966 1978	Patients on oral contraceptive agents	Tryptophan load
Krishnaswany et al (26)	1976	Pellagrins	EGOT, quinolinic acid excretion

Table 1 (cont.). Vitamin B-6 Deficiency in the Human: Historical Development

Author	Date	Subjects	Means of Assessment
Wachstein et al. (29)	1960	Pregnancy	Leukocyte and plasma PLP
Dempsey (30)	1978	Pregnancy	Plasma PLP, tryptophan load
Sauberlich (31)	1978	Pregnancy	EGOT, plasma PLP, tryptophan load

Spannuth et al. (19) provided evidence of vitamin B-6 deficiency in patients with uremia and with liver disease. Abnormal
erythrocyte glutamate-oxaloacetate transaminase (EGOT) activity and
lowered plasma pyridoxal phosphate (PLP) levels were observed.
Evidence of vitamin B-6 deficiency occurring in alcoholic patients
has been provided through the use of the tryptophan load test and
the measurement of plasma PLP levels (20,21).

In 1965, Rose (22) observed that women using estrogen-containing
oral contraceptive agents excreted abnormal levels of tryptophan
metabolites following the ingestion of a tryptophan load. Since
then, considerable investigative efforts have been devoted to whether
or not oral contraceptive agents produced a true vitamin B-6
deficiency. The subject was reviewed recently by Rose (23).

The question of vitamin B-6 deficiency in pellagrins was
investigated again more recently by Krishnaswany et al. (24-27).
With the use of quinolinic acid excretion studies and EGOT activity
measurements and other tests, a vitamin B-6 deficiency was demonstrated in some pellagrins. Recently, Bamji et al. (28) have also
reported evidence of vitamin B-6 deficiency in rural school boys
near Hyderabad, India.

An increased need for vitamin B-6 during pregnancy has been
recognized for many years (29). This has been based largely upon
the observations that with advanced pregnancy, leukocyte and plasma
PLP levels fall and an abnormal tryptophan test frequently occurs
(30,31).

EXPERIMENTALLY INDUCED VITAMIN B-6 DEFICIENCY IN THE HUMAN

Table 2 lists various studies that have been conducted to
induce experimentally a vitamin B-6 deficiency in the human. The
means used to establish the presence of a vitamin B-6 deficiency
are briefly indicated.

Lepkovsky and associates (32) observed in 1943 that animals
deprived of vitamin B-6 excreted abnormal metabolites of tryptophan
which were enhanced following a load of this amino acid. A green
pigment was found in the urine collected in rusty metabolism cages
from pyridoxine-deficient rats. The green pigment was shown to be
the product of a reaction between xanthurenic acid and ferric
ammonium sulfate or other ferric salts. Xanthurenic acid was shown
to originate from dietary tryptophan. Thus, the tryptophan load
test was born. Greenberg et al. utilized the test for the first
time on the human in 1949 (33).

Table 2. Experimental Vitamin B-6 Deficiency Induced in the Human

Authors	Date	Subject	Means of Assessment
Greenberg et al. (33)	1949	Adults	Tryptophan load, xanthurenic acid excretion
Snyderman et al. (34)	1953	Infants	Clinical signs, urinary pyridoxic acid
Mueller et al. (35,36)	1950 1953	Men	Clinical signs
Harding et al. (37)	1959	Men	Tryptophan load
Cheslock & McCully (38)	1960	7 Women 1 Man	Blood vitamin B-6 levels, tryptophan load
Babcock et al. (39)	1960	Men & Women	Serum transaminase activity
Hodges et al. (40)	1962	Men	Antibody formation, tryptophan load
Baker et al. (43)	1964	Men	Tryptophan load, urinary vitamin B-6 levels
Raica & Sauberlich (44)	1964	Men	Erythrocyte, plasma, and leukocyte transaminase activity
Yess et al. (47)	1964	Men	Tryptophan load and urinary metabolites
Brown et al. (49)	1965	Men	Quinolinic acid and niacin metabolites

Table 2 (cont). Experimental Vitamin B-6 Deficiency Induced in the Human

Authors	Date	Subject	Means of Assessment
Kelsay et al. (51)	1968	Men	Blood and urine levels of vitamin B-6 forms
Kelsay et al. (50)	1968	Men	Urinary quinolinic acid and niacin metabolites
Swan et al. (66)	1964	Men	Urinary taurine and sulfate
Baysal et al. (52)	1966	Men	Blood vitamin B-6, plasma PLP, serum transaminases, urinary vitamin B-6 and 4-pyridoxic acid
Park & Linkswiler (53)	1970	Men	Methionine load
Donald et al. (56)	1971	Women	Erythrocyte transaminases, blood vitamin B-6 levels, urinary 4-pyridoxic acid
Canham et al. (61)	1969	Men	Tryptophan load, plasma and urinary amino acid levels, urinary vitamin B-6
Shin & Linkswiler (54)	1974	Women	Methionine load, tryptophan load
Leklem et al. (55)	1975	Women	Methionine and tryptophan loads, plasma PLP, erythrocyte transaminases, urinary 4-pyridoxic acid, kynurenine sulfate load
Ritchey et al. (57)	1978	Boys	Urinary levels of vitamin B-6 and 4-pyridoxic acid

In 1953, Synderman and associates (34) first demonstrated an essential role for vitamin B-6 in human erythropoiesis. An 8-month old boy placed on a vitamin B-6 deficient diet developed microcytic, hypochromic anemia after 130 days. The anemia responded to vitamin B-6 administration. Urinary excretion of 4-pyridoxic acid and pyridoxine fell to low levels. Convulsive seizures that responded to pyridoxine occurred in another infant after 170 days on the deficient diet.

Mueller et al. (35,36) induced a vitamin B-6 deficiency in adults with the associated use of the pyridoxine antagonist, 4-deoxypyridoxine. Clinical findings included the following: lesions resembling seborrhea about the eyes, in the nasolabial fold, face forehead, etc.; occurrence of cheilosis, glossitis, and stomatitis; and peripheral neuropathy and increased irritability.

Harding et al. (37) fed prolonged stored packaged military rations that had a reduced amount of vitamin B-6 present. Xanthurenic acid excretion after a tryptophan load was abnormal. This elevated excretion of xanthurenic acid did not occur in subjects fed rations that provided 2.76 mg of vitamin B-6 per day. Cheslock and McCully (38) used blood vitamin B-6 levels and tryptophan loads to assess the vitamin B-6 status in their subjects.

The initial attempt to use blood transaminase activities in human vitamin B-6 deficiency was made by Babcock and coworkers (39). These investigators were apparently not impressed by the procedure since they indicated that because of the wide normal range of transaminase activity, a single determination, even at the height of deficiency, was not sufficient to assess the degree of deficiency.

Hodges et al. (40) induced a vitamin B-6 deficiency in human subjects also with the use of a deficient diet and deoxypyridoxine. Clinical signs of a deficiency were observed as well as the excretion of excessive amounts of xanthurenic acid after a test dose of tryptophan. Evidence of impaired antibody formation was noted.

Studies conducted in Denver (41-44) on vitamin B-6 depletion and repletion utilized the tryptophan load test; urinary levels of vitamin B-6; transaminase activities of erythrocytes, plasma, and leukocytes; and electroencephalogram measurements as the major means of assessment. Other procedures were investigated but not proven reliable or useful (41,45,46). Clinical signs as previously described were noted in the majority of the experimental subjects (41). Urinary excretion of xanthurenic acid was markedly increased after two weeks on a vitamin B-6 deficiency and was enhanced with the use of a high protein diet. Urinary excretion of free vitamin B-6 fell rapidly when the subjects were on a deficient diet. Upon supplementation with pyridoxine, the urinary excretion of vitamin B-6 was increased and correlated closely with level of intake. Erythrocyte GOT activities combined with an in vitro PLP stimulation effect appeared to be a useful measure in the evaluation of vitamin B-6 nutritional status (44).

Yess et al. (47) studied in detail a number of tryptophan metabolites of the kynurenine pathway. Marked increased in the urinary excretion of kynurenine, 3-hydroxykynurenine, and xanthurenic acid occurred with a vitamin B-6 depletion. Lesser amounts of acetyl-kynurenine and kynurenic acid were excreted. With a tryptophan load, the amount of 3-hydroxykynurenine and kynurenine excreted exceeded that of xanthurenic acid. Nevertheless, the urinary excretion of any one, or all of these compounds was considered suitable for the evaluation of vitamin B-6 nutritional status (48).

Quinolinic acid and niacin metabolites were measured in the urine of vitamin B-6 deficient men following a tryptophan load by Linkswiler and associates (49,50). The reason for the increased excretion of quinolinic acid in a vitamin B-6 deficiency has not been satisfactorily explained. It has been suggested that another unrecognized step may exist in tryptophan metabolism beyond the cleavage of the 3-hydroxykynurenine side chain that is vitamin B-6 dependent (26).

Other studies conducted by the University of Wisconsin investigators to assess a vitamin B-6 deficiency induced in adult humans have utilized measurements of the various forms of vitamin B-6 in the urine and blood (51,52). The urinary excretion of pyridoxal, pyridoxamine, and pyridoxine decreased very rapidly when subjects were placed on a diet deficient in vitamin B-6. Urinary 4-pyridoxic acid excretion also appeared to reflect the level of intake of vitamin B-6 (51,52). Blood levels of vitamin B-6 also fell rapidly when vitamin B-6 was withheld from the subjects.

Linkswiler and associates (53-55) made the initial attempt to use a methionine load to assess an induced vitamin B-6 deficiency. Urinary cystathionine levels were markedly elevated in a vitamin B-6 deficiency. A 3-gram methionine load test increased these excretion levels further.

The studies of Donald et al. (56), Shin and Linkswiler (54), and Leklem et al. (55) have demonstrated the usefulness of various techniques in assessing induced vitamin B-6 deficiency in women. A deficiency caused a rapid fall in the urinary 4-pyridoxic acid and plasma pyridoxal phosphate levels. The quantity of metabolites of tryptophan present in the urine after a tryptophan load increased rapidly with vitamin B-6 depletion. Methionine metabolism was likewise adversely affected in a manner similar to that reported for men.

Few studies have been conducted on vitamin B-6 status in children or adolescents. Ritchey et al. (57) reported on studies with boys on which urinary levels of vitamin B-6 and 4-pyridoxic acid were measured. Urinary vitamin B-6 levels have also been measured in a group of Wainwright Eskimo boys and girls (58).

CLINICAL SIGNS AND SYMPTOMS ASSOCIATED WITH A VITAMIN B-6 DEFICIENCY

The reports listed in Tables 1 and 2 have provided an indication of the clinical signs and symptoms that may be associated with a deficiency of vitamin B-6 in the human. Signs and symptoms most frequently observed with a deficiency of this vitamin are summarized in Table 3. It should be noted, however, that the presence of any of these manifestations may not be considered a reliable indicator of a vitamin B-6 deficiency since such signs or symptoms are not specific to a pyridoxine deficiency. The seborrheic or seborrheid lesion that may occur about the eyes, nose, and mouth can result from causes other than of vitamin B-6 deficiency. The lesions that may develop around the mouth resemble cheilosis of riboflavin deficiency and the glossitis observed resembles a conditions seen in niacin deficiency. The most common clinical manifestations associated with a vitamin B-6 deficiency appear to be the central nervous system changes and the abnormal electroencephalograms. Because of the uncertainty of the use of clinical signs or symptoms in diagnosing a vitamin B-6 deficiency, biochemical laboratory procedures have evolved that are more reliable.

Table 3. Clinical Signs and Symptoms
Associated with a Vitamin
B-6 Deficiency

Eczema and seborrheic dermatitis: ears, nose, mouth

Cheilosis, glossitis, angular stomatitis

Anemia: hypochromic, microcytic

Central nervous system changes: hyper-irritability, convulsive seizures, hyperacusis

Abnormal electroencephalograms

ASSESSMENT OF VITAMIN B-6 STATUS BY DIETARY INTAKE MEASUREMENTS

Few nutrition surveys have made an attempt to perform an assessment of the dietary intake of vitamin B-6. Information on the dietary intakes of nutrients can be helpful in the general evaluation of the nutritional status of a group or of a population. Such information is less reliable in predicting the nutritional status of an individual. Dietary recalls of only 24 hours are of little value for this purpose. Dietary intake data must be collected for a number of days or even for several weeks in order to assess the adequacy of the nutrient intakes by an individual. This procedure is difficult, time consuming, inconvenient, and expensive.

What are our major food sources of vitamin B-6 in our diet? Contributions of the major food groups to the United States food supply of vitamin B-6 are depicted in Fig. 1. The major supply is provided by meats (40.0%), followed by vegetables (22.2%), dairy items (11.6%), and cereals (10.2%).

VITAMIN B₆

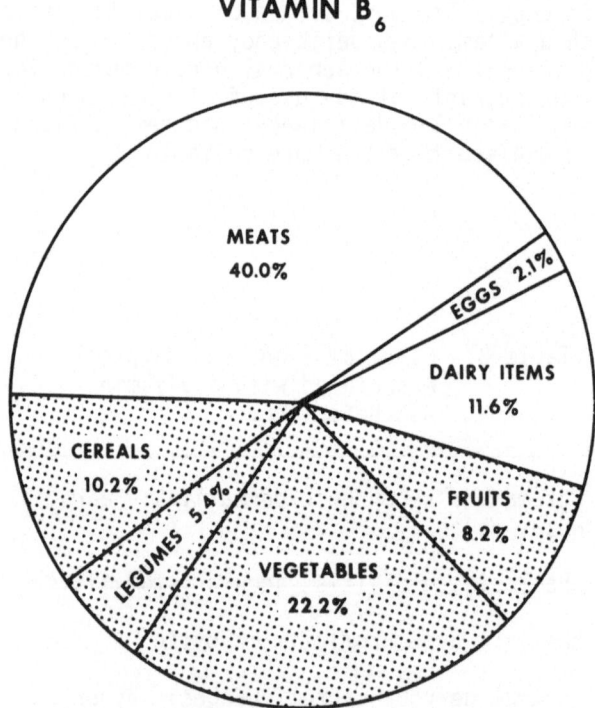

Fig. 1. Contribution of major food groups to the national food supply of vitamin B-6 /adapted from the data of Marston and Peterkin (59)/.

During two nutrition surveys conducted by this Laboratory at the Naval Air Station, Alameda, California, an attempt was made to assess the dietary intakes of vitamin B-6 by the naval personnel. Some of the observations are summarized in Table 4. In the first survey, personnel who ate all three meals at the Naval dining facilities ingested 2.60 mg of vitamin B-6/day and thus received 118% of the Recommended Dietary Allowance. In the second survey, conducted after a menu pricing system had been implemented, vitamin B-6 intakes were somewhat less; namely, 2.22 mg/day, which just met the Recommended Dietary Allowance for vitamin B-6.

The personnel obtained 57% of the vitamin B-6 in their diets from animal products. The remainder was obtained from the consumption of cereals, legumes, fruits and vegetables, and paralleled closely the contribution of major food groups to the national nutrient supplies (59) (Fig. 1).

Recently data were released from the USDA Nationwide Food Consumption Survey of 1977-1978 (60). The mean intakes of vitamin B-6 were only 60 to 65% of the Recommended Dietary Allowances for females age 15 years and above. For men 65 years of age and over, the mean intake of vitamin B-6 was 78% of the Recommended Dietary Allowances. These dietary data would suggest that vitamin B-6 nutriture is inadequate for some individuals and may be reflected

Table 4. Vitamin B-6 Intakes by Naval Personnel, 19-22 Years of Age[a]

Study	Breakfast	Lunch	Supper	Total Intake
Naval Air Station, Alameda, CA (March 1975)				
Vitamin B-6 Intake (mg)	0.80	0.86	0.94	2.60
% RDA	36	39	43	118
Naval Air Station, Alameda, CA (August 1977)				
Vitamin B-6 Intake (mg)	0.51	0.82	0.89	2.22
% RDA	23	37	40	101

[a]RDA of 2.2 mg vitamin B-6 (1980). In study I, consumption data were collected over a 17-day period on an average of 182 subjects for breakfast, 248 for lunch, and 235 for supper. In study II, consumption data were collected over an 18-day period on an average of 221 subjects for breakfast, 215 for lunch, and 225 for supper.

in abnormal biochemical parameters. However, it should be noted
that the lack of reliable and up-to-date values on the vitamin B-6
content of foods has placed uncertainties as to the actual consumption of this vitamin by the American population. Increased attention
needs to be placed on vitamin B-6 analysis of foods as consumed and
on the bioavailability of the nutrient before dietary intake information can be reliably utilized.

ASSESSMENT OF VITAMIN B-6 STATUS BY BIOCHEMICAL PROCEDURES

Table 5 summarizes the main biochemical laboratory procedures
that have been used to evaluate vitamin B-6 nutritional status. The
table provides a brief description of principles involved with each
procedure along with pertinent comments. As may be noted from the
table, numerous and diverse procedures have been utilized. Unfor-
tunately, many of the procedures are unreliable or unsatisfactory
for various reasons. Procedures that appear unsatisfactory, for
the present at least, include the alanine load, urinary oxalate
measurements, o-phosphoryl-ethanolamine levels in the urine, plasma
or urine amino acid alterations, total vitamin B-6 levels in blood
components, and serum or leukocyte transaminase activities.

Laboratory procedures that appear feasible and contain a degree
of reliability for the assessment of vitamin B-6 status are indicated in Table 6. For population groups, urinary vitamin B-6
measurement is the only noninvasive procedure feasible. Although
the tryptophan load test was used during the ICNND survey of Burma
on a limited number of subjects, the test is not a practical means
for evaluating vitamin B-6 status in population groups. Measurements of vitamin B-6 can be performed on morning fasting urine
samples and values expressed on a per gram creatinine basis, which
avoids the use of a 24-hour urine collection. Urinary levels of
vitamin B-6 have the weakness of reflecting only recent intakes of
the nutrient and may not provide an indication of the degree of
deficiency or level of body pool of vitamin B-6. Urinary excretion
of vitamin B-6 decreases proportionately with a decreased intake of
the nutrient to a critical point after which further lowering of
intake results in only minor and variable changes in urinary excretion (45,61). To overcome the limitations of urinary vitamin B-6
measurements, the erythrocyte transaminase and in vitro PLP stimulation procedure provides a functional test of vitamin B-6 status.
For field studies, this entails the inconveniences of blood sample
collection, preparation, and shipment. GOT activities are considerably higher in the red blood cell than that of GPT and, hence,
easier to measure. As noted earlier, improved standardized analytical procedures are needed in order to reduce variations in results.
Plasma PLP measurements would be desirable, but sample stabilization
problems and time requirements to analyze large numbers of samples
currently precludes the general use of this technique.

Table 5. Biochemical Procedures Used to Evaluate Vitamin B-6 Nutritional Status in the Human

Procedure	Principle	Comments
Tryptophan Load	Urine collected for 24 hours after ingestion of 2 or 5 g of L-tryptophan and the excretion of xanthurenic acid, kynurenine, kynurenic acid, 3-hydroxykynurenine, acetylkynurenine, quinolinic acid, or niacin metabolites measured	Xanthurenic acid most readily measured, although greater excretion of some other metabolites may occur in vitamin B-6 deficiency; useful for studies on individuals
Methionine Load	Urine collected for 24 hours after ingestion of 3 g L-methionine and the excretion of cystathionine, cysteine sulfinic acid, taurine, or sulfate measured	Tedious; only cystathionine measurements useful for assessing vitamin B-6 status
Alanine Load	Rise in blood urea nitrogen levels measured after alanine load	Unsatisfactory for assessing vitamin B-6 status
Kynurenine Sulfate Load	Urine collected for 24 hours after ingestion of 0.2 g of L-kynurenine sulfate and the excretion of 3-hydroxykynurenine measured	No apparent advantage over tryptophan load procedure
Oxalic Acid	Amounts in 24-hour urine collection determined	Unsuitable for assessing vitamin B-6 status

Table 5 (cont). Biochemical Procedures Used to Evaluate Vitamin B-6 Nutrition Status in the Human

Procedure	Principle	Comments
0-phosphoryl-ethanolamine	Urine levels measured	Not sufficiently sensitive for assessment of vitamin B-6 status
Amino Acids	Measure levels in plasma or urine samples	Although changes occur in vitamin B-6 deficiency, none appear suitable as a satisfactory basis to assess vitamin B-6 status
4-Pyridoxic Acid	Levels in a 24-hour urine collection determined	A rapid, sensitive, and specific method (e.g., HPLC) would enhance the usefulness and reliability of the procedure
Urinary Vitamin B-6	Random fasting or 24-hour urine samples analyzed for total vitamin B-6, pyridoxine, pyridoxal, or pyridoxamine levels	Excretion levels reflect recent intakes of the vitamin; non-invasive procedure useful with population groups; analytical methods tedious. Pyridoxal major vitamin B-6 form present in urine

Table 5 (cont).   Biochemical Procedures Used to Evaluate Vitamin B-6 Nutritional
Status in the Human

Procedure	Principle	Comments
Blood Levels of Vitamin B-6	Total vitamin B-6 levels measured in plasma, erythrocytes, leuko- cytes, whole blood	Procedure unreliable to assess vitamin B-6 status due to analytical difficulties
Pyridoxal Phosphate	Levels measured in serum, erythrocytes, or leukocytes with use of radioisotopic enzyme assays	Standardized and less tedious analytical methods would improve the reliability and usefulness of the tech- nique for assessing vitamin B-6 status
Serum Transaminases	GOT or GPT activity measured with the use of standardized methods	Variable, insensitive, and unreliable for the assessment of vitamin B-6 status, serum levels of the enzymes normally very low
Leukocyte Transaminases	Leukocytes isolated and enzyme activity measured with the use of standardized methods	Presently, methods for the isolation of leukocytes too tedious for routine use of the procedure, requires larger sample size

Table 5 (cont).   Biochemical Procedures Used to Evaluate Vitamin B-6 Nutrition
                   Status in the Human

Procedure	Principle	Comments
Erythrocyte Transaminases	EGOT and EGPT activity measured and combined with in vitro stimulation with pyridoxal phosphate; EGOT measurements usually preferred since erythrocytes contain consid- erable more GOT than that of GPT	Improved standardized ana- lytical procedures needed in order to reduce vari- ations in reported results, guidelines require further validation

Table 6. Laboratory Procedures Feasible for the Assessment of Vitamin B-6 Status

Subjects	Primary	Secondary	Potential
Population Groups	Erythrocyte transaminase activity and in vitro PLP stimulation	Plasma PLP	HPLC measurement of urinary 4-pyridoxic acid and vitamin B-6
	Urinary vitamin B-6		Radioimmune assays
Individual Subjects	Tryptophan load	Methionine load	HPLC measurement of xanthurenic acid and other tryptophan metabolites
	Erythrocyte transaminase activity and in vitro PLP stimulation	Erythrocyte PLP	Leukocyte measurements
	Plasma PLP	Urinary vitamin B-6	

When the evaluation of the vitamin B-6 status of an individual is involved, then the tryptophan load test becomes more feasible. For a reliable test, however, the inconvenience of providing a 24-hour urine collection exists with this procedure. Xanthurenic acid can be easily measured while the measurement of other metabolites of tryptophan is more involved. At present, only a limited number of research laboratories have at hand services to provide plasma PLP or erythrocyte transaminase measurements. Methods need to be modified to meet the needs of the clinical laboratory before proper attention will be given to the clinical patient that may have a deficiency of vitamin B-6. While HPLC approaches may eventually prove useful in this respect, current methods have been handicapped by inadequate sensitivity and involved sample preparation.

The potential exists for the development of standardized kits for the measurement of erythrocyte GOT activity and in vitro PLP stimulation. The development of a suitable quality control or reference standards would be required for use in such kits.

Another approach would be the development of radioassay procedures to measure PLP in serum or erythrocytes in a manner analogou to the assay kits developed over the past few years to measure folic acid in serum and erythrocytes. A similar approach has been recentl used for the measurement of pantothenic acid in blood and other samples (62,63).

UTILIZATION OF VITAMIN B-6 ASSESSMENT PROCEDURES IN FIELD STUDIES

As noted earlier, few nutrition studies of population groups have included an attempt to assess vitamin B-6 status. The Health and Nutrition Examination Surveys (HANES) did not assess vitamin B-6 status. However, the earlier Ten-State Nutrition Survey did obtain some information. Table 7 presents the mean urinary excretion of free vitamin B-6 (μg/g creatinine) observed for samples collected on adults in five locations. The mean excretion for females was somewhat higher than that for males for each area. The mean urinary levels of vitamin B-6 were the lowest for samples collected on subjects located in South Carolina. Fig. 2 presents the urinary excretion data on all the subjects by age and sex. As has been noted previously for thiamin and riboflavin (45), children had a markedly higher level of vitamin B-6 excretion when expressed on a creatinine basis than adults. These data have served as a basis for a tentative guide for the interpretation of urinary levels of vitamin B-6 for various age groups (45). Using these guides, a number of Wainwright Eskimo children were observed to have unacceptable urine vitamin B-6 levels (58).

Table 7.   Urinary Excretion of Free Vitamin B-6
            by Adults[a]

State	Male	Female
	μg vitamin B-6/g creatinine	
South Carolina	25.4	35.7
New York City	33.0	40.8
S. California	38.6	48.5
N. California	38.9	43.6
Massachusetts	36.0	46.3

[a]Data collected during Ten-State Nutrition
Survey on 1450 females and 921 males, age
16 years and over.

During the past several years, this laboratory has conducted
a series of nutrition surveys that included an attempt to evaluate
the vitamin B-6 status of Arizona Indians and of military personnel.
Some of the findings from the study conducted in 1977 at the Marine
Corps Base at Twentynine Palms, California, will demonstrate the
usefulness of laboratory procedures to assess vitamin B-6 nutritional
status. Fig. 3 presents the distribution of urinary free vitamin
B-6 levels (μg/g creatinine) on 353 subjects studied. Using a
urinary vitamin B-6 value of 20 μg/g of creatinine and above as
acceptable, nearly 10% of the subjects had unacceptable levels of
vitamin B-6 in their urine.

Fig. 4 presents the distribution of erythrocyte GOT activities
(IU/ml red blood cells) for 312 males. A considerable range of
values was observed. Was this a reflection of vitamin B-6 status
or the result of other factors, including methodology? Fig. 5
presents the distribution of erythrocyte GOT in vitro stimulation
by PLP for the same samples used for erythrocyte GOT activity
measurements. Again, a considerable range in percent stimulation
was observed (3-fold).

Fig. 6 is a plot of urinary vitamin B-6 levels versus erythrocyte GOT activity in 41 female subjects studied. Fig. 7 is a plot
of urinary vitamin B-6 levels versus stimulation effect of PLP on
erythrocyte GOT for the same subjects. The surprising degree of
correlation between these independent vitamin B-6 assessment procedures would support the concept that erythrocyte GOT and erythrocyte GOT PLP stimulation effect are related to vitamin B-6 intake
as measured by urinary levels of the vitamin.

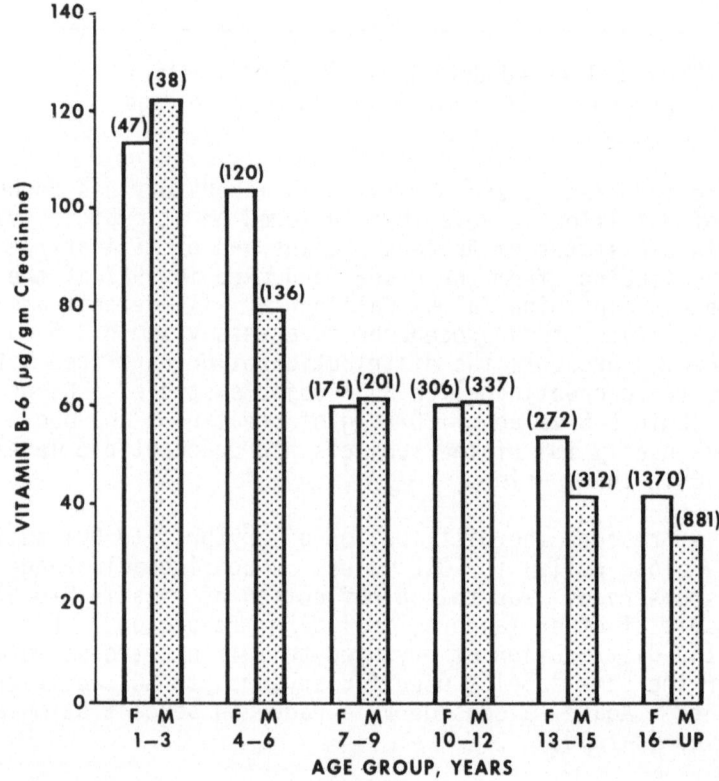

Fig. 2.   Mean urinary excretion of free vitamin B-6 (μg/g creatinine)
          by age and sex.   Data were obtained during the Ten-State
          Nutrition Survey from the areas indicated in the text.
          Values in parentheses indicate the number of subjects
          studied.

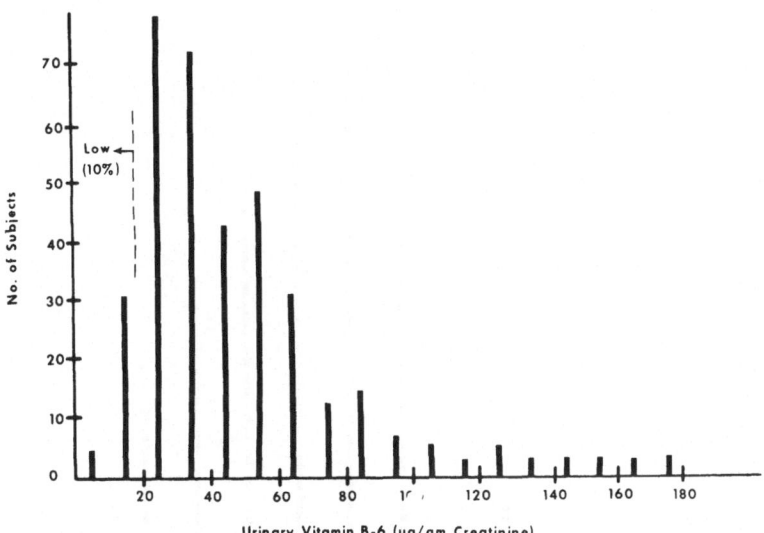

N = 353 Mean = 45.0 ± 26.8

Fig. 3. Distribution plot of urinary levels of vitamin B-6 (µg/gm creatinine) in samples collected on 353 marine personnel during March 1977 at the Marine Corps Base, Twentynine Palms, CA.

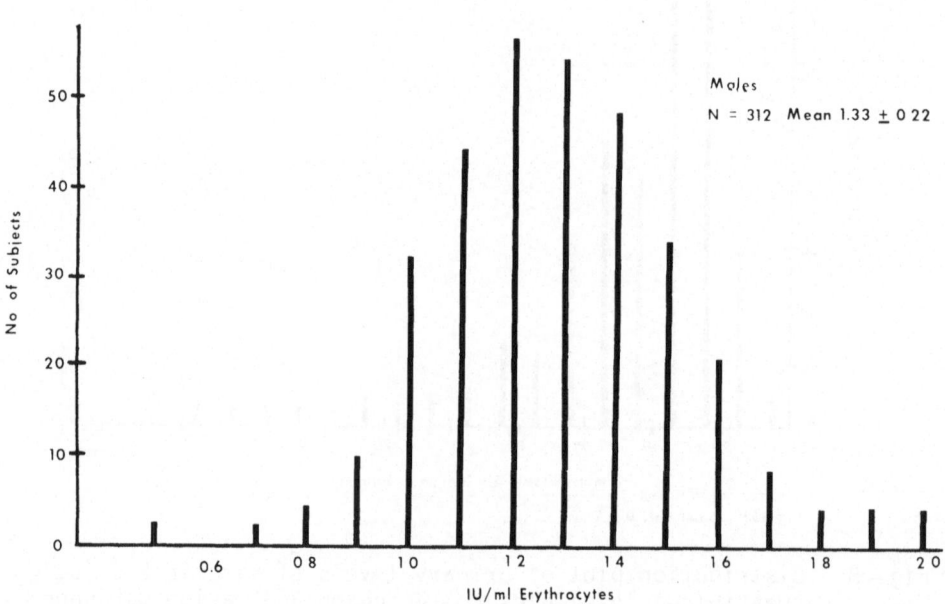

Fig. 4.   Distribution plot of erythrocyte GOT activities in blood
          samples obtained from 312 male marine personnel during
          March 1977 at the Marine Corps Base, Twentynine Palms, CA.

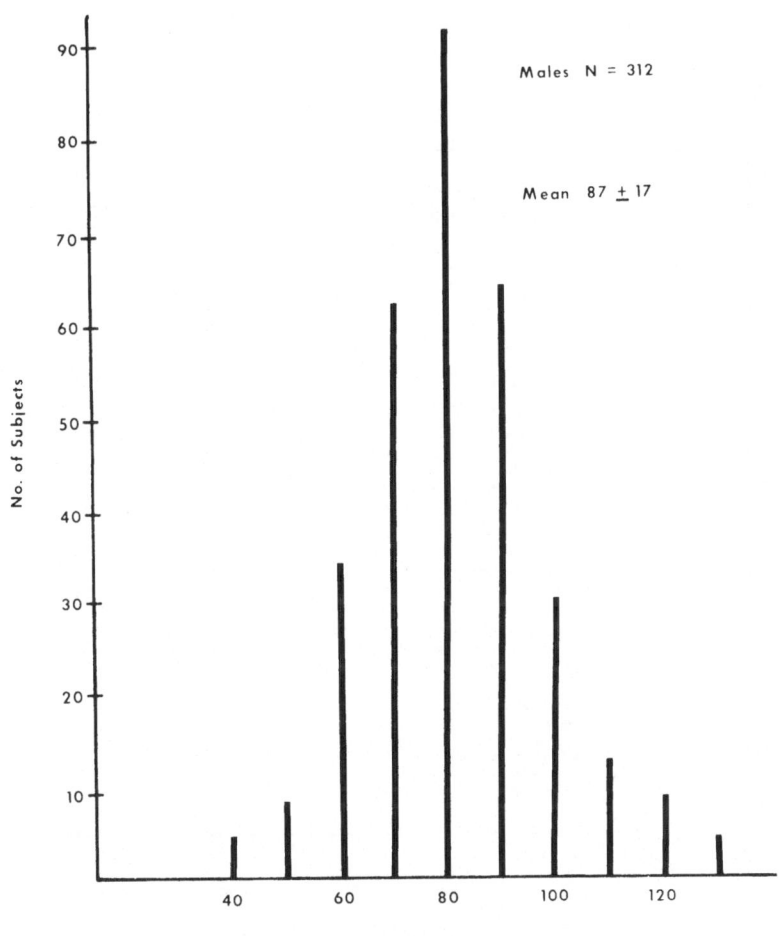

Fig. 5. The in vitro stimulation effect of pyridoxal phosphate on erythrocyte GOT activity of blood samples obtained from 312 male marine personnel during March 1977 at the Marine Corps Base, Twentynine Palms, CA.

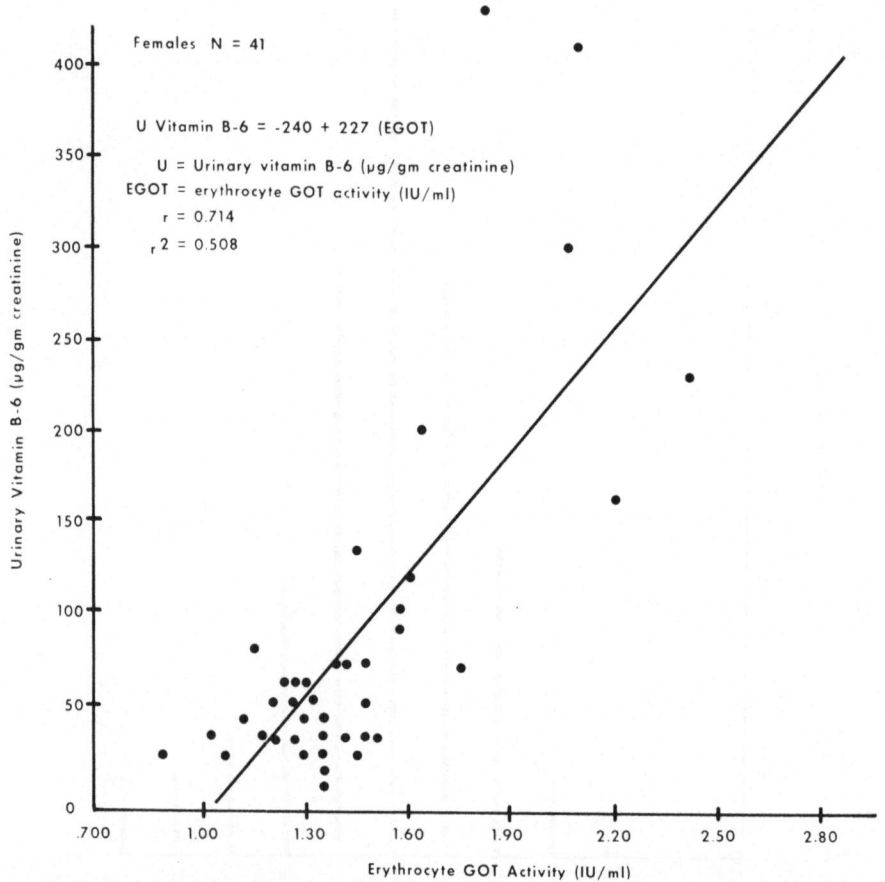

Fig. 6.   Relationship between urinary vitamin B-6 levels and
          erythrocyte GOT activity in 41 samples obtained from
          female marine personnel in March 1977 at the Marine Corps
          Base, Twentynine Palms, CA.

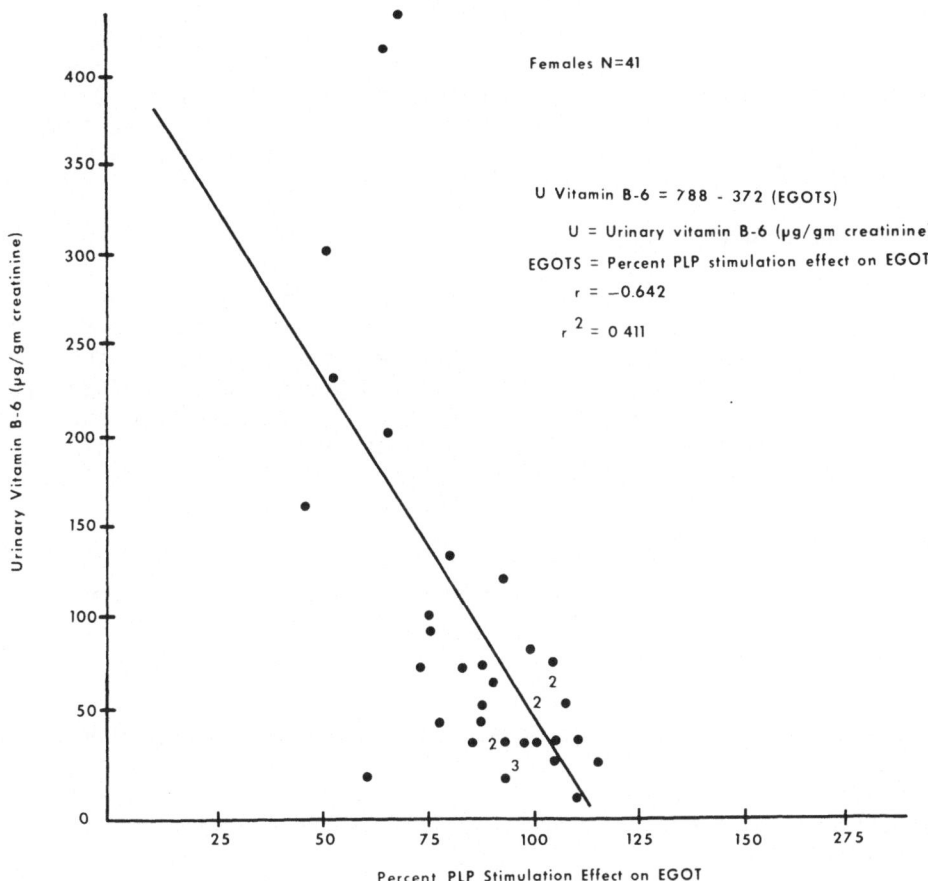

Fig. 7.   Relationship between urinary vitamin B-6 levels and percent in vitro pyridoxal phosphate stimulation effect on
erythrocyte GOT activities in 41 samples obtained from
female marine personnel in March 1977 at the Marine Corps
Base, Twentynine Palms, CA.

FACTORS THAT MAY INFLUENCE VITAMIN B-6 METABOLISM

Numerous factors may influence vitamin B-6 metabolism and in turn may invalidate certain methods used to assess vitamin B-6 status. Some of these factors are listed in Table 8. Various drugs, for example, have vitamin B-6 antagonistic effects. For the subject receiving isoniazid, penicillamine, or cycloserine, urinary measurements for vitamin B-6 would probably not be valid since excessive amounts of vitamin B-6 may be lost in the urine (45,64). Heavy exercise may cause elevated serum transaminase activities. On occasion, a riboflavin deficiency may reduce erythrocyte transaminase activities (24,65). Demographic and clinical information can help to prevent misinterpretation of laboratory data.

ADDITIONAL RESEARCH NEEDS

Table 9 lists some of the areas where additional studies are necessary for the improvement of methods to assess vitamin B-6 nutritional status. As summarized earlier, the majority of the vitamin B-6 studies have been conducted on young adults. Other age groups need increased attention. The need for standardized and simplified assessment procedures cannot be overemphasized. HPLC procedures and radioassay methods may prove fruitful to meet these needs. Is there any justification for the consideration of food fortification with pyridoxine?

Table 8. Factors That May Influence Vitamin B-6 Metabolism

Protein level

Dietary amino acids; e.g., cystine, methionine and tryptophan

Drugs; e.g., L-Dopa, isonicotinic acid hydrazide, cycloserine, hydralazine, linatine, penicillamine, ethanol, agaritine, hydrocortisone

Oral contraceptive agents

Physiological status; e.g., pregnancy, starvation, exercise

Health status; e.g., liver disease, uremia

Pyridoxine-dependencies

Riboflavin deficiency

Table 9.   Areas of Additional Studies for the Improvement
of Methods to Assess Vitamin B-6 Nutrition Status

Application of assessment procedures to younger and
older age groups

Standardization of procedures

Simplification of methods

Development of suitable quality controls

Additional functional tests

Relate analytical data to functional impairment, level
of risk, or body pool of vitamin B-6

HPLC applications to improve specificity and
reliability of methods

Develop radioassay procedures to measure pyridoxal
phosphate in plasma and erythrocytes

Use of leukocytes in assessment of vitamin B-6 status

Additional vitamin B-6 data for food consumption tables

Need for accurate dietary intake data on vitamin B-6

Additional information on the bioavailability of
vitamin B-6 forms present in diet; processing effects;
food fortification benefits

CONCLUSION

How does one define optimal vitamin B-6 nutrition in terms of
biochemical or physiological functions of humans? An overt dietary
deficiency of vitamin B-6 would generally be recognized by current
indicators of vitamin B-6 nutritional status, but the ability to
detect a marginal deficiency of the vitamin remains uncertain. For
many of the assessment procedures, only tentative guides are available to interpret data. Sensitive biochemical, physiological,
immunological, or even behavioral indicators of vitamin B-6 nutritional status need to be developed. What do our present assessment
methods tell us? For example, during pregnancy abnormal metabolites
of tryptophan may appear in the urine and plasma pyridoxal phosphate

levels may fall. Are these changes a reflection of reduction in body pool of vitamin B-6 and signs of a subclinical deficiency of the vitamin or merely the normal response of pregnancies. Yet certain tryptophan metabolites have been demonstrated to have carcinogenic and/or mutagenic properties. Is it desirable then for the body to produce increased quantities of these compounds when their production can be reduced or prevented by increased intakes of vitamin B-6? In terms of vitamin B-6, to what degree of risk should the body be exposed? The adult human has a body pool of only 20-30 mg of vitamin B-6 which can be depleted very rapidly when fed diets devoid of the nutrient (66). Most of the assessment techniques available have not been developed to the state where they may provide an indication of the degree of deficiency of vitamin B-6 or level of depletion of the vitamin B-6 pool.

Table 10 suggests the events that may occur if the supply of vitamin B-6 is inadequate to meet the minimum requirement. Phase 1 provides biochemical and clinical parameters associated with an adequate intake of vitamin B-6.

With an inadequate intake of the nutrient, the body pool of vitamin B-6 would be reduced. Changes observed in phase 3 may not occur if the fall in body pool of vitamin B-6 is only minor or of a temporary nature. Even adaptation or equilibration to this new level of reserves may occur. A continued reduction in body pool size would be expected to result in a lowering in the concentrations of vitamin B-6 or its metabolites in blood, urine, and other tissues as well as in the urine, such as of 4-pyridoxic acid. Lowering of vitamin B-6-dependent enzymes may or may not occur at this stage. Clinical changes will probably not be discernible. With an increased severity or duration of the deficiency, early signs of metabolic disturbances may be observed, which may be detected by tryptophan or methionine load tests and the measurement of activities of vitamin B-6-dependent enzymes. At this stage, central nervous system changes may be detected as well as the appearance of hyper-irritability and abnormal electroencephalograms.

Phase 5 would represent a severe deficiency of vitamin B-6 or one of long duration. At this stage, severe metabolic disturbances would exist and anemia may occur. Both morphological and functional changes are likely to be present.

Table 10. Phases in the Development of a Vitamin B-6 Deficiency

Phases:	1	2	3	4	5
Biochemical Alterations	Normal pool size and concentrations in tissues, blood, urine. Normal metabolite levels and enzyme activities	Reduction in body pool size	Lowering of vitamin concentration in blood, urine, and tissues; lowering of metabolite levels in urine, blood, etc.	Lowering of activity of vitamin B-6-dependent enzmes, early signs of metabolic disturbances	Severe metabolic disturbances, abnormal metabolites present in urine or blood, anemia
Clinical Changes Morphological changes	Normal	Normal	Normal	CNS changes	Seborrheic dermatitis, cheilosis, glossitis, angular stomatitis
Functional changes	Normal	Normal	Normal	Abnormal electroencephalograms, hyperirritability	Convulsive seizures, hyperacusis

Increased Severity or Duration of Deficiency ⟶

Phases 2 and 3 would indicate that the supply of vitamin B-6 is inadequate in terms of a normal body pool of vitamin B-6.   Is phase 3 an acceptable level of risk?   What can be considered an acceptable level of vitamin B-6 in the body, blood, or urine?   What are the normal individual variations that can be identified in a population or age group?   These questions can be asked of other nutrients and have frequently been asked of vitamin C requirements where a functional assessment technique is not available equivalent to the transaminase measurements for vitamin B-6 nutritional status.

SUMMARY

Nutritional assessment of vitamin B-6 is dependent upon satisfactory answers to the following:

1.   What level of vitamin B-6 and associated metabolites, or what activities of vitamin B-6-dependent enzymes corresponds to optimal body stores of vitamin B-6?

2.   What body store, tissue level or metabolite level of vitamin B-6 or vitamin B-6-dependent enzyme activity corresponds to the first metabolic, morphological, or functional disturbance caused by a vitamin B-6 deficiency which would correspond to a borderline deficiency?

To obtain these answers, suitable standardized, reliable, specific, and sensitive methods will be required.   The following papers should provide guidance in resolving these questions.

ACKNOWLEDGMENTS

Appreciation is expressed to Ms. Anne Regh, Mr. Richard Wheeler, and Mr. Richard Nelson for their assistance in the preparation of this manuscript.

LITERATURE CITED

1.   György, P. (1934) Vitamin B-2 and the pellagra-like dermatitis in rats. Nature 133, 498-499.
2.   György, P. (1935) Vitamin B-2 complex. I. Differentiation of lactoflavin and the "rat antipellagra" factor. Biochem. J. 29, 741-759.
3.   Harris, S. A. & Folkers, K. (1939) Synthetic vitamin B-6. Science 89, 347.
4.   György, P. & Eckhardt, R. E. (1939) Vitamin B-6 and skin lesions in rats. Nature 144, 512.
5.   Spies, T. D., Bean, W. B. & Ashe, W. F. (1939) A note on the use of vitamin B-6 in human nutrition. J. Am. Med. Assoc. 112, 2414-2415.

6. Spies, T. D., Ladisch, R. K. & Bean, W. B. (1940) Vitamin B-6 (pyridoxine) deficiency in human beings. J. Am. Med. Assoc. 115, 839-840.
7. Smith, S. G. & Martin, D. W. (1940) Cheilosis successfully treated with synthetic vitamin B-6. Proc. Soc. Expt. Biol. Med. 43, 660-663.
8. Molony, C. J. & Parmelee, A. H. (1954) Convulsions in young infants as a result of pyridoxine (vitamin B-6) deficiency. J. Am. Med. Assoc. 154, 405-406.
9. Coursin, D. B. (1954) Convulsive seizures in infants with pyridoxine-deficient diet. J. Am. Med. Assoc. 154, 406-407.
10. Sauberlich, H. E. & Canham, J. E. (1980) Vitamin B-6. In: Modern Nutrition in Health and Disease (Goodhart, R. S. & Shils, M. E., eds.), 6th ed., pp. 216-229. Lea & Febiger, Philadelphia, PA.
11. Bessey, O. A., Adam, D. J. D. & Hansen, A. E. (1957) Intake of vitamin B-6 and infantile convulsions: A first approximation of requirements of pyridoxine in infants. Pediatrics 20, 33-44.
12. Hunt, A. D., Jr., Stokes, J., Jr., McCrory, W. W. & Stroud, H. H. (1954) Pyridoxine dependency: report of a case of intractable convulsions in an infant controlled by pyridoxine. Pediatrics 13, 140-146.
13. Waldinger, C. & Berg, R. B. (1963) Signs of pyridoxine dependency manifest at birth in siblings. Pediatrics 32, 161-168.
14. Harris, J. W., Whittington, R. M., Weisman, R., Jr., & Horrigan, D. L. (1956) Pyridoxine responsive anemia in the human adult. Proc. Soc. Expt. Biol. Med. 91, 427-432.
15. Hines, J. D. & Harris, J. W. (1964) Pyridoxine-responsive anemia. Am. J. Clin. Nutr. 14, 137-146.
16. Mudd, S. H. (1971) Pyridoxine-responsive genetic disease. Fed. Proc. 30, 970-976.
17. Frimpter, G. W., Andelman, R. J. & George, W. F. (1969) Vitamin B-6-dependency syndromes. Am. J. Clin. Nutr. 22, 794-805.
18. Knapp, A. (1960) Uber eine neue hereditare von vitamin B-6 abhangige storung im tryptophan-stoffwechsel. Clin. Chim. Acta 5, 6-13.
19. Spannuth, C. L., Mitchell, D., Stone, W. J., Schenker, S. & Wagner, C. (1978) Vitamin B-6 nutriture in patients with uremia and with liver disease. In: Human Vitamin B-6 Requirements, pp. 180-192, Nat. Acad. Sci., Washington, DC.
20. Walsh, M. P., Howorth, P. J. N. & Marks, V. (1966) Pyridoxine deficiency and tryptophan metabolism in chronic alcoholics. Am. J. Clin. Nutr. 19, 379-383.

21. Li, T.-K. (1978) Factors influencing vitamin B-6 requirement in alcoholism. In: Human Vitamin B-6 Requirements, pp. 210-225, Nat. Acad. Sci., Washington, DC.

22. Rose, D. P. (1966) The influence of oestrogens upon tryptophan metabolism in man. Clin. Sci. 31, 265-272.

23. Rose, D. P. (1978) Oral contraceptives and vitamin B-6. In: Human Vitamin B-6 Requirements, pp. 193-201, Nat. Acad. Sci., Washington, DC.

24. Krishnaswany, K. (1971) Erythrocyte glutamic oxaloacetic transaminase activity in patients with oral lesions. Internat. J. Vit. Nutr. Res. 41, 247-252.

25. Krishnaswany, K. (1971) Erythrocyte transaminase activity in human vitamin B-6 deficiency. Internat. J. Vit. Nutr. Res. 41, 240-246.

26. Krishnaswany, K., Bapurao, S., Raghuram, T. C. & Srikantia, S. G. (1976) Effect of vitamin B-6 on leucine-induced changes in human subjects. Am. J. Clin. Nutr. 29, 177-181.

27. Bapurao, S. & Krishanswany, K. (1978) Vitamin B-6 nutritional status of pellagrins and their leucine tolerance. Am. J. Clin. Nutr. 31, 819-824.

28. Bamji, M. S., Rameshwar Sarma, K. V. & Radhaiah, G. (1979) Relationship between biochemical and clinical indices of B-vitamin deficiency. A study in rural school boys. Br. J. Nutr. 41, 431-441.

29. Wachstein, M., Kellner, J. D. & Ortiz, J. M. (1960) Pyridoxal phosphate in plasma and leukocytes of normal and pregnant subjects following B-6 load tests. Proc. Soc. Expt. Biol. Med. 103, 350-353.

30. Dempsey, W. B. (1978) Vitamin B-6 and pregnancy. In: Human Vitamin B-6 Requirements, pp. 202-209, Nat. Acad. Sci., Washington, DC.

31. Sauberlich, H. E. (1978) Vitamin indices. In: Laboratory Indices of Nutritional Status in Pregnancy, pp. 109-156, Nat. Acad. Sci., Washington, DC.

32. Lepkovsky, S., Roboz, E. & Hargen-Smith, A. J. (1943) Xanthurenic acid and its role in the tryptophan metabolism of pyridoxine-deficient rats. J. Biol. Chem. 149, 195-201.

33. Greenberg, L. D., Bohr, D. F., McGrath, H. & Rinehart, J. F. (1949) Xanthurenic acid excretion in the human subject on pyridoxine-deficient diet. Arch. Biochem. 21, 237-239.

34. Snyderman, S. E., Holt, L. E., Jr., Carretero, R. & Jacobs, K. (1953) Pyridoxine deficiency in human infant. J. Clin. Nutr. 1, 200-207.

35. Mueller, J. F. & Vilter, R. W. (1950) Pyridoxine deficiency in human beings induced with deoxypyridoxine. J. Clin. Invest. 29, 193-201.

36. Vilter, R. W., Mueller, J. F., Glazer, H. S., Jarrold, T., Abraham, J., Thompson, C. & Hawkins, V. R. (1953) The effect of vitamin B-6 deficiency induced by deoxypyridoxine in human beings. J. Lab. Clin. Med. 42, 335-357.

37. Harding, R. S., Plough, I. C. & Friedemann, T. E. (1959) The effect of storage on the vitamin B-6 content of a packaged Army ration, with a note on the human requirement for the vitamin. J. Nutr. 68, 323-332.

38. Cheslock, K. E. & McCully, M. T. (1960) Response of human beings to a low-vitamin B-6 diet. J. Nutr. 70, 507-513.

39. Babcock, M. J., Brush, M. & Sostman, E. (1960) Evaluation of vitamin B-6 nutrition. J. Nutr. 70, 369-376.

40. Hodges, R. E., Bean, W. B., Ohlson, M. A. & Bleiler, R. E. (1962) Factors affecting human antibody response. IV. Pyridoxine deficiency. Am. J. Clin. Nutr. 11, 180-186.

41. Sauberlich, H. E., Canham, J. R., Baker, E. M., Raica, N., Jr. & Herman, Y. F. (1970) Human vitamin B-6 nutriture. J. Sci. & Ind. Res. 29, 1-10.

42. Sauberlich, H. E. (1964) Human requirements for vitamin B-6. Vit. Hormones 22, 807-823.

43. Baker, E. M., Canham, J. E., Nunes, W. T., Sauberlich, H. E. & McDowell, M. E. (1964) Vitamin B-6 requirement for adult men. Am. J. Clin. Nutr. 15, 59-66.

44. Raica, N., Jr. & Sauberlich, H. E. (1964) Blood cell transaminase activity in human vitamin B-6 deficiency. Am. J. Clin. Nutr. 15, 67-72.

45. Sauberlich, H. E., Dowdy, R. P. & Skala, J. H. (1974) Laboratory tests for the assessment of nutritional status. CRC Press, Inc., Boca Raton, Florida.

46. Sauberlich, H. E., Canham, J. E., Baker, E. M., Raica, N. Jr. & Herman, Y. F. (1972) Biochemical assessment of the nutritional status of vitamin B-6 in the human. Am. J. Clin. Nutr. 25, 629-642.

47. Yess, N., Price, J. M., Brown, R. R., Swan, P. B. & Linkswiler, H. (1964) Vitamin B-6 depletion in man: urinary excretion of tryptophan metabolites. J. Nutr. 84, 229-236.

48. Linkswiler, H. M. (1978) Vitamin B-6 requirements of men. In: Human Vitamin B-6 Requirements, pp. 279-290, Nat. Acad. Sci., Washington, DC.

49. Brown, R. R., Yess, N., Price, J. M., Linkswiler, H., Swan, P. & Hankes, L. V. (1965) Vitamin B-6 depletion in man: Urinary excretion of quinolinic acid and niacin metabolites. J. Nutr. 87, 419-423.

50. Kelsay, J., Miller, L. T. & Linkswiler, H. (1968) Effect of protein intake on the excretion of quinolinic acid and niacin metabolites by men during vitamin B-6 depletion. J. Nutr. 94, 27-31.

51. Kelsay, J., Baysal, A. & Linkswiler, H. (1968) Effect of vitamin B-6 depletion on the pyridoxal, pyridoxamine, and pyridoxine content of the blood and urine of men. J. Nutr. 94, 490-496.

52. Baysal, A., Johnson, B. A. & Linkswiler, H. (1966) Vitamin B-6 depletion in man: blood vitamin B-6, plasma pyridoxal-phosphate, serum cholesterol, serum transaminases and urinary vitamin B-6 and 4-pyridoxic acid. J. Nutr. 89, 19-23.

53. Park, Y. K. & Linkswiler, H. (1970) Effect of vitamin B-6 depletion in adult man on the excretion of cystathionine and other metabolites. J. Nutr. 100, 110-116.

54. Shin, H. K. & Linkswiler, H. (1974) Tryptophan and methionine metabolism of adult females as affected by vitamin B-6 deficiency. J. Nutr. 104, 1348-1355.

55. Leklem, J. E., Brown, R. R., Rose, D. P. & Linkswiler, H. M. (1975) Vitamin B-6 requirements of women using oral contraceptives. Am. J. Clin. Nutr. 28, 535-541.

56. Donald, E. A., McBean, L. D., Simpson. M. H. W., Sun, M. F. & Aly, H. E. (1971) Vitamin B-6 requirement of young adult women. Am. J. Clin. Nutr. 24, 1028-1041.

57. Ritchey, S. J., Johnson, F. S. & Korslund, M. K. (1978) Vitamin B-6 requirements in the preadolescent and adolescent. In: Human Vitamin B-6 Requirements, pp. 272-278, Nat. Acad. Sci., Washington, DC.

58. Sauberlich, H. E., Goad, W., Herman, Y. F., Milan, F. & Jamison, P. (1972) Biochemical assessment of the nutritional status of the Eskimos of Wainwright, Alaska. Am. J. Clin. Nutr. 25, 437-445.

59. Marston, R. M. & Peterkin, B. B. Nutrient content of the national food supply. National Food Review, u.S. Dept. of Agriculture, Economics, Statistics, and Cooperative Serv., Winter 1980, NFR-9, 21.-25.

60. USDA Nationwide Food Consumption Survey, 48 States, Spring 1977 (preliminary). U.S. Dept. of Agriculture.

61. Canham, J. E., Baker, E. M., Harding, R. S., Sauberlich, H. E. & Plough, I. C. (1969) Dietary protein - its relationship to vitamin B-6 requirements and functions. Ann. N.Y. Acad. Sci. 166, 16-29.

62. Howe, J., Wyse, B. W. & Hansen, R. G. (1979) Measurement of pantothenic acid in nursing home meals using a microbiological assay and a radioimmunoassay. Fed. Proc. 38, 452.

63. Wyse, B. W., Wittwer, C. W. & Hansen, R. G. (1979) Radio-immunoassay for pantothenic acid in blood and other tissues. Clin. Chem. 25, 108-111.

64. Sauberlich, H. E. (1968) Vitamin B-6 group. VIII. Active compounds and antagonists. In: The Vitamins, vol. 2, 2nd ed. (Sebulla, W. H., Jr. & Harris, R. S., eds.), pp. 33-44, Academic Press, New York.

65. Lakshmi, A. V. & Bamji, M. S. (1974) Regulation of blood pyridoxal phosphate in riboflavin deficiency in man. Nutr. Metab. 20, 228-233.
66. Tillotson, J. A., Sauberlich, H. E., Baker, E. M. & Canham, J. E. (1966) Use of carbon-14 labeled vitamins in human nutrition studies: pyridoxine. Proc. of the Seventh Intern. Congr. of Nutr. (Hamburg) 5, 554-557.
67. Swan, P., Wentworth, J. & Linkswiler, H. (1964) Vitamin B-6 depletion in man: urinary taurine and sulfate excretion and nitrogen balance. J. Nutr. 84, 220-228.

ESTIMATED DIETARY INTAKES OF VITAMIN B-6

Judy A. Driskell and Barbara M. Chrisley

Virginia Polytechnic Institute
and State University
Blacksburg, VA   24061

Most of the researchers who have estimated dietary intakes
of vitamin B-6 have utilized the composition tables in Home
Economics Research Report No. 36 (1). The values given in this
bulletin as well as those published by others (2-7) were obtained
mainly via microbiological assay, generally Saccharomyces uvarum,
ATCC No. 9080. Vitamin B-6 is found mainly bound to the protein
portion of foods; however, the vitamin may also be present in food
in its free state. Pyridoxal (PL) and pyridoxamine (PM) are the
forms of the vitamin usually found in animal products; whereas
pyridoxine (ol, PN) is the predominant form in plant products (8).
The relative potency of PN, PL, and PM in man has not yet been
determined.

Methods used for the quantitation of vitamin B-6 should be
capable of detecting all forms of the vitamin. Most of the time
in biological systems, the vitamin is bound to protein. Various
types of food samples present unique problems with regard to
hydrolysis and extraction. The methods must be capable of accurately measuring nanogram quantities of the nutrient in the
presence of varying interfering substances.

The following disadvantages are inherent in the microbiological
method for determining the vitamin B-6 content of foods: the procedure is time-consuming, variability exists in the growth response
of various microorganisms to the vitamin, the microorganisms can
mutate, microbiologically unavailable complexes of the vitamin may
be formed as a result of acid extraction, and microbial growth may
be retarded by substances in the food extract. Thirteen collabo-
rators, all using Saccharomyces uvarum, found the vitamin B-6

content of milk to vary almost two-fold and almost three-fold for
flour (9).   Considerable variation in vitamin B-6 content also
exists due to variety, growing conditions, and location (3,5).   All
of these factors must be considered in estimating the vitamin B-6
intakes of individuals in that the values in the composition tables
were obtained in this fashion.   The food composition table values
for vitamin B-6 content are generally given in terms of raw food.
Cooking losses in processed foods are in the range of 0% to 40%
(10).

Researchers must obtain dietary information from their
subjects by using some type of tool(s) such as 24-hour recalls
(best if by a trained interviewer), food or dietary records,
dietary histories, dietary composites, cross-checking lists, and
food models made from plastic or paper "cut-outs".   These methods
are not without their limitations.   Serving sizes must be estimated
or weighed.   Procedures, advantages, and limitations of these
methods are discussed in Nutritional Assessment in Health Programs
(11).   What subjects report eating may not be what they actually
consume.

Few researchers have reported data regarding dietary intakes
of vitamin B-6 particularly relating intake values to biochemical
parameters.

INFANTS

Milk from cows has both a higher vitamin B-6 and protein
content than that from humans; 0.23-0.6 mg vitamin B-6 is found in
a liter of cows' milk (12).   Table 1 lists approximations of the
vitamin B-6 intakes of infants based upon their milk consumption
(13).   The 1980 Recommended Dietary Allowance (RDA) for vitamin
B-6 (14) is also given in the table.   An intake of 0.3-0.4 mg daily
is adequate as judged by xanthurenic acid excretion measurements
(13).   Metabolic requirements of infants seem to be satisfied if
the formula contains 0.015 mg of vitamin B-6 per gram of protein
or 0.04 mg/100 kcal (14).

CHILDREN

The estimated vitamin B-6 intakes of preschool children living
in Virginia are listed in Table 2 (15).   The dietary data were
obtained by a 24-hour interview recall method from a parent; food
models and cross-checking were used.   A 48-hour food record was
also kept by a parent.   Thus, 3 consecutive days of dietary records
were obtained.   Although the 3- and 4-year old subjects consumed
similar quantities of the vitamin, more of the 4-year olds consumed
less than two-thirds of the 1980 RDA as the RDA is higher for
4-year olds as compared to 3-year olds.   Three of the 35 subjects
were found to have plasma pyridoxal phosphate levels below 8.5 ng/ml.

Table 1. Reported Vitamin B-6 Intakes of Infants[a]

Age	Milk Intake	Breast-fed	Formula-fed	1980 RDA
mo	ml/day	µg/day	µg/day	µg/day
Birth	450	45	180	300
3	800	107	307	300
6	850/900	245	520	600
12			820	600

[a]From Ref. 13.

Lewis and Nunn (16) studied 6 female and 16 male 2-9-year olds with regard to vitamin B-6 intakes. The mothers of the children kept food records for 3 consecutive days; the vitamin B-6 intake was 1.10 + 0.47 mg (mean + SD); the 1980 RDA is 0.9-1.6 mg for this age group. Eight of the 18 subjects had intakes less than the 1974 RDA, 2 had intakes less than two-thirds of the 1974 RDA; and 3 had low 4-pyridoxic acid excretion values. Ritchey and Feeley (17), as a result of a 36-day metabolic study involving girls 7 years 10 months to 9 years 5 months, suggested that their minimal daily requirement was about 1.3 to 1.73 mg as indicated by 4-pyridoxic acid excretion values.

ADOLESCENTS

Kirksey et al. (18) found the vitamin B-6 intake of 127 females 12-14 years of age to be 1.24 + 0.70 mg, mean + SD, as calculated from 24-hour recall records. Approximately one-half of these subjects consumed less than two-thirds of the 1974 RDA for the vitamin. The protein intake of these subjects was 71 + 25 g, mean + SD. Coenzyme stimulation of erythrocyte alanine amino-transferase (E-ALAT) activity values equal to or greater than 16% were found in 31% of the subjects and 13% of the subjects had a stimulation index $\geq$1.25.

The vitamin B-6 intake of 6 females, 18 years of age, and living in Florida as obtained by 24-hour recalls followed by 48-hour food records was 1.13 + 0.31 mg, mean + SD (19). One of these 6 subjects had a coenzyme stimulation of E-ALAT value $\geq$16%.

A market basket dietary study in which the vitamin B-6 content of diets typically consumed by 16-19 year old males in August 1962 was measured microbiologically from diet composites (20). The diets typically contained 2.8 mg vitamin B-6, 147 g protein, and 4200 kcal.

Table 2. Estimated Vitamin B-6 Intakes of Preschool Children[a]

Age	Sex	Mean Intake		1980 RDA	Number Subjects	No. having B-6 intakes at	
		Protein	Vitamin B-6			<1980 RDA	<2/3 1980 RDA
yr		g/day	mg/day	mg/day			
3	Female	53.6	1.19	0.9	9	3	1
3	Male	50.9	1.18	0.9	6	2	0
4	Female	58.3	1.14	1.3	10	7	2
4	Male	61.9	1.19	1.3	10	7	3

[a]Dietary data obtained by 24-hr recall (food models and cross-checking) and 48-hr food record kept by a parent--3 consecutive days. Three subjects had plasma pyridoxal phosphate levels < 8.5 ng/ml. From Ref. 15.

The vitamin B-6 content of meals served to college students in 31 states was determined using diet composites of typical serving sizes and S. uvarum (21); 1.43 + 0.52 mg, mean + SD, was served to these students. More than one-fourth of these colleges served meals containing less than 50% of the 1974 RDA for vitamin B-6.

ADULT MALES

Thirty-three males, 19-25 years of age, reported consuming 1.98 + 1.14 mg, mean + SD, vitamin B-6 daily (19). The dietary data were obtained by 24-hour interview recalls (food models and cross-checking) followed by 48-hour food records. The protein intake of these subjects was 106.5 + 45.3 g, mean + SD. Of these subjects, 32% reported consuming less than 70% of the 1974 RDA for vitamin B-6. Thirty percent of the subjects had E-ALAT coenzyme stimulation values greater than 12% and greater than 16% for 12% of these males.

Chrisley and Driskell (22) reported the following estimated vitamin B-6 and protein intakes of males living in Virginia: (mean + SD) 6 males, 19-22 years, 1.88 + 0.72 mg, 104.2 + 32.9 g; 10 males, 23-35 years, 2.02 + 0.76 mg, 135 + 43. Sg; and 10 males, 36-59 years, 1.60 + 0.48 mg, 103.0 + 34.7 g. The dietary data were obtained as described previously by these researchers. Nine percent of the subjects reported consuming less than two-thirds of the 1980 RDA for vitamin B-6. Two subjects had E-ALAT coenzyme stimulation values above 12%.

Baker et al. (23) fed 8 males, 18-22 years old, diets containing different levels of vitamin B-6 and protein; the optimal requirement as judged by xanthurenic acid excretion after a tryptophan load was 1.75-2.0 mg for the high protein (100 g) diet and 1.25-1.5 mg for the low protein (30 g). A daily intake of 2.16 mg vitamin B-6 appeared to barely meet the requirement when males consumed 150 g protein (24). The vitamin B-6 requirement appeared to be >1.9 mg when packaged Army rations containing 165 g protein were used (25).

ADULT FEMALES

Driskell and coworkers (19) estimated the reported vitamin B-6 intakes of 73 females 18-25 years of age living in Florida. Twenty-four-hour recalls (food models and cross-checking) followed by 48-hour food records were used to obtain the data. The vitamin B-6 and protein intakes of these subjects were 1.24 + 0.50 mg and 73.0 + 31.3 g, mean + SD, respectively. The reported vitamin B-6 intakes of 72% of the subjects were less than 70% of the 1980 RDA. Fifteen percent of the subjects had >12% E-ALAT coenzyme stimulation and 5% had values >16% stimulation.

Recently Chrisley and Driskell (22) estimated the vitamin B-6 intakes of females living in Virginia; the same methods were used for obtaining the dietary information as were discussed previously. The vitamin B-6 and protein intakes were as follows: (mean $\pm$ SD) 29 females, 19-22 years, 1.38 $\pm$ 0.60 mg, 76.8 $\pm$ 30.4 g; 22 females, 23-35 years, 1.48 $\pm$ 0.58 mg, 79.1 $\pm$ 35.4 g; and 12 females, 36-59 years, 1.60 $\pm$ 0.70 mg, 84.6 $\pm$ 28.5 g. No differences in dietary or other data were observed between females taking oral contraceptives (OC's) for more than 6 months and those who had never taken OC's; hence their data were combined. Forty-one percent of the subjects reported consuming less than two-thirds of the 1980 RDA for vitamin B-6, yet only one subject had >12% coenzyme stimulation of E-ALAT. A metabolic study involving another nutrient was also described in this report; 35 females 18-27 years of age consumed approximately 1.37 mg vitamin B-6 (estimated using food composition tables) and 70.6 g protein for 4 weeks; all of these subjects had E-ALAT coenzyme stimulation values <12%.

Miller and coworkers (26) estimated that 4 females 20-29 years of age consumed 1.5 $\pm$ 0.5 mg (mean $\pm$ SD) vitamin B-6 daily and 5 females, same age, on OC's, 1.6 $\pm$ 0.4 mg; these researchers used 3-day dietary records and food composition tables to obtain their data. One control female and 3 females on OC's reported consuming less than two-thirds of the 1980 RDA for vitamin B-6; 3 of the females on OC's had normal-low plasma vitamin B-6 values. Prasad et al. (27) reported that the calculated vitamin B-6 intake of 19 females in the higher socioeconomic group not receiving supplementation was 1.19 $\pm$ 0.57 mg (mean $\pm$ SEM) and 1.02 $\pm$ 0.54 mg for the 36 females in the lower socioeconomic group.

Donald et al. (28) reported that 8 women were fed a diet containing 0.34 mg vitamin B-6 plus 0.6, 1.2, and 30 mg of the vitamin for 7, 3, and 1 days. The vitamin B-6 requirement of these women on a moderate protein diet as assessed by 4-pyridoxic acid excretion was 1.5 mg. Cheslock and McCully (29) found that the vitamin B-6 requirement of 8 college females maintained on a metabolic diet for 52 days was >0.5 mg as measured by xanthurenic acid excretion values. Several researchers (28,30-32) using various status parameters found that a vitamin B-6 intake of 1.5 mg daily was borderline for women consuming diets containing 78 g protein, yet intakes of 2.2 mg seemed to be excessive.

Driskell et al. (19) estimated the vitamin B-6 intakes of 46 females 18-25 years of age that reported taking OC's for over one year. Twenty-four hour interview recalls (food models and cross-checking) followed by 48-hour food records were obtained. The estimated daily vitamin B-6 and protein intakes were 1.26 $\pm$ 0.53 mg (mean $\pm$ SD) and 76.1 $\pm$ 35.2 g, respectively. Sixty-seven percent

of the subjects reported consuming less than 70% of the 1980 RDA
for vitamin B-6. E-ALAT coenzyme stimulation values >12% were
observed in 41% of the subjects and >16% for 17% of the subjects.
Prasad et al. (27) also estimated the vitamin B-6 intakes of females
18-45 years of age taking OC's but not supplementation. These
intakes were as follows: (mean + SEM) higher socioeconomic group
on Norinyl 1/50 and Ovral, 1.31 + 0.65 mg, 23 subjects, and 0.98 +
0.63 mg, 20 subjects respectively, and lower socioeconomic group
on Norinyl 1/50 and Ovral, 0.88 + 0.47 mg, 39 subjects, and 0.97 +
0.59 mg, 39 subjects, respectively. Dietary intakes of females on
OC's seem to be similar to those not on OC's; these intakes seem
to vary widely within the groups of all researchers.

ELDERLY

     Hampton et al. (33) estimated the reported vitamin B-6 intakes
of 17 males and 20 females above the age of 60 years living in
Virginia. Twenty-four hour interview recalls (food models and
cross-checking) followed by 48-hour food records were obtained.
The estimated vitamin B-6 and protein intakes of the males were
1.46 + 0.64 mg, mean + SD, and 88.0 + 48.5 g and of females, 1.06
+ 0.34 mg and 53.0 + 19.4 g. Approximately half of the females and
one-fifth of the males reported consuming less than 50% of the
1974 RDA for vitamin B-6, 90% of the females and 47% of the males
reported consuming less than 70% of the 1974 RDA, and all the
females and 88% of the males reported consuming less than the 1974
RDA. About one-fourth of the males and females had high E-ALAT
coenzyme stimulation values.

     Vir and Love (34) found that 102 hospitalized aged males
consumed 0.8 + 0.2 mg, mean + SD, vitamin B-6 and females 0.8 + 0.2
mg as indicated by 3-day weighing records; 18.6% of the subjects
consumed <0.66 mg vitamin B-6 daily. E-ALAT coenzyme stimulation
values greater than 15% were observed in 28.4% of the subjects.
Jacobs et al. (35) found that males and females over 65 years of
age consumed about 1.45 mg vitamin B-6 and 79.8 g protein over a
one week period.

PREGNANCY

     Unsupplemented diets consumed by 106 pregnant females 18-37
years of age contained an average of 1.24 mg vitamin B-6 (36).
Dietary information was obtained by 24-hour recalls and 3-day diet
records. Intakes less than the 1974 RDA seemed to result in lower
levels of vitamin B-6 as measured by S. uvarum in maternal serum
at delivery and cord serum than did higher intakes.

Eighteen of 26 pregnant subjects consumed ≤1.9 mg vitamin B-6 daily as indicated by 3 consecutive day food records (37). These subjects received 2.5, 4, and 10 mg pyridoxine hydrochloride supplementation. Plasma pyridoxal phosphate levels were maintained at the 4 mg supplementation level.

McGanity et al. (38) reported that pregnant women consumed 1.0 ± 0.5 mg, mean ± SD, vitamin B-6 daily. The usual diet of pregnant women according to Coursin and Brown contains about 1.5 mg of the vitamin (39). A large proportion of apparently normal pregnant women do not have adequate vitamin B-6 status as judged by standards for nonpregnant adults. These biochemical findings can usually be prevented by 6 or 10 mg pyridoxine hydrochloride supplementation (36,37,39-42). Inadequate data are available regarding vitamin B-6 requirements of pregnant women. The 1980 RDA, 2.6 mg, for vitamin B-6 takes into account the additional protein allowance of pregnancy. A higher vitamin B-6 allowance would necessitate supplementation. Presently available data are not considered as being sufficient to justify a higher recommendation (14).

LACTATION

West and Kirksey (43) found the dietary intake of vitamin B-6 to be 2.0 ± 0.6 mg, mean ± SD, for 19 females at various stages of lactation as indicated by 3 consecutive days of records; 6 subjects consumed less than the 1974 RDA for the vitamin. The vitamin B-6 status of the lactating female seems to be reflected in the vitamin content of her milk (43,44). Based upon vitamin B-6/protein ratios, the RDA of 2.5 mg allows the breast-fed infant to obtain an adequate amount of the vitamin (14).

A few other estimates of vitamin B-6 intakes have been published. Food mixtures representative of adult United States consumption contain about 1.5 mg of the vitamin (45). The adult human requirement can be satisfactorily met with 2-3 mg vitamin B-6 daily (46).

The nationwide food consumption survey of spring 1977 indicated that the mean vitamin B-6 intakes of females ≥15 years was 35-40% less than the RDA while boys and girls 12-14 years of age had mean intakes 7-22% less than the RDA (47). To the knowledge of this author, more specific data regarding these intakes are not yet available.

The consumption of diets containing suboptimal levels of vitamin B-6 is prevalent particularly in the elderly and in females of all ages. Most individuals reportly consume less vitamin B-6 than the RDA.

Few researchers studying vitamin B-6 status or requirements have estimated dietary intakes of the nutrient. The studies which have been published indicate that the vitamin B-6 requirements of individuals in the same age-sex group as reflected by various biochemical parameters varies greatly. This requirement seems also to be increased when diets high in protein are consumed. A ratio of 0.02 mg vitamin B-6/g protein consumed has been suggested for use in calculating allowances for the vitamin (48).

A few researchers (49-51) are now proposing that high performance liquid chromatographic (HPLC) techniques may more accurately quantitate the vitamin B-6 found in foods than the standard microbiological method thus making possible better estimates of dietary intakes. These newer methods would also allow for more valid estimates of human vitamin B-6 requirements.

LITERATURE CITED

1. Orr, M. L. (1969) Pantothenic acid, vitamin B-6, and vitamin B-12 in foods. USDA Home Econ. Res. Rep. No. 36, U.S. Government Printing Office, Washington, DC.
2. Meder, H. & Wiss, O. (1968) Vitamin B-6 group: Occurrence in foods. In: The Vitamins: Chemistry, Physiology, Pathology, Methods (Sebrell, W. H. & Harris, R. S., ed.), vol. 2, pp. 21-29, Academic Press, NY.
3. Polansky, M. M., Murphy, E. W. & Toepfer, E. W. (1964) Components of vitamin B-6 in grains and cereal products. J. Assoc. Off. Agric. Chem. 47, 750-753.
4. Toepfer, E. W., Polansky, M. M., Richardson, L. R. & Wilkes, S. (1963) Comparison of vitamin B-6 values of selected food samples by bioassay and microbiological assay. Agric. Food Chem. 11, 523-525.
5. Polansky, M. M. (1969) Vitamin B-6 components in fresh and dried vegetables. J. Am. Dietet. Assoc. 54, 118-121.
6. Meyer, B. H., Mysinger, M. A. & Wodarski, L. A. (1969) Pantothenic acid and vitamin B-6 in beef. J. Am. Dietet. Assoc. 54, 122-125.
7. Polansky, M. M. & Murphy, E. W. (1966) Vitamin B-6 components in fruits and nuts. J. Am. Dietet. Assoc. 48, 109-111.
8. Brin, M. (1978) Vitamin B-6: Chemistry, absorption, metabolism, catabolism, and toxicity. In: Human Vitamin B-6 Requirements, pp. 1-20, Nat. Acad. Sci., Washington, DC.
9. Edwards, M., Benson, E. & Storvick, C. A. (1963) Collaborative study of vitamin B-6 methodology. J. Assoc. Off. Agric. Chem. 46, 396-399.
10. Birdsall, J. J. (1975) Stability and availability of nutrients. In: Technology of Fortification of Foods, pp. 19-31, Nat. Acad. Sci., Washington, DC.

11. Christakis, G., ed. (1979) Nutritional assessment in health
     programs. Am. Public Health Assoc., Washington, DC.
12. Coursin, D. B. (1955) Symposium on frontiers of human nutri-
     tion in relation to milk; vitamin B-6 (pyridoxine) in milk.
     Q. Rev. Pediatr. 10, 2-9.
13. McCoy, E. E. (1978) Vitamin B-6 requirements of infants and
     children. In: Human Vitamin B-6 Requirements, pp. 257-271,
     Nat. Acad. Sci., Washington, DC.
14. Food & Nutrition Board, Nat. Res. Council, Nat. Acad. Sci.
     (1980) Recommended Dietary Allowances, 9th ed., pp. 96-106,
     Nat. Acad. Sci., Washington, DC.
15. Fries, M., Chrisley, B. & Driskell, J. Unpublished data.
16. Lewis, J. S. & Nunn, K. P. (1977) Vitamin B-6 intakes and
     24-hour 4-pyridoxic acid excretions of children. Am. J. Clin.
     Nutr. 30, 2023-2027.
17. Ritchey, S. J. & Feeley, R. M. (1966) The excretion patterns
     of vitamin B-6 and B-12 in preadolescent girls. J. Nutr. 89,
     411-413.
18. Kirksey, A., Keaton, K., Abernathy, R. P. & Greger, J. L.
     (1978) Vitamin B-6 nutritional status of a group of female
     adolescents. Am. J. Clin. Nutr. 31, 946-954.
19. Driskell, J. A., Geders, J. M. & Urban, M. C. (1976) Vitamin
     B-6 status of young men, women, and women using oral contra-
     ceptives. J. Lab. Clin. Med. 87, 813-821.
20. Deutsch, M. J., Duffy, D., Pillsbury, H. C. & Loy, H. W. (1963)
     Total diet study: B. Nutrient content. J. Assoc. Off. Agric.
     Chem. 46, 759-762.
21. Walker, M. A. & Page, L. (1975) Nutritive content of college
     meals. J. Am. Dietet. Assoc. 66, 146-152.
22. Chrisley, B. M. & Driskell, J. A. (1979) Vitamin B-6 status
     of adults in Virginia. Nutr. Rep. Intern. 19, 553-560.
23. Baker, E. M., Canham, J. E., Nunes, W. T., Sauberlich, H. E.
     & McDowell, M. E. (1964) Vitamin B-6 requirement for adult
     men. Am. J. Clin. Nutr. 15, 59-66.
24. Linkswiler, H. M. (1978) Vitamin B-6 requirements of men.
     In: Human Vitamin B-6 Requirements, pp. 279-290, Nat. Acad.
     Sci., Washington, DC.
25. Harding, R. S., Plough, I. C. & Friedmann, T. E. (1959) The
     effect of storage on the vitamin B-6 content of a packaged
     Army ration, with a note on the human requirement for the
     vitamin. J. Nutr. 68, 323-331.
26. Miller, L. T., Dow, M. J. & Kokkler, S. C. (1978) Methionine
     metabolism and vitamin B-6 status in women using oral contra-
     ceptives. Am. J. Clin. Nutr. 31, 619-625.
27. Prasad, A. S., Lei, K. Y., Oberleas, D., Moghissi, K. S. &
     Stryker, J. C. (1975) Effect of oral contraceptive agents
     on nutrients: II. Vitamins. Am. J. Clin. Nutr. 28, 385-391.
     (Number of subjects in each group obtained by personal commu-
     nication of June 24, 1980, with Lei.)

28. Donald, E. A., McBean, L. D., Simpson, M. H. W., Sun, M. F. &
     Aly, H. E. (1971) Vitamin B-6 requirement of young adult
     women. Am. J. Clin. Nutr. 24, 1028-1041.
29. Cheslock, K. E. & McCully, M. T. (1960) Response of human
     beings to low-vitamin B-6 diet. J. Nutr. 70, 507-513.
30. Shin, H. K. & Linkswiler, H. (1974) Tryptophan and methionine
     metabolism of adult females as affected by vitamin B-6
     deficiency. J. Nutr. 104, 1348-1355.
31. Brown, R. R., Rose, D. P., Leklem, J. E., Linkswiler, H. &
     Anand, R. (1975) Urinary 4-pyridoxic acid, plasma pyridoxal
     phosphate, and erythrocyte aminotransferase levels in oral
     contraceptive users receiving controlled intakes of vitamin
     B-6. Am. J. Clin. Nutr. 28, 10-19.
32. Leklem, J. E., Linkswiler, H. M., Brown, R. R., Rose, D. P. &
     Anand, C. R. (1977) Metabolism of methionine in oral contra-
     ceptive users and control women receiving controlled intakes
     of vitamin B-6. Am. J. Clin. Nutr. 30, 1122-1128.
33. Hampton, D. J., Chrisley, B. M. & Driskell, J. A. (1977)
     Vitamin B-6 status of the elderly in Montgomery County, VA.
     Nutr. Rep. Intern. 16, 743-750.
34. Vir, S. C. & Love, A. H. G. (1978) Vitamin B-6 status of the
     hospitalized aged. Am. J. Clin. Nutr. 31, 1383-1391.
35. Jacobs, A., Cavill, I. A. J. & Hughes, J. N. P. (1968)
     Erythrocyte transaminase activity: Effect of age, sex, and
     vitamin B-6 supplementation. Am. J. Clin. Nutr. 21, 502-507.
36. Roepke, J. L. B. & Kirksey, A. (1979) Vitamin B-6 nutriture
     during pregnancy and lactation: I. Vitamin B-6 intake, levels
     of the vitamin in biological fluids, and condition of the
     infant at birth. Am. J. Clin. Nutr. 32, 2249-2256.
37. Lumeng, L., Cleary, R. E., Wagner, R., Yu, P.-L. & Li, T.-K.
     (1976) Adequacy of vitamin B-6 supplementation during
     pregnancy: A prospective study. Am. J. Clin. Nutr. 29,
     1376-1383.
38. McGanity, W. J., Cannon, R. O., Bridgforth, E. B., Martin,
     M. P., Densen, P. M., Newbill, J. A., McClellan, G. S.,
     Christie, A., Peterson, J. C. & Darby, W. J. (1954) The
     Vanderbilt cooperative study of maternal and infant nutrition:
     VI. Relationship of obstetric performance to nutrition. Am.
     J. Obst. Gynec. 67, 501-527.
39. Coursin, D. B. & Brown, V. C. (1961) Changes in vitamin B-6
     during pregnancy. Am. J. Obstet. Gynecol. 82, 1207-1211.
40. Hamfelt, A. & Tuvemo, T. (1972) Pyridoxal phosphate and
     folic acid concentration in blood and erythrocyte aspartate
     aminotransferase activity during pregnancy. Clin. Chem. Acta
     41, 287-298.
41. Brown, R. R., Thornton, J. & Price, J. M. (1961) The effect
     of vitamin supplementation on the urinary excretion of trypto-
     phan metabolites by pregnant women. J. Clin. Invest. 40,
     617-623.

42. Cleary, R. E., Lumeng, L. & Li, T.-K. (1975) Maternal and fetal plasma levels of pyridoxal phosphate at term: Adequacy of vitamin B-6 supplementation during pregnancy. Am. J. Obstet. Gynecol. 121, 25-28.

43. West, K. D. & Kirksey, A. (1976) Influence of vitamin B-6 intake on the content of the vitamin in human milk. Am. J. Clin. Nutr. 29., 961-969.

44. Roepke, J. L. B. & Kirksey, A. (1979) Vitamin B-6 nutriture during pregnancy and lactation. II. The effect of long term use of oral contraceptives. Am. J. Clin. Nutr. 32, 2257-2264.

45. Booher, L. E. & Behan, I. T. (1949) Nutrient analyses of United States food supplies: Analyses of composited samples of our national food supplies and of the white flour and non-white flour components thereof in terms of various nutrients. J. Nutr. 39, 495-515.

46. Vilter, R. W., Mueller, J. F., Glazer, H. S., Jarrold, T., Abraham, J., Thompson, C. & Hawkins, V. R. (1953) The effect of vitamin B-6 deficiency induced by desoxypyridoxine in human beings. J. Lab. Clin. Med. 42, 335-357.

47. Pao, E. M. (1980) Nutrient consumption patterns of individuals, 1977 and 1965. Family Econ. Rev., Spring, 1980, pp. 16-20.

48. Dietary Standard for Canada (1975) Bureau of Nutr. Sci., Dept. Nat. Health & Welfare, Ottawa, Canada.

49. Gregory, J. F. (1980) Comparison of high-performance liquid chromatographic and Saccharomyces uvarum methods of the determination of vitamin B-6 in fortified breakfast cereals. J. Agr. Food Chem. 28, 486-489.

50. Lim, K. L., Young, R. W. & Driskell, J. A. (1980) Separation of vitamin B-6 components by high-performance chromatography. J. Chromatog. 188, 285-288.

51. Vanderslice, J. T., Maire, C. E. & Takupkovic, J. (1980) High performance liquid chromatographic analysis of vitamin B-6 in ready-to-eat breakfast cereals. Program of Institute of Food Technologists annual meetings, June 10, 139 abs.

ASSESSMENT OF VITAMIN B-6 STATUS IN INFANTS AND CHILDREN: SERIAL

PYRIDOXAL PHOSPHATE LEVELS IN PREMATURE INFANTS

Ernest E. McCoy, Robert Drebit, Ken Strynadka and
David Schiff

Department of Pediatrics
University of Alberta School of Medicine
Edmonton, Alberta, Canada

At the 1976 Workshop on Human Vitamin B-6 Requirements,
material was presented on which the present recommended allowances
for vitamin B-6 are based. As an introduction, parts of that work
will be presented, followed by work we have done over the past year
on plasma pyridoxal phosphate levels in premature infants.

Adult recommended dietary allowances (RDA) for vitamin B-6 are
based on studies where individuals were placed on vitamin B-6
restricted diets with varying protein intake until biochemical evidence of deficiency was present. The excretion of xanthurenic acid
after a tryptophan load was the principal test used for evidence
of vitamin B-6 deficiency. The amount of daily intake of vitamin
B-6 that normalized xanthurenic acid excretion was judged to be
adequate. The daily quantity of vitamin B-6 with varying protein
intake that normalized xanthurenic acid excretion and other biochemical tests of vitamin B-6 function was used in determining the
recommended dietary allowances for vitamin B-6 in adults (1-4). It
is not unexpected that similar types of studies have not been
carried out in children for determination of RDA despite the differences in rates of metabolism, growth, and body surface area that
exist.

One study was carried out which took advantage of accidental
vitamin B-6 depletion in a group of young infants due to a manu-
facturing process which resulted in a low vitamin B-6 content in
the formula (5). The principal signs of vitamin B-6 deficiency in
these infants were convulsions and irritability. The results of
providing formulas with normal vitamin B-6 content alone or with

additional vitamin B-6 supplementation showed that 0.26 mg/day
stopped seizures but that 1.0 to 1.2 mg/day were required to reduce
xanthurenic acid excretion to normal values for age. Two breast-
fed infants who developed vitamin B-6 responsive seizures required
1.0 to 1.4 mg/day of pyridoxine to reduce xanthurenic acid excretion
to normal values. In these limited number of vitamin B-6 deficient
infants, the amount of vitamin B-6 required to normalize xanthurenic
acid excretion was larger than current recommended dietary allowances for this age group, but the amount required to prevent
convulsions was similar to recommended allowances. These data are
shown in Table 1.

There are several publications which contain plasma pyridoxal
phosphate (PLP) values for children of varying ages (6-9). These
are random samples without information on vitamin B-6 intake. The
values are generally similar to accepted normal levels for adults
(10-12). For children, these have ranged from 6.2 ± 2.2 to $16.3 \pm$
5.6 ng/ml while for adults the values range from 7.5 ± 3.2 to
13.9 ± 2.4 ng PLP/ml plasma.

Recommended dietary allowance for infants and children range
from 0.015 to 0.025 mg vitamin B-6/g of protein intake (13). From
published values of vitamin B-6 content of breast milk and the
expected volume of milk consumed at varying ages, one can calculate
the vitamin B-6 intake of such infants. An illustrative calculation
is shown in Table 2 for breast-fed infants and in Table 3 for formula-
fed infants. Infants 0-3 months of age who are breast-fed, assuming
a vitamin B-6 content of 0.10 mg/l (14), would receive 0.006 mg/g
protein while formula-fed infants would receive 0.016 mg/g protein.
Data to be presented in the following section show that formula-fed
premature infants have higher plasma PLP values than breast-fed
infants. As the dietary intake of vitamin B-6 of the nursing
mother may vary, a longitudinal study relating maternal vitamin B-6
intake, breast milk vitamin B-6 content, and infant plasma PLP levels
would be of value to determine what are actual vitamin B-6 requirements for the breast-fed infant.

Although there are limitations to the use of plasma pyridoxal
phosphate levels as a reflection of adequacy of vitamin B-6 intake,
it is a more direct indicator of vitamin B-6 intake than the excretion of metabolites that have both vitamin B-6 dependent and non-
dependent steps in their formation.

Table 1. Summary of Biochemical Data Relative to the Nutritive Status of Vitamin B-6 in Infants With and Without Convulsions[a]

Group	Case No.	Diet	Vitamin B-6 Intake mg/day	Vitamin B-6 Required to Relieve Convulsions mg/day	Xanthurenic Acid Excretion mg/18 hr	Vitamin B-6 Required to Normalize Xanthurenic Acid Excretion mg/day
		Convulsions Related to Intake of Vitamin B-6				
A	1	SMA	0.085	0.26[b]	no test	no test
	2	SMA	0.085	0.26[b]	no test	no test
	3	SMA	0.085	0.26[b]	no test	no test
	4	SMA	0.085	0.26[b]	8[c]	no test
	5	SMA	0.085	0.26[b]	20-63	1.0-1.2
		Breast-Fed Infants				
B	6	human milk	?	0.26[b]	25-110	1.2-1.4
	7	human milk	0.067	0.26[b]	35-43	1.0
		Apparent Vitamin B-6 Dependent Seizures				
C	8	evaporated milk and pureed foods	0.3-0.4	5	18	0.4
	9	evaporated milk and pureed foods	0.3-0.4	2	c	

Table 1 (cont). Summary of Biochemical Data Relative to the Nutritive Status of Vitamin B-6 in Infants With and Without Convulsions[a]

Group	Case No.	Diet	Vitamin B-6 Intake	Vitamin B-6 Required to Relieve Convulsions	Xanthurenic Acid Excretion	Vitamin B-6 Required to Normalize Xanthurenic Acid Excretion
			mg/day	mg/day	mg/18 hr	mg/day
		Nonvitamin B-6 Related Seizures				
D	10	evaporated milk	0.26	ineffective	0	0.3-0.4
	10	SMA	0.085	ineffective	35-40	0.3-0.4
	11	evaporated milk and pureed foods	0.3-0.4	ineffective	0	
	12	evaporated milk and pureed foods	0.3-0.4	ineffective	0	
		Control Group				
E	13	evaporated milk	0.26		0	
	13	SMA	0.085		3-0	0.3-0.4
	14	evaporated milk	0.26		0	
	15	evaporated milk	0.26		0	
	16	evaporated milk and pureed foods	0.3-0.4		0	
	17	Mull-Soy	0.20		0	
	18	evaporated milk	0.26		0	
	19	fresh skim milk	0.50		0	
	20	Mull-Soy	0.20		53	5.0

Table 2.   Vitamin B-6 Intake of Breast-Fed Infants

Age	Milk Received	Protein Intake[a]	Milk Vitamin B-6 Content	Other Sources Vitamin B-6	Ratio Vitamin B-6/ Protein
	ml/day	g/day	µg/day	µg/day	mg/g
Birth	450	6.7	45	-	0.006
3 months	800	8.1 $\begin{cases} 8.1 \\ 0.5^b \end{cases}$	80 80	27	0.010 0.012
6 months	850	$\begin{cases} 7.4 \\ 7.0^c \end{cases}$	85	160	0.017

[a]Based on protein content in breast milk of 0.8 to 1.5 g/100 ml at ages shown.
[b]Protein content based on additional intake of three tablespoons (approximately 10 g) of rice cereal per day.
[c]Protein content based on average intake of cereal, meat, commercially prepared meat and vegetables, vegetables and fruit. Calculations based on nutrient content from Orr (17) and Foman (18).

Table 3.   Vitamin B-6 Intake of Formula-Fed Infants

Age	Milk Intake	Protein Intake[a]	Vitamin B-6 in Milk	Other Sources Vitamin B-6	Ratio Vitamin B-6/ Protein
	ml/day	g/day	µg/day	µg/day	mg/g
Birth	450	11.2	180	-	0.016
3 months	700	17.5 17.5[b] 0.5	280 280	- 27	0.016 0.017
6 months	900	22.5 7.0[c]	360	160	0.017
1 year	900	22.5 18.5[d]	360	460	0.020

[a]Based on average protein content of prepared infant formulas.
[b]Three tablespoons (approximately 10 g) of rice cereal.
[c]Based on intake of commercial infant foods of meat, meat and vegetables, and fruit.
[d]Based on intake of table foods: cereal, meat, vegetables, and fruit. Calculations based on nutrient content from Orr (17) and Church and Church (19).

The present study was undertaken to answer the question: what are the levels of plasma PLP in premature infants over a period of time when they are growing, being cared for, and fed in the usual manner in an intensive care unit? Premature infants were chosen for initial studies as they presented a variety of clinical problems within a facility which has the ability to accurately record their intake, medications, and clinical course. This regional center cares for small but otherwise well infants, infants with various congenital abnormalities, and infants with a variety of acute illnesses. In this nursery, the first choice for feeding is breast milk from the infant's mother, then pooled breast milk, and then the proprietory formulas PM 60/40 or Similac. The manufacturers state that vitamin B-6 content of PM 60/40 is 0.33 mg/l while for Similac it is 0.40 mg/l.

METHODS

Subjects and Selection

Blood was collected from a total of 46 infants. The majority of infants were sampled initially at day 3 and then sequentially on days 7, 10, 17, and 24. A few infants had samples taken on days 1-2 or 7-8. The size of the blood sample taken was approximately 0.2 ml, usually taken between 0700 and 1100 hours. The infants were either premature but well, premature but ill, small for gestational age but well and ranged in weight from 1100 to 2500 g. Full term ill infants were also studied.

Materials

The L-tyrosine apodecarboxylase method as described by Bhagavan et al. (15) for plasma PLP was used. A saturated 500 ml solution of unlabeled L-tyrosine was prepared in water and to this 20 μCi of L-(1-^{14}C) tyrosine (50 mCi/mM) was added. The solution was chilled, sonicated, and stored in the cold. A standard solution of PLP (Calbiochem) was prepared (1 mg to 20 ml water), the concentration determined in 0.1N NaOH by extinction coefficient, then stored in aliquots at -70° prior to use. The apodecarboxylase was prepared from freeze-dried Streptococcus faecalis cells (Worthington Biochem) by treatment of a slurry of 1 g of cells with 150 ml saturated $(NH_4)_2SO_4$ for 30 minutes, centrifugation of the cells, resuspension, and recentrifugation, then resuspension in buffer A (1.5 M potassium acetate, pH 5.5, 5 mM Na$_4$EDTA), brought to a final concentration of 0.5% β-mercaptoethanol, 0.033% L-tyrosine, and 20% glycerol. Aliquots of the suspension are frozen at -70° prior to use.

Collection and Preparation of Plasma

Blood is collected in heparinized tubes in a volume of 0.2-0.4 ml between 0800 and 1200 hours. The blood is stored in covered containers and processed within one hour. The plasma obtained is stored in a -70° freezer and assayed for PLP within a 2-week period. The specimens were extracted as described (15) in the cold and in subdued light. To 0.1 ml of plasma was added 20 μl of 50% perchloric acid (PCA) while vortexing. The precipitate obtained by centrifuging at 12,000 g for 10 minutes was homogenized with a loose-fitting pestle with 20 μl of 0.3 N PCA. The supernatants were combined and brought to pH of 5.5 with KOH to remove the perchlorate ion as potassium perchlorate. The mixture was chilled on ice for 45 minutes and the precipitate removed by centrifugation. The precipitate was washed once with buffer B (0.01 M potassium acetate, pH 5.5, 5 mM Na_4EDTA) and final volume of the combined supernatants recorded.

Assay

To ensure accuracy and reproducibility, the components of the assay are kept at $0-4^{\circ}$. Samples are run in duplicate and an enzyme blank is included to correct for endogenous PLP present in the enzyme test system.

The samples and standards are placed into 20 ml Erlenmeyer flasks, in a Dubnoff water bath. A final volume of 0.3 ml is obtained by the addition of H_2O. This is followed by 0.2 ml of enzyme-buffer solution (the enzyme solution is diluted with buffer A to get the desired enzyme activity in the aliquot used for the assay). The mixture of apoenzyme and PLP is incubated for 30 minutes at 37° in order to permit the penetration of PLP into the S. faecalis cells. After chilling in an ice-water bath, 0.5 ml of the L-(1-^{14}C) tyrosine suspension is then added and the flask is immediately stoppered with a septum containing a center well (both obtained from Kontes Glass Co.). The septums are folded down, the rack is removed from the icebath and incubated with shaking at 37° for 20 minutes in an AO shaking incubator. The flasks are removed at the end of the incubation and chilled immediately. The reaction is stopped by the injection of 1 ml 10% TCA to the mixture through the septum. NCS (0.3 ml; Amersham/Searle) is injected into the center well through the septum and the flasks are shaken for 30 minutes at 37° in the incubator. Following this, the flasks are removed, the septum taken out, and the center wells with the NCS are snipped off into plastic scintillation vials containing 10 ml of OCS (Amersham/Searle) counting fluid. The samples are counted in a liquid scintillation spectrometer. The sensitivity of the method is 50 picograms per reaction flask.

After correcting for the blank, the counts are plotted on a linear graph paper against the amount of PLP in the standard flasks.

RESULTS

Comparison of Breast- and Formula-Fed Infants

A comparison of PLP levels, a total of 46, in breast- or formula-fed infants at 3, 10, or 17 days after birth shows that at each of these days, plasma PLP levels are higher in formula compared to breast-fed infants. At day 3, the level of PLP in breast-fed infants was 2.28 ± 0.26 compared to 4.34 ± 0.87 ng/ml plasma in formula-fed infants ($P < .05$). Infants fed both breast and formula milk had PLP levels of 3.98 ± 1.13 ng/ml. By day 10, the plasma PLP level in breast-fed infants was 1.41 ± 0.34 while for formula-fed infants it had risen to 13.25 ± 3.29 ng/ml ($p < .005$). On day 17, PLP for breast-fed infants was 1.75 ± 0.70 and 25.84 ± 4.13 ng/ml for formula-fed infants ($p < .001$). These results are shown in Table 4.

Serial PLP Levels in Individual Infants

Baby Ha was born at 32 weeks gestation with a birth weight of 1531 g. An early onset of respiratory distress occurred, characterized by a respiratory rate of 50-60/minute with grunting. Cultures were taken from the throat and blood and were negative. The baby received supplemental oxygen, 20-30%, for 2 days. Recurrent periods of apnea occurred during the first 2 days, which were treated with intermittent iv aminophylline. The infant received partial maintenance for fluids with iv two-thirds saline solution. On day 1, small amounts of breast milk were taken; day 2, small amounts of PM 60/40; day 3 to day 10, breast milk; days 11 and 12, Similac 60/40; and days 13 to 24, breast milk. As shown in Fig. 1, plasma PLP varied from 1.1 to 3.8 ng/ml up to day 24. Similac replaced breast milk on day 25, and by day 31 PLP had risen to 17.3 ng/ml and to 36.4 ng/ml by day 38.

Baby Mac was born at 29 weeks gestation with a birth weight of 1300 g. At birth, severe bruising of face and head was noted. Within an hour, grunting respirations developed which required assisted ventilation. At 15 hours of age, severe cyanosis was noted and a bulging fontanelle. An intracranial hemorrhage was confirmed by CAT scan. He was given part of his fluid requirements by iv two-thirds glucose, one-third saline solution. Cardiac decompensation occurred on day 4 due to patent ductus arteriosus, which did not respond well to medical therapy and required ligation at age 10 days. Following the operation, his condition stabilized and the course was satisfactory. Feeding history showed breast milk was started at 24 hours of age and continued plus iv fluids to age

Table 4. Plasma PLP in Breast- and Formula-Fed Premature Infants

Source of Milk	Day 3	Day 10	Day 17
	ng/ml	ng/ml	ng/ml
Breast	2.28+0.26(N=15)	1.41+0.34(N= 9)	1.75+0.70(N=4)
Formula	4.34+0.87(N=11)	13.25+3.29(N=12)	25.8 +4.13(N=7)
Signif. B vs F	P <.05	P <.005	P <.001
Breast & Formula	3.98+1.13(N=11)	4.14+1.33(N=11)	8.31+1.91(N=7)

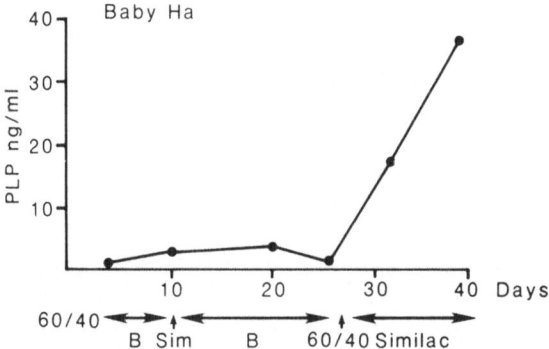

Fig. 1.   Baby Ha.   Determinations of plasma PLP were carried out
          on days marked by ● . Type of feeding given at different
          times is shown below the figure.

6 days. He received only iv fluids to day 10, then was on breast
milk without formula until day 56. Until Similac was started on
day 56, as shown in Fig. 2, PLP varied from undetectable to 2.1 ng/ml.
Eight days after starting Similac, plasma PLP level was 7.9 ng/ml.

Baby P was born at 37 weeks gestation with a birth weight of
2170 g. A gastroschisis which involved the whole bowel outside
the abdominal cavity was present. The infant underwent surgery on
the first day of life and had a primary repair on day 6. Parenteral
alimentation with glucose, lipids, and amino acids was started on
day 2 and continued until day 32. Oral feedings were then gradually
introduced and tolerated. A multivitamin solution containing from
1-3 mg/day of pyridoxine was administered. Plasma PLP level, as
shown in Fig. 3, on day 3 was 2.3 ng/ml; on day 10, 6.8 ng/ml;
day 17, 20.7 ng/ml; day 24, 38.4 ng/ml; and on day 32, 21.9 ng
PLP/ml plasma. This infant illustrates that when intravenous
alimentation is given under usual nursery conditions, adequate
amounts of vitamin B-6 are received to maintain normal plasma PLP
values.

Baby S "B" (Fig. 4) was one of twins of 30 weeks gestation,
with a birth weight of 1410 g. The infant had an uneventful course.
Breast milk was given for first day, PM 60/40 from day 2 to day 17,
Similac from day 17 onwards. Plasma PLP level on days 3 and 17
was 1.7 ng/ml; day 10, 5.5 ng/ml; day 17, 13.3 ng/ml; day 24, 29.4
ng/ml; and day 30, 41.4 ng/ml. These results show that formula
feeding will give PLP values seen in older infants and above normal
values by 3 weeks of age.

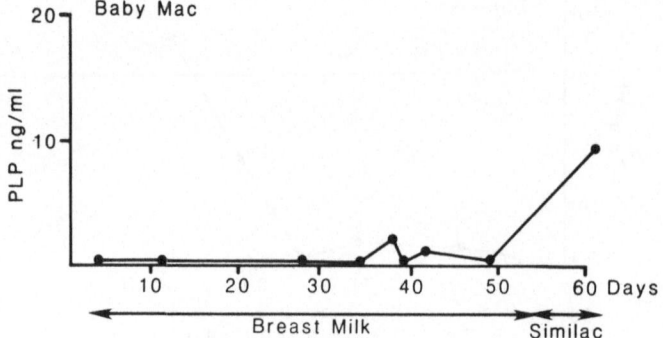

Fig. 2. Baby Mac. Serial plasma PLP determinations at times shown
by •. Duration of breast milk feeding is shown below the
figure.

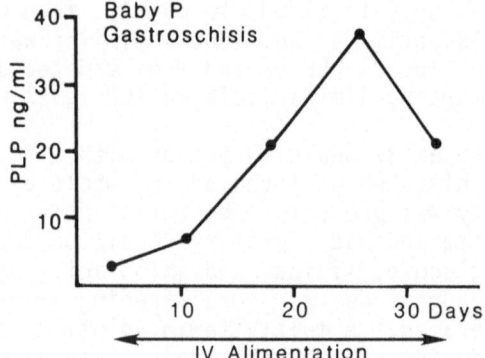

Fig. 3. Baby P. Serial plasma PLP determinations as shown by •
in an infant whose calorie intake was by parenteral
alimentation over the period shown.

DISCUSSION

The 1980 edition of Recommended Dietary Allowances (13) suggests
a vitamin B-6 intake of 0.3 mg/day for infants to 6 months of age
and 0.6 mg/day from 6 months to 1 year. At 3 months of age, an
infant totally breast-fed will receive between 80-100 µg of vitamin
B-6/day which will provide approximately 0.010 µg/g protein. The
totally formula-fed infant will receive approximately 0.3 mg of
vitamin B-6/day or 0.015 mg/g protein. Because of normal growth
and development of most breast-fed infants, serial determination of
plasma PLP would be of value with the view of determining whether
vitamin B-6 requirements for breast-fed infants are lower in the

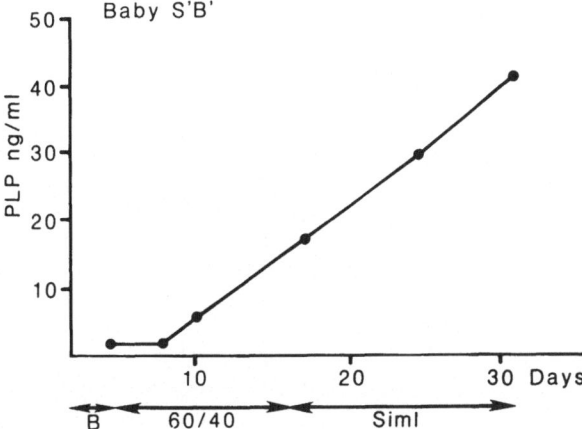

Fig. 4. Baby S "B". One of twins with uneventful course. Serial
         plasma PLP determinations on days as shown by ●. Duration
         of different types of feeding shown below the figure.

early months of life compared to formula-fed infants. The provi-
sion of optimal amount of vitamin B-6 to young infants is important
because of their rapid growth--particularly of brain in view of
neural defects produced by vitamin B-6 deficiency in developing
rats (16).

     The objective of the study of premature infants was to deter-
mine serial plasma PLP levels under the usual conditions in which
these infants are cared for and fed. The studies are of benefit to
the infant in determining whether supplemental vitamin B-6 be given.
The studies are done in a controlled environment where careful
recording of data pertaining to intake and clinical condition of
the infant as well as optimal care is carried out.

     The level of plasma PLP in formula-fed infants by 3 weeks of
age generally exceeded 20 ng/ml and frequently went as high as 30-
40 ng/ml compared to published values for children of 5-16 ng/ml.
There is no apparent toxicity due to these levels of PLP in infants
and indeed much higher levels have been reported in children
receiving pharmacological amounts of vitamin B-6 for hyperactivity
(6,9) without evident ill effects.

     Further studies will be required for longer time periods in
these formula-fed premature infants as well as in full-term infants
to determine whether these observed high levels of PLP in plasma
may be due to immaturity in storage or metabolism of PLP, or is
associated with the amounts of vitamin B-6 present in commercial
formulas.

It was an unexpected finding that the majority of breast-fed infants had plasma PLP levels under 2.0 ng/ml. One infant had a level of 3.2 ng/ml but another infant did not exceed 2.0 for a month, and for more than a week had undetectable plasma PLP levels. All but one infant increased plasma PLP when placed on commercial formula, indicating there was not a problem in absorption of the vitamin. These observations raise a troublesome question whether the observed PLP levels are physiologically correct for premature infants or whether the amount of vitamin B-6 in breast milk is insufficient for the majority of premature infants. Further studies will be necessary to answer this question.

Individual case studies during which the infant developed sepsis or other types of severe illness were accompanied by a decrease in plasma PLP levels. These findings suggest that there may be an increased requirement for vitamin B-6 during such periods of stress. If further studies confirm these individual observations, consideration may need to be given to increase vitamin B-6 intake during such periods.

These initial studies indicate that although controlled studies in which vitamin B-6 depletion is induced and then replenishment carried out are not ethically possible in children; clinical observations and serial sampling may provide data which may be used to confirm the present recommendations for vitamin B-6 requirements or suggested changes for specific age groups.

LITERATURE CITED

1. Baker, E. M., Canham, J. E., Nunes, W. T., Sauberlich, H. E. & McDowell, M. E. (1964) Vitamin B-6 requirements for adult men. Am. J. Clin. Nutr. 15, 59-66.
2. Canham, J. E., Baker, E. M., Hardin, R. S., Sauberlich, H. E. & Plough, I. C. (1969) Dietary protein - Its relation to vitamin B-6 requirements and function. Ann. N.Y. Acad. Sci. 166, 16-29.
3. Cinnamon, A. D. & Beaton, J. R. (1970) Biochemical assessment of vitamin B-6 status in man. Am. J. Clin. Nutr. 23, 696-702.
4. Miller, L. & Linkswiler, H. (1967) Effect of protein intake in the development of abnormal tryptophan metabolism by men during vitamin B-6 depletion. J. Nutr. 93, 53-59.
5. Bessey, O. A., Adam, D. J. D. & Hansen, A. E. (1957) Intake of vitamin B-6 and infantile convulsions: A first approximation of vitamin B-6 requirements of pyridoxine in infants. Pediatrics 20, 33-44.

6. Bhagavan, H. N., Coleman, M. & Coursin, D. B. (1975) Distribution of pyridoxal-5-phosphate in human blood between the cells and plasma: Effect of oral administration of pyridoxine on the ratio in Down's and hyperactive patients. Biochem. Med. 14, 201-208.

7. Reinken, L., Zieglauer, H. & Berger, H. (1976) Vitamin B-6 nutriture of children with acute celiac disease, celiac disease in remission and of children with normal duodenal mucosa. Am. J. Clin. Nutr. 29, 750-753.

8. Barlow, G. B. & Wilkinson, A. W. (1975) Plasma pyridoxal phosphate levels and tryptophan metabolism in children with burns and scalds. Clin. Chim. Acta 64, 78-82.

9. Bhagavan, H. G., Coleman, M. & Coursin, D. B. (1975) The effect of pyridoxine hydrochloride on blood serotonin and pyridoxal phosphate content in hyperactive children. Pediatrics 55, 437-441.

10. Cleary, R. E., Lumeng, L. & Li, T.-K. (1975) Maternal and fetal levels of pyridoxal phosphate at term: Adequacy of vitamin B-6 supplementation during pregnancy. Am. J. Obst. & Gyn. 121, 25-28.

11. Spannuth, C. L., Warnock, L. G., Wagner, C. & Stone, W. J. (1977) Increased plasma clearance of pyridoxal-5-phosphate in vitamin B-6 deficient uremic men. J. Lab. Clin. Med. 90, 632-637.

12. Hamfelt, A. (1967) Pyridoxal phosphate concentration and aminotransferase activity in human blood cells. Clin. Chim. Acta 16, 19-28.

13. Recommended Dietary Allowances (1980) 9th ed., p. 96, Nat. Acad. Sci., Washington, DC.

14. Roepke, J. & Kirksey, A. (1979) Vitamin B-6 nutriture during pregnancy. II. The effect of long-term use of oral contraceptives. Am. J. Clin. Nutr. 32, 2257-2264.

15. Bhagavan, H. N., Koogler, J. M. & Coursin, D. B. (1976) Enzymic microassay of pyridoxal-5'-phosphate using L-tyrosine apodecarboxylase and L-(1-^{14}C) tyrosine. Internat. J. Vit. Nutr. Res. 46, 160-164.

16. Davis, S. D., Nelson, T. & Shepard, T. H. (1970) Teratogenicity of vitamin B-6 deficiency: Omphalocoele, skeletal and neural defects and splenic hypoplasia. Science 169, 1329-1330.

17. Orr, M. L. (1969) Pantothenic acid, vitamin B-6 and vitamin B-12 in foods. Consumer and Food Economics Research Division, ARS/USDA Home Econ. Res. Rep. No. 36, U.S. Government Printing Office, Washington, DC.

18. Foman, S. J. (1974) Infant Nutrition, W. B. Saunders Co., Philadelphia, PA.

19. Church, C. F. & Church, H. N. (1975) Food Values of Portions Commonly Used, 12th ed., J. B. Lippincott Co., Philadelphia, PA.

THE VITAMIN B-6 CONTENT IN HUMAN MILK

Avanelle Kirksey, Judith L.B. Roepke and Lynn M. Styslinger

Department of Foods and Nutrition
Purdue University
West Lafayette, IN 47907

Vitamin B-6 is known to be a critical dietary factor, especially during the development of the central nervous system in human infants (1-4). Findings from rat experiments in our laboratory showed decreased vitamin B-6 content in brain of progeny of vitamin B-6 deficient mothers and this paralleled low levels of vitamin B-6 in the mother's milk (5). The content of myelin lipids, gangliosides, and cerebrosides in brain of progeny during the suckling period paralleled maternal intake of vitamin B-6 (6). Myelination in the mediodorsal portion of the pyramidal tract was reduced (7) and Purkinje cell monolayer arrangement in cerebellum was abnormal (8) during early postnatal development in progeny of vitamin B-6 deficient rats. Quantitative electron microscopy of axon diameters in the ventral funiculus portion of spinal cord of suckling progeny of deficient rats showed fewer large axons with decreased number of myelin lamellae compared to controls (9). The far-reaching consequences of vitamin B-6 inadequacy during early infancy on the developing central nervous system are evident from both human and animal studies. More data are needed concerning the level of vitamin B-6 provided to the infant in human milk and the factors which can influence the level. Recently, the American Academy of Pediatrics (10) recommended that human milk be used as the sole source of nutrients for the infant during the first four to six months. In view of this recommendation, efforts should be intensified to assess the nutrient composition and volume of human milk as it relates to infant needs.

Current information concerning the level of vitamin B-6 in human milk and the effect of changes in vitamin B-6 on the concentration of the vitamin in milk is based on data from six published investigations (11-16). These studies show that the vitamin B-6 content of human milk is influenced by vitamin B-6 intake (11-16), stage of lactation (14,16), and vitamin B-6 nutritional status (14, 15, Kirksey et al., unpublished data).

RESPONSE TO CHANGES IN VITAMIN B-6 INTAKE

Vitamin B-6 content in human milk responds rapidly to changes in vitamin B-6 intake since regulatory mechanisms are apparently not present for maintaining the concentration of the vitamin within definite limits. Karlin (11) observed that within one hour after an intramuscular injection of pyridoxine was given to five lactating women, the level of the vitamin in milk rose to six times the initial level. The highest concentration, ten times the original level, was reached three hours after the injection. After 24 hours, the concentration of vitamin B-6 in milk was more than three times the initial level and did not return to the original level for 5 to 7 days. Similarly, Karlin (11) found that following oral administration of a single large dose of pyridoxine (500 and 1000 mg) to three lactating subjects, the vitamin passed rapidly into milk. Approximately three hours after the oral dose, a peak of 9,000 to 11,500 μg vitamin B-6/l milk was reached or about 100 times the initial level. The vitamin content decreased rapidly in the next 9 hours but remained elevated for 2 to 7 days at about twice its original level. The investigator postulated that reserves of vitamin B-6 were reduced by pregnancy and that this resulted in low levels of the vitamin in milk and modified the effect of excess vitamin. She suggested that a continued saturation with the vitamin resulted in accumulation in the milk before the concentration decreased if vitamin administration was continued.

In contrast to the high elevations of vitamin B-6 in milk following a large dose of the vitamin, extremely low levels of the vitamin have been observed in milk when the intake of vitamin B-6 is low. In this laboratory, West and Kirksey (12) observed that vitamin B-6 was less than 50 μg/l in milk of a subject whose dietary intake of vitamin B-6 was estimated to be 1.4 mg/day, and who did not take extra-dietary sources of the vitamin. At birth the infant of this woman suffered mild periodic seizures which were diagnosed as resulting from hypoglycemia. The mother had used oral contraceptives for a period of 3-1/2 years prior to her pregnancy, and this, in addition to the low dietary intake of vitamin B-6, could have interfered with the coenzyme functions of pyridoxal phosphate resulting in vitamin B-6 inadequacy that was reflected in milk.

This woman secreted less than 4% of her daily intake of vitamin B-6 (1.4 mg) into milk (0.05 mg/1). The inability of mammary gland to concentrate vitamin B-6 in milk when the intake of the vitamin is deficient seems evident from these data.

Preliminary studies from our laboratory (Kirksey and Styslinger, unpublished data) suggest, as Karlin (11) postulated earlier, that vitamin B-6 reserves modified the effect of excess vitamin B-6 by a prolonged period of elevation of the vitamin level in milk before returning to baseline. Data for subjects D and E (Table 1) from Karlin's study (11) showed elevations of vitamin B-6 in milk, ten times the initial level, at 12 to 13 hours after a large oral dose of pyridoxine. These subjects were reported to have low reserves of vitamin B-6 following pregnancy. Similarly, data from our laboratory (Table 1) showed differences in the elevation of the vitamin in milk 12-13 hours after a 20 mg dose of pyridoxine was given to subject B compared to subject C. Since early gestation, subject B took a 2 mg/day pyridoxine supplement which possibly increased her vitamin B-6 reserve, whereas subject C had no extra-dietary sources of vitamin B-6 prior to the supplement. Vitamin B-6 levels in milk from subject B elevated more slowly and peaked at a lower level on the first day a 20 mg oral dose of the vitamin was taken compared to the response of subject C. The level of vitamin B-6 in milk of subject B was near baseline 12-13 hours after the dose, whereas the level for subject C was twice the original level (Figs. 1 and 2).

Rat experiments (6) also indicate that the vitamin B-6 content in milk responds rapidly to changes in vitamin B-6 intake. Low levels of vitamin B-6 in milk of deficient rats were restored to control levels or higher within 30 minutes following an ip injection of 600 g pyridoxine, within 6 hours following a change from a deficient diet to one containing 60 mg pyridoxine/kg or within 24 hours following a change to 30 mg pyridoxine/kg diet. In deficient animals, the elevation of the vitamin was prolonged after a single large dose of pyridoxine was given ip. Furthermore, 5 days after 30 to 60 mg pyridoxine/kg diet was fed to deficient dams, the elevation of vitamin B-6 in their milk was almost twice control levels.

INFLUENCE ON VITAMIN B-6 INTAKE OF INFANTS

Kirksey and Styslinger (unpublished data) determined infant intakes of vitamin B-6 from volume measurements estimated by differences in infant weights prior to and after a feeding (Figs. 1 and 2). The increase in weight of infants was taken to represent the weight of milk consumed and from specific gravity measurements of the milk samples, volume was calculated. Samples of milk from each

Table 1. Vitamin B-6 Content in Milk of Individual Subjects Before and After Receiving Different Doses of Pyridoxine

Subject	Day	Pyridoxine Dose mg	Vitamin B-6 Content of Milk					Investigator
			Before Dose µg/l	Peak			After Dose 12-13 Hr µg/l	
				µg/l	Δ µg/l	hr		
A		IM 50	135	1300	1165	3	475	Karlin[a]
		Oral						
B		2	200	425	225	5-1/2	300	Kirksey & Styslinger[b]
	1	20	450	1325	875	5-1/2	525	
	2	20	400	1175	775	5-1/2	475	
C	1	20	450	1475	1025	4-1/2	900	Kirksey & Styslinger[b]
	2	20	375	1375	1000	3-1/2	510	
D		500	100	9750	9650	3	1000	Karlin[a]
E		1000	100	11,500	11,400	3	1000	Karlin[a]

[a]Reference 11.
[b]Unpublished data.

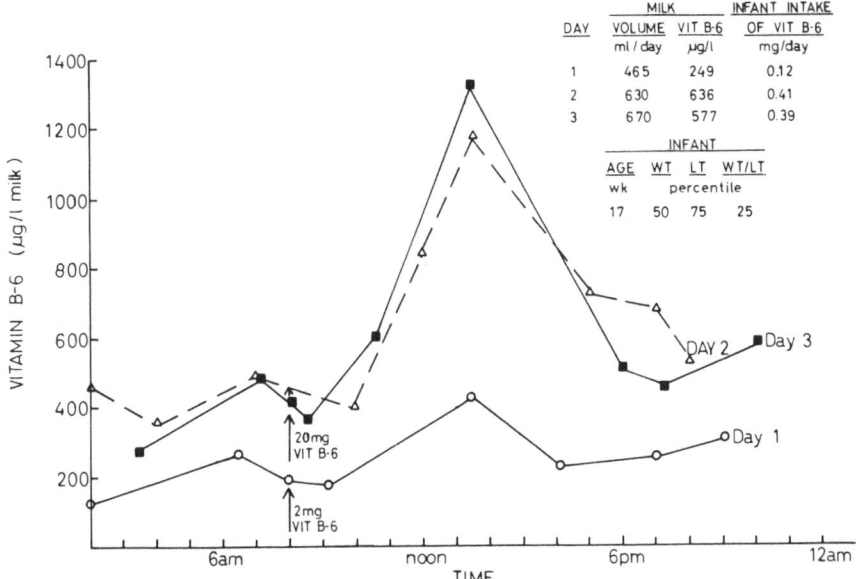

Fig. 1. Vitamin B-6 content in milk of subject B obtained at each infant feeding time for 24 hours after taking 2 or 20 mg oral supplements of pyridoxine.

feeding were analyzed for vitamin B-6 content, and this was multiplied by volume of intake to obtain vitamin B-6 intakes of infants. The infant of subject B had an estimated vitamin B-6 intake of 0.12 mg/day when a maternal supplement of 2 mg of pyridoxine was taken. The infant's intake was increased to 0.39 and 0.41 mg vitamin B-6/day on two days when the mother took a 20 mg pyridoxine supplement (Fig. 1). Subject C's infant consumed only 0.05 and 0.08 mg vitamin B-6/day on two days when no maternal supplement was taken, whereas the infant's intake was 0.50 and 0.37 mg/day on the two days when the mother took a 20 mg pyridoxine supplement (Fig. 2). When single samples of milk, obtained at an early morning feeding, were analyzed for vitamin B-6 content and an assumed milk volume of 850 ml was used for calculation of the infant's daily intake of vitamin B-6, the values approximated those obtained by test-weighing the infant at each feeding for 24 hours to estimate milk volume and measurement of the vitamin B-6 content in samples from each feeding during the 24-hr period. The maternal supplement appeared to affect significantly the level of vitamin B-6 for 2 to 3 feedings of the infant's 6 to 8 feedings during a 24-hr period (Figs. 1 and 2). The baseline for vitamin B-6 content of milk before and after the peak level following supplementation was higher for mothers who took vitamin supplements compared to values observed when supplements were not taken.

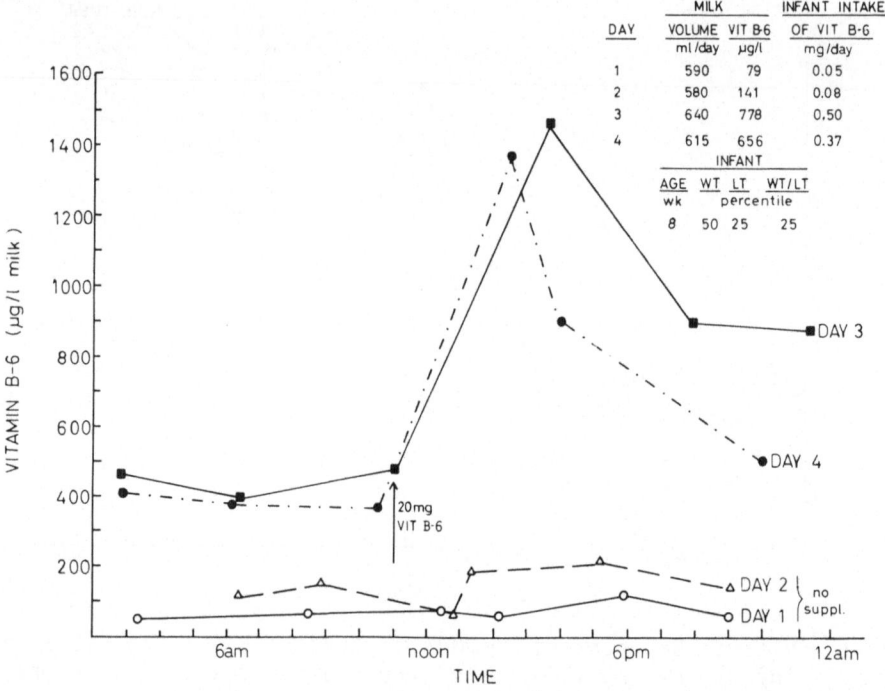

Fig. 2.   Vitamin B-6 content in milk of subject C obtained at each
          infant feeding time for 2 days prior to pyridoxine supple-
          mentation and for 2 days after taking a 20 mg oral
          supplement.

Milk volume for subjects B or C was not altered by the 20 mg
pyridoxine supplement. This is in contrast to Greentree's (17)
warning that vitamin B-6 is a lactation-inhibiting vitamin and
should be excluded from multi-vitamin supplements for nursing
mothers. His warning was based on pharmacological doses of pyridoxine (200 to 600 mg orally or 300 mg iv) which have been purported
to have hypoprolactinemic effects in the suppression of lactation
(18). However, reports are conflicting as to whether even pharmacologic doses of pyridoxine decrease prolactin levels in normal
women or those with galactorrhea-amenorrhea syndrome (19-21). Two
studies were done during the puerperium in women who chose not to
breast-feed their infants. One study showed that 600 mg pyridoxine
daily was more effective than a placebo in suppressing lactation
(20), whereas another study using the same dose failed to show any
effect (21). Prolactin levels were not measured in either study.
Rivlin (22) points out that there is no evidence that physiologic
doses of vitamin B-6 (2 to 10 mg) as contained in major prenatal
formulations have hypoprolactinemic or antilactogenic effects and

that it is misleading to refer to vitamin B-6 as a lactation-inhibitor. Findings from our laboratory in which 20 mg pyridoxine supplements were used are in agreement with this opinion.

INFLUENCE OF STAGE OF LACTATION

Kirksey and West (13) reported that the vitamin B-6 content in human milk was not significantly affected by the stage of lactation. However, all of the subjects who participated in their study were at 6 weeks or a later stage of lactation when milk would be mature, except one subject who was at 4 weeks lactation. In subsequent experiments in this laboratory, Roepke and Kirksey (14) observed that the vitamin B-6 content in milk was reduced markedly in colostrum at 3 days postpartum and in transitional milk at 14 days postpartum compared to values for mature milk obtained after 4 to 6 weeks lactation (Table 2). The mean level of vitamin B-6 in milk increased from 16 µg/l on day 3 to 57 µg/l on day 14 and then to ≂200 µg/l at 6 weeks. Karlin (11) reported that milk contained only 10-20 g vitamin B-6/l during the first few days of lactation and noted that levels rose to 100 µg/l in mature milk. Thomas et al. (16) reported that levels of vitamin B-6 in milk at 5-7 days postpartum (128 µg/l) were lower than values for mature milk at 43-45 days (204 µg/l) when no vitamin B-6 supplements were taken by the subjects. The values reported by these investigators at 5 to 7 days were higher than those reported by Karlin (11) or Kirksey and West (13).

The ratio of vitamin B-6 to protein content in milk was markedly lower at 3 and 14 days lactation than at 4 weeks or later stages of lactation (Table 2). The ratio of vitamin B-6/protein (µg/g) increased from ≤ 1.0 at 3 days to >15 at 6 weeks or later stages of lactation. The relationship between the amounts of these nutrients in milk is important in infant feeding since vitamin B-6 needs are known to increase with increments in dietary protein. During early lactation when levels of vitamin B-6 are low in milk, the infant appears to be protected by high concentrations of the vitamin in blood. Levels of vitamin B-6 in cord serum were observed to be 2- to 3-fold that in maternal serum at delivery (14,15).

Relationships between the levels of vitamin B-6 in plasma and milk at two stages of lactation, 3 days and 6 weeks, are shown in Table 3. The ratio of vitamin B-6 concentration in milk to that in plasma was less than 1 in colostrum at 3 days, whereas at 6 weeks the ratio exceeded 7. This indicated a greater concentration of vitamin B-6 by mammary gland in later lactation compared to earlier stages.

Table 2.   Effect of Stage of Lactation on Vitamin B-6
           Content in Human Milk When Intakes Were
           ≥2.5 mg Vitamin B-6 Per Day

Stage of Lactation	Subjects	Vitamin B-6 Content	
		Milk	Protein
	No.	µg/l	µg/g
Days[a]			
3	42	16 + 3	0.8 + 0.2
14	35	57 + 7	4.6 + 0.7
Weeks[b]			
4	27	186 + 30	13 + 2
6	25	226 + 30	16 + 3
Months[c]			
3	6	257 + 31	26 + 2
3-7	6	294 + 60	26 + 11
7	4	248 + 59	26 + 3

[a]Reference 14.
[b]Kirksey et al., unpublished data.
[c]Reference 13.

Table 3.   Effect of Stage of Lactation on the Levels
           of Vitamin B-6 in Plasma, Milk and Milk/
           Plasma Ratio When Vitamin B-6 Intakes Were
           ≥2.5 mg Per Day

Vitamin B-6 Measurements	Stage of Lactation	
	3 Days[a]	6 Weeks[b]
Plasma, ng/ml	16.5[c] +2.4	40.4[d] +7.0
Milk, µg/l	16.1 +3.0	226 +38
Milk/Plasma Ratio	0.98 +0.12	7.6 +1.3

[a]Reference 14.
[b]Kirksey and Roepke, unpublished data.
[c]Mean + SE for 33 subjects.
[d]Mean + SE for 27 subjects.

Kirksey and Styslinger (unpublished data) found that the vitamin B-6 content in milk from mothers of preterm infants (27-36 week gestational age at birth) was similar to that in milk from mothers of term infants (40 week gestational age at birth) (Table 4). However, during early lactation, milk of mothers of preterm infants appeared more resistant to concentration changes in response to vitamin B-6 supplementation. All values represented a 24-hr pooled milk collection. After 14 days postpartum, the effects of vitamin B-6 supplements in increasing the vitamin content of milk were demonstrated clearly in all 24-hr pooled milk samples.

INFLUENCE OF LEVEL OF VITAMIN B-6 INTAKE

West and Kirksey (12) classified 19 human subjects according to three levels of vitamin B-6 intake <2.5, 2.5-5.0, and >5.0 mg/day in order to determine whether the level of vitamin B-6 intake influenced the content of the vitamin in milk. All subjects were ≥4 week stage of lactation. Subjects consuming the lowest intake of vitamin B-6 (<2.5 mg/day) had the lowest mean level of vitamin B-6 in milk (129 + 37 µg/l). This level of vitamin B-6 in milk was significantly lower than the means of the other groups but was higher than the average level of vitamin B-6 in human milk (100 µg/l) reported by Karlin (11) and Macy and Kelly (23). However, investigators are not in agreement regarding the average level of vitamin B-6 in human milk. Values are generally higher in milk from women who take vitamin B-6 supplements than for those who do not take supplements. West and Kirksey (12) observed a significant correlation (r = 0.65) between levels of vitamin B-6 intake ranging from 1.3 to 12.5 mg/day and concentrations of the vitamin in milk. The mean vitamin B-6/protein ratio in milk was significantly lower for subjects with the lowest vitamin intake. The mean ratio was <13 µg vitamin B-6/g protein for subjects who consumed <2.5 mg vitamin B-6 daily. In order to satisfy the metabolic requirements of infants, a vitamin B-6/protein ratio of 15 µg/g has been recommended. West and Kirksey (12) observed that four of six subjects consuming less than 2.5 mg vitamin B-6/day had ratios less than 15 µg vitamin B-6/g protein.

Kirksey and West (13) found no significant differences in the mean values of vitamin B-6 content in the milk of five subjects who took no pyridoxine supplements and who were grouped according to six different times of feeding on two consecutive days. However, marked diurnal changes in vitamin B-6 content in milk were found among subjects who took vitamin B-6 supplements. Minimal and maximal values of individual subjects who took supplements ranged from 100 to 447 µg vitamin B-6 per liter of milk at different feedings. When the dietary intake of vitamin B-6 was inadequate and no extra dietary sources of the vitamin were taken, this was reflected in low levels of the vitamin in milk.

Table 4. Vitamin B-6 Concentration in Milk at Different Stages of Lactation of Vitamin B-6 Unsupplemented and Supplemented Mothers of Term and Preterm Infants

Vitamin B-6 Supplement	Gestational Age	Subjects	Stage of Lactation					
			Day				Week	
			7	14	21	28	6	8
mg/day		no.	vitamin B-6 concentration, μg/l milk					
none	term[a]	7	63 ±10	104 ±22	114 ±16	110 ±13		
none	preterm[b]	7	77 ±12	104 ±13	144 ±16	129 ±18	199 ±22	186 ±23
5	term	6	143[c] ±16	278[d] ±27	327[d] ±37	213[d] ±30		
5	preterm	5	84[c] ±18	132[c] ±17	264[d] ±40	280[d] ±36	302[d] ±40	357[d] ±35

[a] 40 weeks gestational age at birth.
[b] 27-36 weeks gestational age at birth
[c] P < 0.05 different from later stages of lactation.
[d] P < 0.05 different from corresponding unsupplemented group.

Work from this laboratory (15) indicated that vitamin B-6 intakes $\leq$ 2.5 mg/day resulted in significantly lower levels of vitamin B-6 in both maternal serum and milk at 3 days without a significant effect on the milk/serum ratio compared to values for women whose vitamin intakes exceeded 2.5 mg/day. The milk/serum ratio was maintained at approximately one. By 14 days postpartum, the level of vitamin in milk was lower in the group with low vitamin intake but the mean was not significantly different from that of mothers whose intake of the vitamin was higher. These findings suggested that an intake of vitamin B-6 $\geq$ 2.5 mg/day was needed to ensure optimal infant nutrition without compromising maternal resources.

Recently, Kirksey and Roepke (unpublished data) determined the vitamin B-6 content in milk at 2, 4, and 6 weeks of lactation for subjects who took daily supplements of vitamins containing 2.5, 5, 10, or 15 mg pyridoxine (Table 5). Dietary intakes of vitamin B-6 were not assessed but these could increase vitamin B-6 intake by 1.5-2.5 mg/day. Milk samples were obtained at an early morning feeding before vitamin B-6 supplements were taken. At 2 and 4 weeks lactation, vitamin B-6 content in milk was significantly less for subjects taking 2.5 mg/day pyridoxine supplements compared to those taking 15 mg/day supplements. At 2 weeks all supplemented groups, excepting the 15 mg group, had significantly lower levels of vitamin B-6 in milk compared to values for the same subjects taking the same level of supplement at 6 weeks of lactation when milk was mature. Pyridoxine supplements ranging from 2.5 to 15 mg/day did not significantly alter the vitamin B-6 content in milk at 6 weeks (Table 5). Also, plasma vitamin B-6 and milk/plasma ratios of the vitamin were not significantly affected by the four levels of pyridoxine supplementation. The reason for the apparent lack of effect of the level of pyridoxine supplements on milk values at 6 weeks lactation is related to the time of obtaining the milk samples. All samples were obtained at an early morning feeding before vitamin supplements were taken. Hence, only the residual effects of pyridoxine supplements on the level of vitamin B-6 in milk were evident. The residual effects were similar among levels of supplements ranging from 2.5 to 15 mg pyridoxine/day. These findings are in agreement with those of Kirksey and West (13) that levels of vitamin B-6 observed in mature milk, obtained at an early morning feeding, did not differ when intakes of vitamin B-6 ranged from 2.5 to 12.5 mg/ day. However, recent studies (Kirksey and Styslinger, unpublished data) of vitamin B-6 content in 24-hr pooled milk samples (Table 4) and of daily vitamin B-6 intakes of breast-fed infants indicated that different levels of maternal supplements of vitamin B-6 ranging from 2 to 20 mg resulted in significant differences in infant intakes (Figs. 1 and 2).

Table 5. Vitamin B-6 Content in Milk and Plasma of Women Taking Different Levels of Pyridoxine·HCl Supplements at Various Stages of Lactation

Stage of Lactation	Pyridoxine·HCl Supplement (mg/day)			
	2.5	5	10	15
Week	μg vitamin B-6/1 milk[a]			
2	$75^{b,c}$ ±15	122^{c} ±21	147^{c} ±25	220 ±30
4	106^{b} ±26	147 ±21	231 ±48	307 ±79
6	160 ±57	214 ±23	246 ±41	294 ±30
	ng vitamin B-6/ml plasma[a]			
6	34.5 ±11.1	26.9 ±3.3	43.4 ±10.4	46.6 ±8.3
	milk/plasma ratio[a]			
6	4.5 ±0.9	9.9 ±2.3	6.5 ±1.8	6.9 ±0.3

[a]Mean $\pm$ SE for $\geq$ 6 subjects.
[b]$P<0.05$ different from corresponding 15 mg supplemented group.
[c]$P<0.05$ different from 6 week stage of lactation.

INFLUENCE OF VITAMIN B-6 NUTRITIONAL STATUS

Kirksey and Susten (24,25) examined the effects of five different levels of dietary pyridoxine (1.2, 2.4, 4.8, 9.6, or 19.6 mg/kg) fed to rats during growth, gestation, and lactation on milk composition and on the vitamin saturation of muscle, liver, and milk. Three major components of milk--fat, carbohydrate, casein or non-casein protein--were not affected by the levels of pyridoxine fed. The lowest level, 1.2 mg pyridoxine/kg diet, appeared adequate for synthesis of these macronutrients in milk. Vitamin B-6 concentration in muscle reached apparent saturation at 2.4 mg pyridoxine/kg diet and in liver at 4.8 mg vitamin/kg diet, the values were almost twice those in muscle and liver of rats fed 1.2 mg vitamin/kg. However, milk continued to increase in vitamin B-6 content to 9.6 mg vitamin/ kg diet and at this intake, levels of the vitamin in milk were threefold that of rats fed the lowest level of vitamin. Vitamin B-6 content in milk continued to increase when vitamin intake was 2- to 4-fold that needed for saturation of liver or muscle. Conversely, when the diet was inadequate, milk appeared to have less priority for vitamin B-6 than liver or muscle tissue and was an earlier indicator of vitamin B-6 inadequacy.

Subsequent experiments with lactating rats (Felice and Kirksey, unpublished data) indicated that following a short period (6 days) of vitamin B-6 deficiency during lactation, the vitamin B-6 content in milk decreased to less than 20% of control values. In muscle, the concentration was not significantly altered by the short period of dietary inadequacy and in liver, the content was only slightly decreased (Fig. 3). Liver and muscle tissues of lactating rats apparently failed to release vitamin B-6 to milk following the short period of deficiency of the vitamin. The early failure of these tissues to supply vitamin B-6 to milk, when vitamin B-6 intake is inadequate, supported our previous postulation that milk was an earlier indicator of impending vitamin B-6 inadequacy than liver or muscle tissue.

Vitamin B-6 nutritional status appears to influence significantly the vitamin B-6 content in human milk. This is supported by the findings of Roepke and Kirksey (15) that maternal nutritional status, assessed by the level of vitamin B-6 in maternal serum at 5 months gestation, was significantly correlated ($r = 0.51$) with the level of vitamin B-6 in milk at 14 days postpartum (Fig. 4). These data suggested that the fifth month of gestation was an appropriate time for assessment of maternal vitamin B-6 nutriture. This period in gestation precedes the peak of hemodilution (26) that is known to alter the concentration of the vitamin in serum and also precedes the period of most rapid growth of the central nervous system when vitamin B-6 is known to be crucial to normal development.

Previous long-term use (>30 months) of oral contraceptives (OCA) was associated with reduced levels of vitamin B-6 in maternal serum, cord serum, and milk (14). Low levels of vitamin B-6 in both maternal serum at delivery and in cord serum were found among women who had used OCA for >30 months (Fig. 5). The mean level of vitamin B-6 in maternal serum in early postpartum was only 4.8 ng/ml for long-term OCA users or 30% that of nonusers, 15.7 ng/ml. The ratio of vitamin B-6 in cord serum to maternal serum was higher at delivery for long-term OCA users (4.2) compared to values for nonusers (3.4). This suggested a drain of maternal reserves of vitamin B-6 to the fetus, and this was reflected in a significant decrease in levels

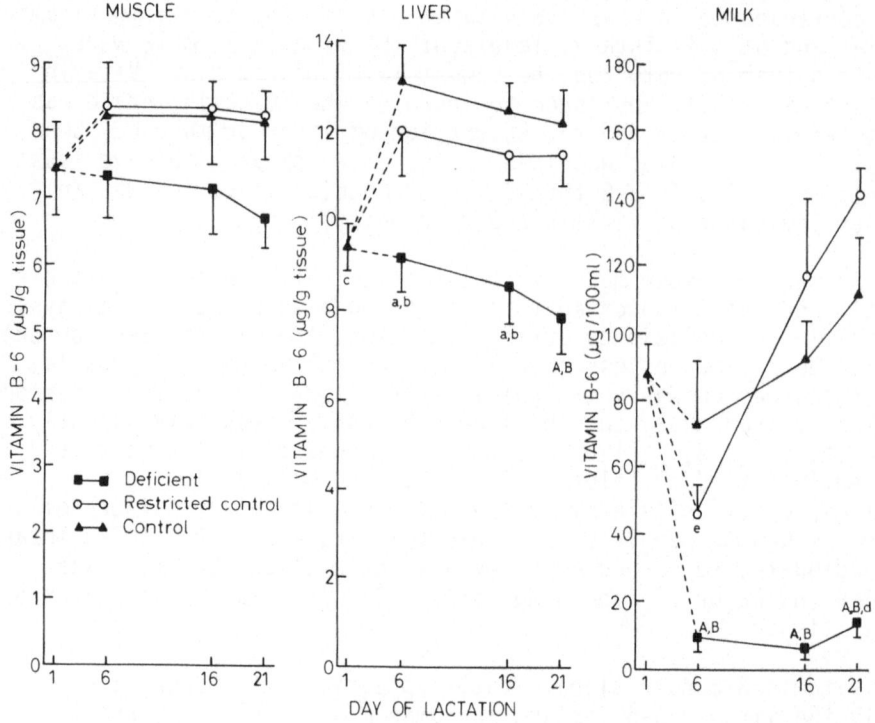

Fig. 3.   Vitamin B-6 concentrations in muscle, liver, and milk on
          1, 6, 16, and 21 days of lactation in rats fed control,
          restricted control, or vitamin B-6 deficient diets from
          day 1 of lactation. Vertical bars represent mean ± SE
          for seven rats.

of vitamin B-6 in maternal serum. The shunting of vitamin B-6 from
maternal serum to the fetus by women, who were long-term users of
OCA, suggested an adaptive response to vitamin B-6 inadequacy in
an attempt to protect the developing fetus.

     Levels of vitamin B-6 in milk were not significantly different
in the early postpartum period (3 days) among women grouped according
to OCA use but were significantly different at 14 days postpartum.
At this time, levels of vitamin B-6/liter of milk were 65'.4 µg for
nonusers, 48.7 µg for short-term OCA users, and 26.6 µg for long-
term OCA users (Fig. 6). Levels of vitamin B-6 in milk were significantly lower for long-term OCA users than short-term users or
nonusers of OCA. Vitamin B-6 content in milk of long-term OCA users
was approximately one-half that of nonusers. At 14 days postpartum,

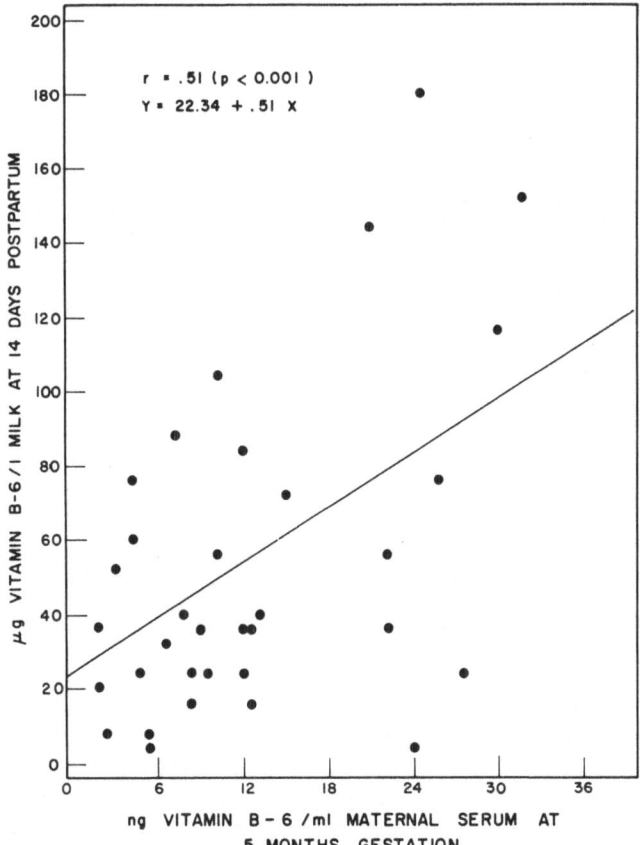

Fig. 4.   Relationship between levels of vitamin B-6 in milk at 14
          days postpartum and in serum at 5 months gestation of 34
          subjects (from Ref. 14 with permission).

the ratio of vitamin B-6/protein in milk was significantly lower for
long-term OCA users than nonusers. The ratio was only 2.2 for OCA
users compared to 5.3 for nonusers, and this raises questions about
the adequacy of vitamin B-6 to protein content in milk of long-term
OCA users.

     Roepke and Kirksey (14) observed that levels of vitamin B-6 in
milk at 3 and 14 days postpartum were significantly lower for mothers
whose infants had unsatisfactory Apgar scores (<7) at 1 minute after
birth compared to values for mothers whose infants had satisfactory
ratings (Table 6). These data strongly suggested that vitamin B-6
nutritional status was poorer for mothers whose infants had low
Apgar scores than for mothers whose infants received acceptable
ratings. Vitamin B-6 levels in maternal serum at delivery were

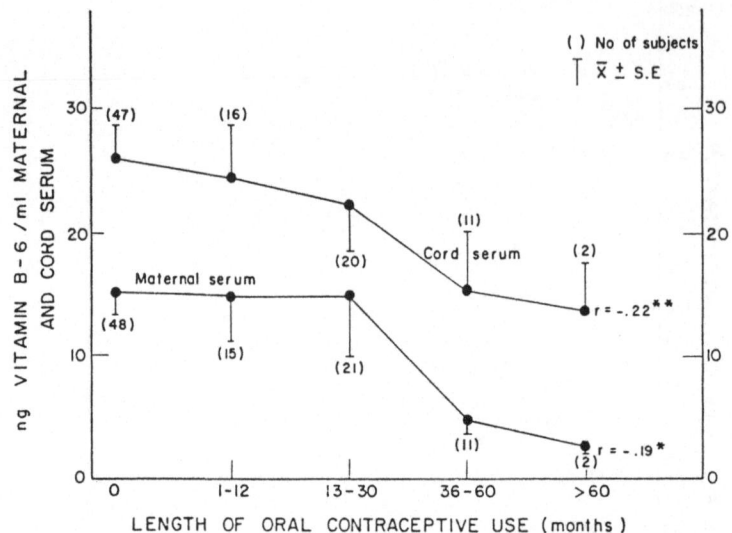

Fig. 5. Levels of vitamin B-6 in maternal and cord serum at delivery
         associated with length of oral contraceptive (OCA) use.
         *p < 0.03 maternal serum and OCA use; **p < 0.01 cord serum
         and length of OCA use (from Ref. 15 with permission).

significantly lower among women whose infants had low Apgar score
at 1 minute after birth compared to values for mothers whose infants
had acceptable scores. The significantly higher cord/maternal serum
ratio of vitamin B-6 among mothers of infants with low Apgar scores
suggested a shunting of maternal reserves to the fetus. The mean
intake of vitamin B-6 (4.2 mg/day) by the 16 women whose infants
had low Apgar scores was considerably greater than the RDA of
2.5 mg/day. These findings suggested that intakes of vitamin B-6
greater than 4 mg/day may be needed on a regular basis by some
women during pregnancy.

SUMMARY

      The vitamin B-6 content in human milk responds quickly to
changes in vitamin B-6 intake since regulatory mechanisms are
apparently not present for maintaining the concentration of the
vitamin within definite limits. Concentrations of the vitamin in
milk are influenced by stage of lactation, vitamin B-6 intake, and
by vitamin B-6 nutritional status. In future investigations of the
vitamin B-6 content in human milk, some factors which should be
ascertained are: (1) Stage of lactation; (2) Quantity and time
of ingestion of foods rich in vitamin B-6; (3) Use, quantity, and
time of vitamin B-6 supplementation; (4) Time of milk sampling

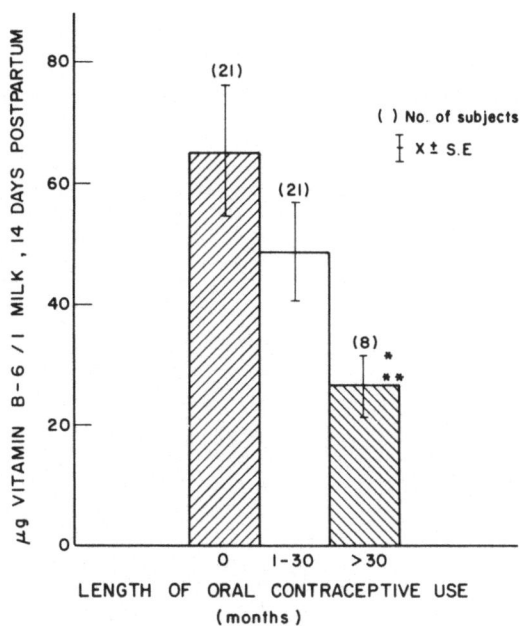

Fig. 6. Levels of vitamin B-6 in milk at 14 days postpartum in
         relation to length of OCA use. *p <0.02 different from
         1-30 months OCA use; **p<0.003 different from no OCA use
         (from Ref. 15 with permission).

particularly in relation to vitamin B-6 intake (diet and/or supplements); (5) Use of oral contraceptives or other drugs which may
interfere with the normal function of vitamin B-6; and (6) Vitamin
B-6 nutritional status.

ACKNOWLEDGMENT

     Supported in part by USPH Grant HD-11996.

Table 6.   Maternal Vitamin B-6 Intake and Levels of the Vitamin
in Biological Fluids Associated with Apgar Scores < 7
and ≥7 for the Infant[a]

	Apgar Scores at 1 Minute		Significance
	< 7	≥ 7	
	mg/day		
Vitamin B-6 Intake	4.2[b] +0.7	6.7[c] +0.7	P <0.01
	ng vitamin B-6/ml		
Maternal Serum, Delivery	7.8 +2.5	15.5 +2.0	P <0.02
Cord Serum	19.6 +3.1	24.8 +1.9	ns
Cord/Maternal Serum Ratio	5.1 +1.4	2.9 +0.3	P <0.01
	µg vitamin B-6/l		
Milk 3 days postpartum	8.6 +1.3	16.0 +3.1	P <0.03
14 days postpartum	31.1 +7.9	57.4 +7.0	P <0.01

[a] Reference 14 with permission.
[b] Mean for 16 to 18 subjects.
[c] Mean for 73 to 81 subjects.

LITERATURE CITED

1. Snyderman, S. E., Holt, E., Carretero, R. & Jacobs, K. (1953) Pyridoxine deficiency in the human infant. Am. J. Clin. Nutr. 1, 200-207.
2. Coursin, D. B. (1954) Convulsive seizures in infants with pyridoxine-deficient diets. J. Am. Med. Assoc. 154, 406-408.
3. Coursin, D. B. (1955) Vitamin B-6 deficiency in infants. Am. J. Dis. Child. 90, 344-348.
4. Molony, C. J. & Parmelee, A. H. (1954) Convulsions in young infants as a result of pyridoxine deficiency. J. Am. Med. Assoc. 154, 405-406.
5. Pang, R. L. & Kirksey, A. (1974) Early postnatal changes in brain composition in progeny of rats fed different levels of dietary pyridoxine. J. Nutr. 104, 111-117.
6. Thomas, M. R. & Kirksey, A. (1976) Influence of pyridoxine supplementation on vitamin B-6 levels in milk of rats deficient in the vitamin. J. Nutr. 106, 509-514.
7. Morré, D. M., Kirksey, A. & Das, G. D. (1978) Effects of vitamin B-6 deficiency on the developing central nervous system of the rat. Myelination. J. Nutr. 108, 1260-1265.
8. Morré, D. M., Kirksey, A. & Das, G. D. (1978) Effects of vitamin B-6 deficiency on the developing central nervous system of the rat. Gross measurements and cytoarchitectural alterations. J. Nutr. 108, 1250-1259.
9. Kirksey, A., Morré, D. M., Rohrer, S. & Wasynczuk, A. (1980) Effect of vitamin B-6 deficiency on the developing spinal cord of the rat: myelination. Fed. Proc. 39, 797.
10. American Academy of Pediatrics, Nutrition Committee of the Canadian Paediatric Society and the Committee on Nutrition of the American Academy of Pediatrics. (1978) Breast-Feeding. Pediatrics 62, 591-601.
11. Karlin, R. (1959) Effet d'un enrichissement en pyridoxine sur la teneur en vitamin B-6 du lait de femme. Bull. Soc. Chim. Biol. 41, 1085-1091.
12. West, K. D. & Kirksey, A. (1976) Influence of vitamin B-6 intake on the content of the vitamin in human milk. Am. J. Clin. Nutr. 29, 961-969.
13. Kirksey, A. & West, K. D. (1978) Relationship between vitamin B-6 intake and the content of the vitamin in human milk. In: Human Vitamin B-6 Requirements, pp. 238-251, Nat. Acad. Sci., Washington, DC.
14. Roepke, J. L. B. & Kirksey, A. (1979) Vitamin B-6 nutriture during pregnancy and lactation. I. Vitamin B-6 intake, levels of the vitamin in biological fluids, and condition of the infant at birth. Am. J. Clin. Nutr. 32, 2249-2256.

15. Roepke, J. L. B. & Kirksey, A. (1979) Vitamin B-6 nutriture during pregnancy and lactation. II. The effect of long-term use of oral contraceptives. Am. J. Clin. Nutr. 32, 2257-2264. 2264.

16. Thomas, M. R., Kawaimoto, J., Sneed, S. M. & Eakin, R. (1979) The effects of vitamin C, vitamin B-6, and vitamin B-12 supplementation on the breast milk and maternal status of well-nourished women. Am. J. Clin. Nutr. 32, 1679-1685.

17. Greentree, L. B. (1979) Dangers of vitamin B-6 in nursing mothers. New Eng. J. Med. 300, 141-142.

18. Foukas, M. D. (1973) An antilactogenic effect of pyridoxine. J. Obstet. & Gynaecol. Br. Commonw. 80, 718-720.

19. De Waal, J. M., Steyn, A. F., Harms, J. H. K., slabber, C. F. & Pannall, P. R. (1978) Failure of pyridoxine to suppress raised serum prolactin levels. S. African Med. J. 53, 293-294.

20. McIntosh, E. N. (1976) Treatment of women with the galactorrhea-amenorrhea syndrome with pyridoxine (vitamin B-6). J. Clin. Endocrinol. & Metab. 42, 1192-1195.

21. Goodenow, T. J. & Malarkey, W. B. (1979) Ineffectiveness of pyridoxine in evaluation and treatment of the hyperprolactinemic amenorrhea-galactorrhea syndrome. Am. J. Obstet. Gynecol. 133, 161-164.

22. Rivlin, R. S. (1979) Letter to the Editor. New Eng. J. Med. 300, 927.

23. Macy, I. C. & Kelly, H. J. (1961) Human milk and cow's milk in infant nutrition. In: Milk: The Mammary Gland and Milk Secretion (Koh, S. A. & Cowle, A. T., eds.), vol. 2, pp. 265-304, Academic Press, New York.

24. Kirksey, A. & Susten, S. S. (1978) Influence of dietary pyridoxine on lactation in the rat. J. Nutr. 108, 104-112.

25. Kirksey, A. & Susten, S. S. (1978) Influence of different levels of dietary pyridoxine on milk composition in the rat. J. Nutr. 108, 113-119.

26. Hytten, F. E. & Thomson, A. M. (1970) Maternal physiological adjustments. In: Maternal Nutrition and the Course of Pregnancy, p. 43, Nat. Acad. Sci., Washington, DC.

PLASMA PLP AS INDICATOR OF NUTRITION STATUS: RELATIONSHIP TO TISSUE VITAMIN B-6 CONTENT AND HEPATIC METABOLISM

Ting-Kai Li and Lawrence Lumeng

VA Medical Center & Departments of
Medicine and Biochemistry
Indiana University School of Medicine
Indianapolis, IN 46223

In assessment of nutritional status, diagnostic indicators should correlate in a well-defined manner not only with tissue content but also with the functional adequacy of the substance in question. Ideally, they would measure undernutrition as well as storage capacity. It is fortunate in the instance of vitamin B-6 that both the storage and the coenzyme (functional) forms are the same compounds, viz., the phosphorylated derivatives, pyridoxal phosphate (PLP) and pyridoxamine phosphate (PMP). These coenzyme forms are interconvertible via transamination reactions, but different tissues and body fluid compartments contain different amounts and ratios of PLP and PMP, presumedly reflecting regional peculiarities and dependence for the function of certain PLP-specific enzymes and binding proteins. Accordingly, if plasma PLP concentration is to serve as a diagnostic indicator, its relationship to the PLP (and PMP) content of tissues and to the activities of representative PLP-dependent enzymes must be delineated under conditions of both vitamin B-6 deficiency and excess. Furthermore, because the liver is the principal, if not the sole, organ that supplies blood plasma with PLP (1), the dependence of PLP and other B-6 vitamers in plasma upon hepatic metabolism needs to be understood. This communication summarizes recent studies from our laboratory and those of others that address these issues.

TISSUE AND PLASMA PLP CONTENT DURING VITAMIN B-6 DEFICIENCY AND EXCESS

It has been demonstrated by a number of investigators that PLP and PMP are the predominant forms of vitamin B-6 in mammalian tissues (2-4). Pyridoxine-P normally occurs in trace amounts and the non-phosphorylated B-6 vitamers constitute less than 10% of the total vitamin B-6 content. The liver is particularly rich in both PLP and PMP, but skeletal muscle, by virtue of its total mass, represents the single, largest repository of vitamin B-6 in the body. Of note, the PMP/PLP ratio varies widely from one tissue to another: that in brain, liver, and skeletal muscle of male rats fed regular laboratory chow is 1.9, 1.0, and 0.2, respectively (Table 1). Similar data have been reported for mice (4). In contrast to these tissues, the PLP and PMP content of blood plasma is considerably lower. The concentration of PLP in the plasma of human subjects ingesting a regular diet is approximately 75 nM or 75 pmol/ml. That for PMP is only about 5 nM (Table 1). The PMP/PLP ratio of blood plasma, therefore, more closely resembles that of skeletal muscle than that of liver and brain.

The relationship of plasma PLP concentration to the PLP content of liver, brain, and skeletal muscle has been studied in the rat as a function of vitamin B-6 intake (5). Male weanling rats were fed ad libitum for 9 weeks purified diets that supplied 0, 4, 12, 24, and 100 µg of PN daily. Growth increased with increasing PN intake to a maximum plateau at 24 µg/day. Liver and brain PLP content also increased, attaining maximal values at 12 µg/day intake. By contrast, muscle and plasma PLP content did not saturate even

Table 1. PLP and PMP Content of Liver, Skeletal Muscle, Brain, and Blood Plasma

	n	PLP	PMP	PMP/PLP
		nmol/g	nmol/g	
B-6-Sufficient Rat				
Liver	8	30.8 ± 7.1^a	32.0 ± 7.4	1.0
Muscle	6	21.8 ± 6.1	4.6 ± 2.1	0.2
Brain	5	5.7 ± 1.6	9.8 ± 1.1	1.9
		pmol/ml	pmol/ml	
Human				
Blood plasma	6	75.1 ± 19.6	3.0 ± 6.0	0.1

[a]Mean $\pm$ SD.

when PN intake was 100 µg/day. A strong linear correlation between the PLP content of plasma and muscle was obtained. The difference in the PLP content of brain, liver, muscle, and plasma between the groups with the most deficient (0 µg/day) and the highest intake (100 µg/day) was 37%, 56%, 70%, and 92%, respectively. Thus, brain was the most refractory to change in PLP content, whereas, plasma PLP concentration was the most responsive to changes in B-6 nutritional status. These data are consistent with the notion that both plasma and skeletal muscle function as repositories for vitamin B-6, capable of storing PLP during excessive intake and of releasing it to other issues, such as brain and liver, during dietary deprivation.

The plasma pool of PLP is unique in this regard, since it is also the major transport form of the B-6 vitamers in the circulation.

The above study also examined the effect of dietary PN deficiency and excess upon the holo- and apoenzyme activities of erythrocytic and hepatic aspartate and alanine aminotransferases and of hepatic tyrosine aminotransferase and serine dehydratase. Different patterns of change in enzyme activity and coenzyme saturability were observed, suggesting that factors other than coenzyme availability, such as apoenzyme stability and coenzyme affinity, also importantly affect activity. The holoenzyme activity of erythrocytic alanine aminotransferase was found to correlate best with the changes in plasma and muscle PLP content and PN intake (5).

Certain proteins appear to function uniquely in vitamin B-6 storage and transport. In blood plasma, almost all of PLP is bound to albumin. The binding capacity of albumin in plasma greatly exceeds the levels of PLP attainable even with pharmacologic doses of vitamin B-6 intake (1). In skeletal muscle, 90% or more of the PLP is associated with glycogen phosphorylase (6,7). Muscle phosphorylase activity is lowered in B-6-deficient animals (8-10) and, with an excess intake of PN, both muscle PLP content and glycogen phosphorylase activity increase proportionately (6). Interestingly, however, it was found recently that muscle glycogen phosphorylase activity of PN-loaded rats does not decrease with vitamin B-6 depletion until signs and symptoms (e.g., anorexia) of deficiency become severe. Rather, total or partial starvation elicited a prompt decline in activity, indicating responsiveness to signals from catabolic demand (11). Therefore, unlike PLP in plasma, muscle PLP cannot be readily mobilized for transfer to other tissues during periods of vitamin B-6 deprivation unless there is a concurrent caloric deficit. In contrast to plasma and muscle wherein almost all of the PLP is bound to single proteins, the liver contains a number of major PLP-binding proteins. It has been determined that only about 10% of the PLP in liver is associated with glycogen phosphorylase and that cytosolic aspartate and alanine aminotransferases account for 7-16% of total hepatic PLP content (7). Vitamin B-6 deficiency preferentially depletes PLP in cytosolic fraction (7).

DEPENDENCE OF PLASMA B-6 VITAMER COMPOSITION AND CONTENT ON HEPATIC METABOLISM

Although PLP constitutes more than 50% of the B-6 vitamers in human blood plasma, substantial quantities of nonphosphorylated forms, in particular PL, are also present as well as 4PA, the metabolically inactive degradation product of vitamin B-6. In a recent study (12), the B-6 compounds in the plasma of 6 healthy human subjects were measured before and after the oral administration of 100 mg PN·HCl daily for 1-3 weeks (Table 2). In individuals consuming an unsupplemented, regular diet, PLP and 4PA were the most abundant B-6 compounds in plasma, followed by PL and PN. Very little PMP and PM were detected. After one week of PN supplementation, the plasma concentrations of PLP, PL, and 4PA all increased 5-fold or more, whereas little or no change in the concentration of PM, PN, and PMP were observed. Similar results were obtained after 3 weeks of PN supplementation. These data indicate that orally administered PN is rapidly metabolized and converted to PLP, PL, and 4PA, and that all 3 of these compounds in plasma rapidly attain new steady-state levels, commensurate with the increased intake.

Table 2. Plasma B-6 Compounds in Human Blood Plasma
Before and After Oral Supplementation with
Pyridoxine (100 mg daily for 1 week)

	Before Supplementation	After Supplementation
	nM	nM
PLP	75.1 ± 19.6^a	406.0 ± 27.1
PL	19.0 ± 7.7	119.7 ± 19.3
PMP	3.0 ± 6.0	5.3 ± 4.1
PM	6.3 ± 2.9	7.0 ± 6.1
PN	20.3 ± 14.9	16.7 ± 14.8
4PA	51.6 ± 13.0	274.2 ± 29.3

[a]Mean $\pm$ SD, N = 6.

Because the liver plays a pivotal role not only as the supplier of PLP for circulation but also in PLP degradation (1,13), the hepatic metabolism and release of vitamin B-6 compounds were studied in isolated rat hepatocytes prepared from fed, B-6-sufficient rats (12). The cells, 1 g/15 ml, were incubated for 2 hours in Krebs-Henseleit medium containing 2.5% bovine serum albumin and 10 mM glucose, in the presence of 3.3 µM PN. At zero time, the cells contained about 35 nmol PLP and 25 nmol PMP. The content of all other B-6 compounds was very low. When the hepatocytes were incubated in the absence of PN, the cellular PLP content decreased slightly, accountable almost entirely by the PLP (6 nmol) and small amounts of PL and 4PA released into the medium. PMP content did not change. Incubation in the presence of PN prevented the decline in cellular PLP, and 6-8 nmol each of PLP, 4PA, and PL were released into the medium. The amounts of PMP and PM in the medium remained negligible. Thus, of the 50 nmol of PN added to the incubation mixture, about 21 nmol were converted to PLP, PL, and 4PA, and about 26 nmol remained unmetabolized. These results in vitro with isolated hepatocytes, therefore, mimic the changes in plasma PLP, PL, and 4PA concentrations seen with PN supplementation of human subjects.

Studies employing ^{14}C-PN confirmed the above results but allowed, in addition, the evaluation of miscibility of endogenous and newly synthesized pools of the B-6 compounds in liver. It was found that the specific radioactivity of PLP and PMP within the hepatocytes was less than 20% of that of PN added to the medium. This enormous dilution of radioactive counts indicates that the intracellular endogenous pools of PLP and PMP are not readily miscible with newly synthesized compounds. By contrast, the specific radioactivity of PLP in the medium was the same as that of PN, indicating that newly synthesized PLP is preferentially released into the ambient medium by hepatocytes from B-6-sufficient animals. The specific radioactivity of PL and 4PA in the medium was approximately two-thirds that of PN and 3- to 4-fold higher than that of endogenous PLP. Thus, newly synthesized PLP is more susceptible than endogenous PLP to degradation to PL and 4PA, both of which are also released into the medium.

The above studies permit the following conclusions: (a) PLP and PMP are the major endogenous B-6 compounds in liver cells and their intracellular content is tightly regulated such that excess amounts of these coenzymes do not accumulate in the presence of nonphosphoylated B-6 precursors. Previous experiments in vivo have yielded the same conclusion for both liver and brain (5). (b) Newly synthesized PLP and PMP do not exchange freely with the endogenous pools of the coenzymes in B-6-sufficient animals and, to a large extent, constitute a rapidly mobilizable pool destined for degradation to PL and 4PA and for secretion into the circulation. PLP, PL, and 4PA, but not PMP and PM, are the principal B-6 compounds released by liver.

PLASMA PLP MEASUREMENTS IN HUMAN NUTRITION STUDIES

Plasma PLP measurements have been considered by many investigators to be a sensitive and reliable indicator of vitamin B-6 nutritional status (14-18). The concentration in plasma remains constant over time with little fluctuation when subjects are ingesting regular (unsupplemented), restricted, or B-6-supplemented diets (1,12,18). It is not affected by the menstrual cycle or by the chronic use of oral contraceptive agents in most individuals (18,19). When the dietary content of vitamin B-6 is altered, the plasma PLP concentration decreases or increases commensurate with dietary intake to reach new steady-state levels within 3-4 weeks (18). The $t_{1/2}$ of intravenously administered PLP in normal man is 8.0 ± 1.6 h ($\pm$ SEM) and plasma clearance rate is 31.7 ± 2.7 ml/min (20).

The plasma PLP concentration of apparently healthy subjects ingesting unregulated and unsupplemented "normal" diets is 49.8 $\pm$

1.2 ($\pm$ SEM) pmol/ml (21,22). An age-related decline has been
observed in these population studies. It is decreased during pregnancy and supplementation with 10 mg of PN daily is required in
order to maintain normal values during the third trimester of pregnancy (23,24). The plasma clearance rate of PLP is increased in
liver disease (20,25) and uremia (26). The underlying basis of
these abnormalities is presently unknown. In liver disease, the
rate of synthesis of PLP, as measured by the appearance of PLP in
plasma, from orally administered PN also appears to be decreased
(21,26). decreased plasma PLP levels have been reported to occur
with chronic alcoholism (21), Hodgkin's disease (16), metastatic
cancer (27), celiac disease (28) and chronic hemodialysis (29).

Clearly both nutritional and metabolic factors play roles in
the determination of the plasma concentration of PLP as they do
also for the activities of PLP-dependent enzymes and for urinary
or plasma 4PA levels. The use of any of these measurements as
indicators of vitamin B-6 nutritional status must take into consideration both these factors. Furthermore, attention must be paid
to the state of metabolic balance of the subjects under study.
Values obtained between states of equilibration may be misleading.
Finally, while simple nutritional deficiency may be diagnosed by
any of several measurements; e.g., plasma PLP concentration, PLP-
dependent enzyme activity, or urinary and plasma 4PA concentrations,
the diagnosis of vitamin B-6 deficiency in disease states may require
the use of multiple assessment procedures, including the study of
synthesis and degradation rates, storage, transport, and excretion
of PLP, PL, and 4PA.

LITERATURE CITED

1. Lumeng, L., Brashear, R. E. & Li, T.-K. (1974) Pyridoxal
    5'-phosphate in plasma. Source, protein-binding, and cellular
    transport. J. Lab. Clin. Med. 84, 334-343.
2. Bain, J. A. & Williams, H. L. (1960) Concentrations of B-6
    vitamers in tissues and tissue fluids. In: Inhibition in
    the Nervous System and Gamma-aminobutyric Acid. (Roberts, E,
    Baxter, C. F., Harreveld, A. V., Wiersma, C.A.G., Adey, W. R.
    & Killam, K. F., eds.) Pergamon Press, New York, NY.
3. Lyon, J. B., Jr., Bain, J. A. & Williams, H. L. (1962) The
    distribution of vitamin B-6 in the tissues of two inbred
    strains of mice fed complete and vitamin B-6-deficient rations.
    J. Biol. Chem. 237, 1989-1991.
4. Bell, R. R. & Haskell, B. E. (1971) Metabolism of vitamin B-6
    in the I-strain mouse. I. Absorption, excretion, and conversion
    of vitamin to enzyme co-factor. Arch. Biochem. Biophys. 147,
    588-601.
5. Lumeng, L., Ryan, M. P. & Li, T.-K. (1978) Validation of the
    diagnostic value of plasma pyridoxal 5'-phosphate measurements
    in vitamin B-6 nutrition of the rat. J. Nutr. 108, 545-553.

6.   Black, A. L., Guirard, B. M. & Snell, E. E. (1977) Increased
     muscle phosphorylase in rats fed high levels of vitamin B-6.
     J. Nutr. 107, 1962-1968.
7.   Bosron, W. F., Veitch, R. L., Lumeng, L. & Li, T.-K. (1978)
     Subcellular localization and identification of pyridoxal 5'-
     phosphate-binding proteins in rat liver. J. Biol. Chem. 253,
     1488-1492.
8.   Illingworth, B., Kornfeld, R. & Brown, D. H. (1960) Phos-
     phorylase and uridine diphospho-glucose-glycogen transferase
     in pyridoxine deficiency. Biochim. Biophys. Acta 42, 486-489.
9.   Eisenstein, A. B. (1962) The effect of pyridoxine deficiency
     on liver and muscle phosphorylase. Biochim. Biophys. Acta 58,
     244-247.
10. Takami, M., Fujioka, M., Wada, M. & Taguchi, T. (1968)
     Studies on pyridoxine deficiency in rats. Proc. Soc. Exp.
     Biol. Med. 129, 110-117.
11. Black, A. L., Guirard, M. B. & Snell, E. E. (1978) The
     behavior of muscle phosphorylase as a reservoir for vitamin
     B-6 in the rat. J. Nutr. 108, 670-677.
12. Lumeng, L., Lui, A. & Li, T.-K. (1980) Plasma content of
     B-6 vitamers and its relationship to hepatic vitamin B-6
     metabolism. J. Clin. Invest. 66, 688-695.
13. Li, T.-K., Lumeng, L. & Veitch, R. L. (1974) Regulation of
     pyridoxal 5'-phosphate metabolism in liver. Biochem. Biophys.
     Res. Commun. 61, 667-684.
14. Baysal, A., Johnson, B. A. & Linkswiler, H. (1966) Vitamin
     B-6 depletion in man. Blood vitamin B-6, plasma pyridoxal-
     phosphate, serum cholesterol, serum transaminases, and urinary
     vitamin B-6 and 4-pyridoxic acid. J. Nutr. 89, 19-23.
15. Hamfelt, A. (1967) Enzymatic determination of pyridoxal
     phosphate in plasma by decarboxylation of L-tyrosine-^{14}C(U)
     and a comparison with the tryptophan load test. Scand. J.
     Clin. Lab. Invest. 20, 1-10.
16. Chabner, B. A., DeVita, V. T., Livingston, D. M. & Oliverio,
     V. T. (1970) Abnormalities of tryptophan metabolism and
     plasma pyridoxal phosphate in Hodgkin's disease. New Eng.
     J. Med. 282, 838-843.
17. Sauberlich, H. E., Canham, J. E., Baker, E. M., Raica, N., Jr.
     & Herman, Y. F. (1972) Biochemical assessment of the nutri-
     tional status of vitamin B-6 in the human. Am. J. Clin. Nutr.
     25, 629-642.
18. Brown, R. R., Rose, D.P., Leklem, J. E., Linkswiler, H. &
     Anand, R. (1975) Urinary pyridoxic acid, plasma pyridoxal
     phosphate, and erythrocyte aminotransferase levels in oral
     contraceptive users receiving controlled intakes of vitamin
     B-6. Am. J. Clin. Nutr. 28, 10-19.
19. Lumeng, L., Cleary, R. E. & Li, T.-K. (1974) Effect of oral
     contraceptives on the plasma concentration of pyridoxal
     phosphate. Am. J. Clin. Nutr. 27, 326-333.

20. Mitchell, D., Wagner, C., Stone, W. J., Wilkinson, G. R. &
     Schenker, S. (1976) Abnormal regulation of plasma pyridoxal
     5'-phosphate in patients with liver disease. Gastroenterology
     71, 1043-1049.
21. Lumeng, L. & Li, T.-K. (1974) Vitamin B-6 metabolism in
     chronic alcohol abuse. J. Clin. Invest. 53, 693-704.
22. Rose, C. S., György, P., Butler, M., Andres, R., Norris, A. H.,
     Shock, N. W., Tobin, J., Brin, M. & Spiegel, H. (1976) Age
     differences in vitamin B-6 status of 617 men. Am. J. Clin.
     Nutr. 29, 847-853.
23. Cleary, R. E., Lumeng, L. & Li, T.-K. (1975) Maternal and
     fetal plasma levels of pyridoxal phosphate at term: adequacy
     of vitamin B-6 supplementation during pregnancy. Am. J. Obstet.
     Gynecol. 121, 25-28.
24. Lumeng, L., Cleary, R. E., Wagner, R., Yu, P. L. & Li, T.-K.
     (1976) Adequacy of vitamin B-6 supplementation during pregnancy:
     a prospective study. Am. J. Clin. Nutr. 29, 1376-1383.
25. Labadarios, D., Rossouw, J. E., McConnell, J. B., Davis, M.
     & Williams, R. (1977) Vitamin B-6 deficiency in chronic
     liver disease - evidence for increased degradation of
     pyridoxal 5'-phosphate. Gut 18, 23-27.
26. Spannuth, C. L., Jr., Warnock, L. G., Wagner, C. & Stone, W. J.
     (1977) Increased plasma clearance of pyridoxal 5'-phosphate
     in vitamin B-6-deficient uremic man. J. Lab. Clin. Med. 90,
     632-637.
27. Potera, C., Rose, D. P. & Brown, R. R. (1977) Vitamin B-6
     deficiency in cancer patients. Am. J. Clin. Nutr. 30,
     1677-1679.
28. Reinken, L., Zieglauer, H. & Berger, H. (1976) Vitamin B-6
     nutriture of children with acute celiac disease, celiac
     disease in remission and of children with normal duodenal
     mucosa. Am. J. Clin. Nutr. 29, 750-753.
29. Teehan, B. P., Smith, L. J., Sigler, M. H., Gilgore, G. S. &
     Schleifer, C. R. (1978) Plasma pyridoxal phosphate levels
     and clinical correlations in chronic hemodialysis patients.
     Am. J. Clin. Nutr. 31, 1932-1936.

URINARY 4-PYRIDOXIC ACID, URINARY VITAMIN B-6 AND PLASMA PYRIDOXAL PHOSPHATE AS MEASURES OF VITAMIN B-6 STATUS AND DIETARY INTAKE IN ADULTS[1]

Terry D. Shultz and James E. Leklem

Department of Foods and Nutrition
Oregon State University
Corvallis, OR 97331

As reviewed by Sauberlich (1), a number of studies have been conducted to determine the efficacy of measuring urinary 4-pyridoxic acid and vitamin B-6 excretion levels, as well as plasma pyridoxal phosphate levels, as criteria for assessing vitamin B-6 nutritional status. It has been suggested that urinary vitamin B-6 excretion levels may be reflective only of recent dietary vitamin B-6 intake and may not be indicative of the severity of the deficiency (1). The question then arises as to whether or not urinary 4-pyridoxic acid and plasma pyridoxal phosphate levels are only an indication of recent dietary intake; although, plasma pyridoxal phosphate behaves as a mobilizable storage pool and is thought to be a sensitive indicator of the state of vitamin B-6 nutrition (2). A further important consideration would be to what extent urinary 4-pyridoxic acid, urinary vitamin B-6, plasma pyridoxal phosphate, and dietary vitamin B-6 intake are interrelated. If a significant interrelationship does exist among the aforementioned parameters, perhaps it would be necessary to determine only one parameter in order to assess vitamin B-6 status. Further, if a significant interrelationship does exist, dietary vitamin B-6 intake levels could be estimated by interpolation of urinary and blood vitamin B-6 metabolites.

---

[1]Paper No. 5572 from the Oregon State University Agricultural Experiment Station.

Additional indications of an inadequate dietary vitamin B-6
intake or depleted tissue reserves may be obtained from vitamin B-6
related tests that reveal metabolic changes. These tests are
indirect measures of vitamin B-6 levels in the body. The tryptophan
load test is one such sensitive method of detecting vitamin B-6
deficiency (3). Individuals consuming adequate levels of vitamin
B-6 exhibit little or no increase in metabolite excretion after a
load test (4-12). Numerous investigators have shown urinary tryptophan metabolites to be increased in vitamin B-6 deficiency (4,7,8,
13-15). Pyridoxine intakes of 1.25 to 1.50 mg/day seem to adequately
meet the dietary vitamin B-6 requirement of adult men and women
(4-6,8-10,12,13,16), and elevated levels of tryptophan metabolites
following a tryptophan load test are usually prevented by these
intakes (4,5,8-10,12,13,16). Also, these intakes correct 4-pyridoxic
acid (4PA) and/or urinary vitamin B-6 levels in depleted individuals
to pre-depletion excretion levels (6,12,16).

Another factor to be considered in assessing vitamin B-6 status
is the dietary intake of protein. The protein content of the diet
has been shown to be important in determining the rate at which a
vitamin B-6 deficiency appears (6,8,9). The mechanism(s) whereby
high protein diets cause a higher requirement for vitamin B-6 is
not clearly understood, but it may be due to an increased need of
the cofactor by many vitamin B-6 requiring enzymes necessary for
amino acid metabolism (17,18). The various studies in which the
relationship among tryptophan metabolism, dietary vitamin B-6, and
dietary protein have been examined are summarized in Table 1.

This paper is concerned with evaluating interrelationships
among urine and blood vitamin B-6 metabolites and dietary vitamin
B-6 intake as criteria for assessing vitamin B-6 nutritional status
in adults. Tentative guidelines are also included for evaluating
vitamin B-6 nutritional status as related to studies previously
showing relationships among vitamin B-6 intake, tryptophan metabolites and vitamin B-6 status.

MATERIALS AND METHODS

Thirty-five male and 41 female healthy adult Seventh-day
Adventist (SDA) vegetarians (SV; 14,17), SDA non-vegetarians (SNV;
7,3), and general population non-SDA, non-vegetarians (NV; 14,21)
served as participants. A fasting blood sample, a 24-hour urine
collection made the day prior to blood sampling, and a 3-day dietary
intake record was obtained from each subject. All samples were
stored frozen (-40°) until analyzed. None of the subjects were
taking vitamin B-6 supplements or drugs known to adversely affect
vitamin B-6 metabolism (19). Subjects were classified as vegetarians if they ate meat, fish, or poultry no more than 1-2 times per
month and had followed this type of dietary regimen for at least

Table 1.   Relationship of Tryptophan Load Test, Levels of Dietary Protein, Dietary Vitamin B-6, and B-6/Protein Ratios to the Vitamin B-6 Requirement of Adult Men and Women

Reference	Amino Acid Load	Protein Intake	Vitamin B-6 Intake		Vitamin B-6/Protein Ratios	
			Inadequate	Adequate	Inadequate	Adequate
	g	g/day	mg			
Baker et al. (1964)	10.0 DL-Tryptophan	30		1.25		0.042
	10.0 DL-Tryptophan	100	1.25	1.50	0.012	0.015
Yess et al. (1964)	2.0 L-Tryptophan	100	1.06		0.010	
Miller & Linkswiler (1967)	2.0 L-Tryptophan	54	0.76	1.66	0.014	0.030
	2.0 L-Tryptophan	150	0.76	1.66	0.005	0.011
Canham et al. (1969)	10.0 DL-Tryptophan	40		2.00		0.050
	10.0 DL-Tryptophan	80		2.00		0.025
		80		1.00		0.012
		100		1.30		0.013
Sauberlich et al. (1970)	10.0 DL-Tryptophan	100		1.50		0.015
Donald et al. (1971)		57		1.50		0.026
Leklem et al. (1975)	2.0 L-Tryptophan	78	0.80	2.00	0.010	0.026
Donald et al. (1979)	2.0 L-Tryptophan	57	0.96	1.56	0.016	0.027

1 year. The SV men and women had been practicing vegetarianism for an average of 20.6 + 16.2 years, ranging from 1-62 years. This group was comprised of 26 lacto-ovo (12 men, 14 women), 1 male lacto, and 4 vegan (1 man, 3 women) vegetarians. In addition, 10 male and 26 female vitamin users (SV; 6,13: SNV; 2,1: NV; 2,12) were studied.

Completeness of daily 24-hour urine collections was checked by measuring creatinine by an automated modification (Technicon Autoanalyzer, Technicon Corp., Tarrytown, NY) of the Jaffé reaction (20). Urinary 4PA was determined fluorometrically following separation of 4PA from interfering compounds by ion-exchange chromatography (21). Recoveries of 4PA averaged 96 + 8%. Urinary total vitamin B-6 was determined by a microbiological assay with Saccharomyces uvarum (carlsbergensis) ATCC 9080 (22). The microbiological analysis of urinary vitamin B-6 required an initial hydrolysis step with 0.1 N HCl at 102 kPa for 30 minutes. Plasma pyridoxal phosphate (PLP) was measured enzymatically with tyrosine decarboxylase apoenzyme by the method of Chabner and Livingston (23) with slight modifications. Recoveries of PLP added to plasma averaged 95 + 8% for this method. The urinary vitamin B-6 and PLP assays were carried out in subdued light. Urinary creatinine, 4PA, vitamin B-6, and plasma PLP samples were assayed in duplicate.

All subjects were carefully instructed in keeping a 3-day dietary record. Instructions were provided with the record sheets and included procedures for reporting intake, estimating portions, and describing food combinations. Dietary vitamin B-6 and protein intakes were determined from a computerized nutrient data base (24). Additional nutrient values for dietary vitamin B-6 were taken from published sources (25-28).

The data were statistically analyzed by use of the unpaired t-test and Pearson correlation coefficients (29).

RESULTS AND DISCUSSION

The male and female subjects averaged 38.3 + 13.6 and 49.6 + 14.2 years of age, while ranging in age from 20-78 and 25-79 years, respectively (Table 2). As expected, males were taller and heavier than their female counterparts. There were no significant differences in body weight or height among the SV, SNV, and NV male or female groups, respectively.

Table 2. Vital Statistics of Male and Female Non-Vitamin Users

Combined Groups[a]	Number of Subjects	Age		Height		Weight	
		$\overline{X} \pm SD$[b]	Range	$\overline{X} \pm SD$	Range	$\overline{X} \pm SD$	Range
		yrs		cm		kg	
Males	35	38.3+13.6	20-78	179.0+8.8	142.2-198.1	76.6+11.2	58.6-102.6
Females	41	49.6+14.2	25-79	166.0+6.4	151.0-179.1	66.8+11.0	46.8-102.8

[a] Seventh-day Adventist (SDA) vegetarians (14 males, 17 females); SDA non-vegetarians (7 males, 3 females); non-SDA nor-vegetarians (14 males, 21 females).
[b] Mean ± Standard Deviation.

Virtually no significant differences were found between SV, SNV, and NV male or female groups for 4PA, urinary vitamin B-6, plasma PLP, vitamin B-6 intakes, vitamin B-6/dietary protein intake ratios and percent of vitamin B-6 dietary intake excreted as 4-pyridoxic acid. Also, no significant differences were observed when considering age categories within the individual groups. From a dietary standpoint, the dietary intakes for 13 nutrients were generally the same for either the male or female groups; however, the male and female SNV and NV subjects were consuming more protein, total fat, and cholesterol than the SV subjects. Therefore, all subjects were combined into their respective male or female groups. A consistent sex difference was evident, since all male 4PA (μmol/24 hr), urinary vitamin B-6 (mol/24 hr), PLP (ng/ml), and vitamin B-6 (mg/day) intake mean values were higher than female levels. The values for males and females were as follows: (4PA, μmol/24) 7.46 $\pm$ 4.34 vs 5.57 $\pm$ 3.09, P$\leq$0.05; (urinary vitamin B-6, μmol/24 hr) 0.$\overline{9}$2 $\pm$ 0.49 vs 0.$\overline{7}$6 $\pm$ 0.24; (PLP, ng/ml) 12.82 $\pm$ 4.78 vs 9.31 $\pm$ 3.64, P$\leq$0.001; (vitamin B-6 intake, mg/day) 2.0 $\pm$ 0.8 vs 1.6 $\pm$ 0.$\overline{5}$, P$\leq$0.02, respectively (Tables 3 and 4). Sex differences for $\overline{4}$PA and PLP levels have also been reported by other investigators (30,31). In male and female groups, 4PA (Fig. 1), PLP (Fig. 2), vitamin B-6 and protein intakes tended to decrease slightly with increasing age, but not significantly. Urinary vitamin B-6 (Fig. 3) tended to decrease in male, but not in female subjects with increasing age. These results are in accord with other reports (1,31-34) which also indicate that urinary vitamin B-6 and plasma PLP decrease with increasing age. In males, but not females, B-6/protein ratios tended to decline with increasing age. In contrast, the percent 4PA excretion of females, but not males tended to decrease with increasing age.

Sex differences were not evident between males and females for B-6/protein ratios or percent 4PA excretion (Table 3) and combined averages were 0.024 $\pm$ 0.007 and 60 $\pm$ 26%, respectively. In 1975, the Dietary Standard for Canada (35) recommended a B-6/protein ratio of 0.020 as being an adequate vitamin B-6 nutritional standard for both adult males and females. This ratio was calculated from studies reporting both dietary vitamin B-6 and protein intakes (6,8,16,36,37). Recently, the United States Recommended Dietary Allowances (38) suggested that the requirement for young adult women consuming 100 g protein/day be 2.0 mg of vitamin B-6 (B-6/protein ratio-0.020), and for adult males consuming 110 g protein/day, the allowance be 2.2 mg of vitamin B-6 (B-6/protein ratio-0.022). In the present study, 76% of the subjects were consuming vitamin B-6 and protein such that the ratio was greater than 0.020. Twenty percent to 50% of ingested vitamin B-6 is reported to be converted to 4PA in the adult male and female (16,21,39-41), these values are similar to the combined average which we found.

Table 3.   Male and Female Non-Vitamin User Dietary Protein and Vitamin B-6 Intake, Vitamin B-6/Protein Dietary Intake Ratio, and Percent of Dietary Vitamin B-6 Excreted as 4-pyridoxic Acid (%4PA)

Combined groups[a]	Number of Subjects	Dietary Protein (g/day)		Dietary Vitamin B-6 (mg/day)		Vitamin B-6/Protein Ratio		%4PA[e]	
		$\overline{X}$+SD[b]	Range	$\overline{X}$+SD	Range	$\overline{X}$+SD	Range	$\overline{X}$+SD	Range
Males	35	89+28[c]	43-180	2.0+0.8[d]	1.0-3.8	0.024+0.007	0.016-0.048	62+32	22-168
Females	41	62+12[c]	32- 90	1.6+0.5[d]	0.8-3.2	0.025+0.007	0.014-0.044	59+22	24-142

[a]Seventh-day Adventist (SDA) vegetarians (14 males, 17 females), SDA non-vegetarians (7 males, 3 females), non-SDA non-vegetarians (14 males, 21 females).
[b]Mean + Standard Deviation.
[c]$P \leq 0.001$
[d]$P \leq 0.02$
[e]Relationship of vitamin B-6 intake to urinary 4-pyridoxic acid (4PA) excretion. The percent of intake excreted as 4PA was calculated as follows: μmoles 4PA excreted x 100/μmoles of pyridoxine ingested.

Table 4. Male and Female Non-Vitamin User Urinary 4-pyridoxic Acid (4PA), Urinary Vitamin B-6, and Plasma Pyridoxal Phosphate (PLP) Levels

Combined Groups[a]	Number of Subjects	4PA		Acceptable Level of 4PA Excretion		Number of Subjects with Marginal 4PA Excretion Levels	
		$\overline{X}$+SD[b]	Range	B-6 Intake[c]	B-6/Protein Ratio[c]	B-6 Intake	B-6/Protein Ratio
		μmol/24 hr		μmol/24 hr			
Males	35	7.46+4.34[d]	2.30-25.52	>5.00-5.67	>3.05-4.00	SV=6 SNV=2 NV=6	SV=3 SNV=0 NV=2
Females	41	5.57+3.09[d]	2.76-20.22	>4.60-5.20	>2.78-3.20	SV=10 SNV=2 NV=12	SV=1 SNV=0 NV=4

Combined Groups[a]		Urinary Vitamin B-6	Acceptable Level of Vitamin B-6 Excretion		Number of Subjects with Marginal Vitamin B-6 Excretion Levels	
		μmol/24 hr	μmol/24 hr			
Males	35	0.92+0.49	>0.60-0.69	>0.40-0.52	SV=5 SNV=1 NV=6	SV=2 SNV=0 NV=2
Females	41	0.76+0.24	>0.64-0.72	>0.49-0.54	SV=8 SNV=2 NV=10	SV=3 SNV=2 NV=5

Table 4 (cont).   Male and Female Non-Vitamin User Urinary 4-pyridoxic Acid (4PA), Urinary Vitamin B-6, and Plasma Pyridoxal Phosphate (PLP) Levels

Combined Groups[a]	Number of Subjects	PLP ng/ml	Acceptable Level of PLP ng/ml			Number of Subjects with Marginal PLP Levels	
Males	35	12.82±4.78[e]	5.14-23.16	>9.20-10.20	>9.50-10.20	SV= 5 SNV= 2 NV= 6	SV=5 SNV=2 NV=6
Females	41	9.31±3.64[e]	3.52-19.67	>7.82- 8.79	>5.53- 6.25	SV= 8 SNV= 1 NV=12	SV=3 SNV=0 NV=4

[a] Seventh-day Adventist (SDA) vegetarians (14 males, 17 females), SDA non-vegetarians (7 males, 3 females), non-SDA non-vegetarians (14 males, 21 females).
[b] Mean ± Standard Deviation.
[c] Dietary vitamin B-6 intakes or B-6/protein ratios were correlated with 4PA, urinary vitamin B-6, and PLP levels and extrapolations from these were used to obtain lower and upper range limits using intakes of 1.25 and 1.50 mg of vitamin B-6/day, respectively.
[d] $P \leq 0.05$.
[e] $P \leq 0.001$.

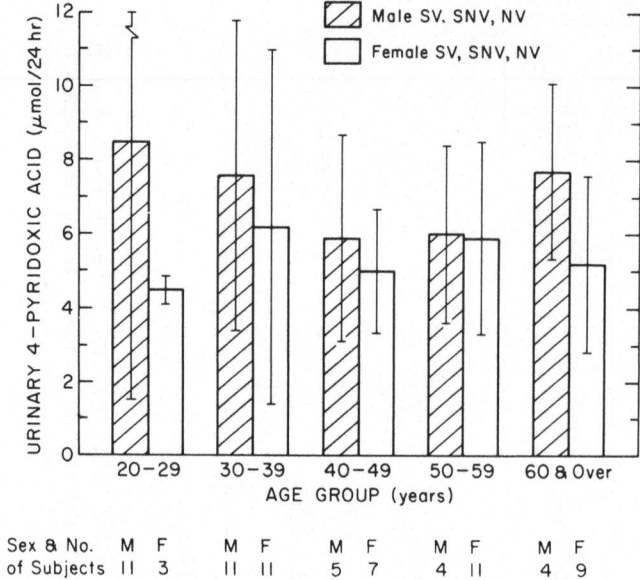

Fig. 1.   Male and female non-vitamin user Seventh-day Adventist
          (SDA) vegetarians (SV), SDA non-vegetarians (SNV), and
          non-SDA non-vegetarians (NV) urinary 4-pyridoxic acid
          excretion levels for the respective age groups. Male
          and female within and between age group mean level
          comparisons were not significantly different. The
          standard deviations are represented by the vertical lines.

        Overall, the SNV and NV were consuming greater amounts of
protein (g/day) than the SV subjects. Combining both into male and
female groups (Table 3), revealed that the males averaged significantly higher intakes than the females (89 ± 28 vs 62 ± 12, P≤0.001,
respectively). Combined male and female, as well as male protein
intake levels were significantly correlated with PLP levels (P≤0.001;
P≤0.05), but not with 4PA or urinary vitamin B-6 levels, respectively.
Male and female groups had vitamin B-6 and protein intakes which
were significantly related (P≤0.001; P≤0.001). Also, combining of
male and female groups separately, revealed dietary vitamin B-6
and B-6/protein ratios to be significantly related (P≤0.001;
P≤0.001). Our findings suggest that PLP levels are more intimately
related to the combination of vitamin B-6 and protein intake than
are 4PA and urinary vitamin B-6.

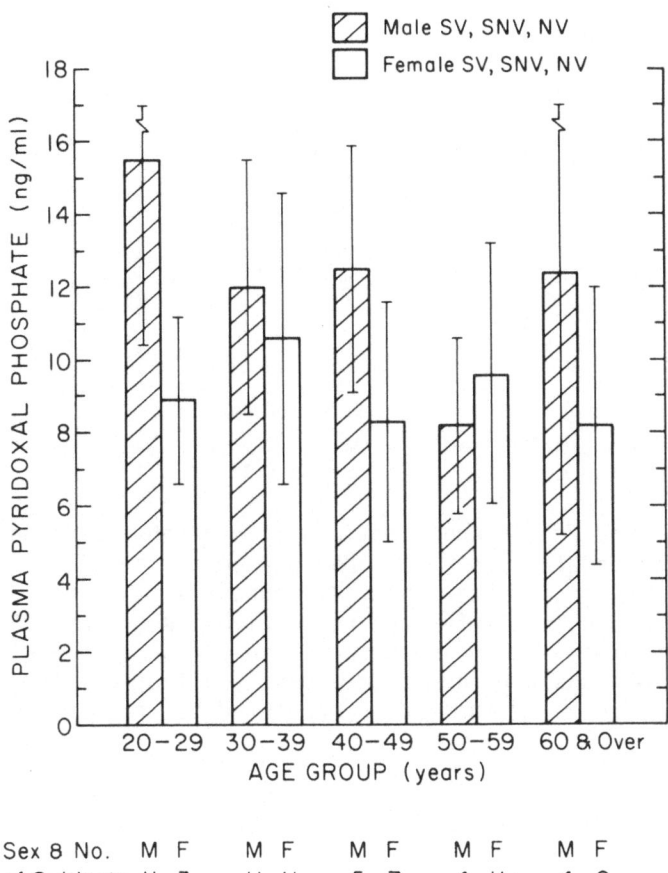

Sex 8 No. of Subjects

	M F	M F	M F	M F	M F
	II 3	II II	5 7	4 II	4 9

20-29 30-39 40-49 50-59 60 & Over

AGE GROUP (years)

Fig. 2. Male and female non-vitamin user Seventh-day Adventist
(SDA) vegetarians (SV), SDA non-vegetarians (SNV), and
non-SDA non-vegetarians (NV) plasma pyridoxal phosphate
levels for the respective age groups. Male and female
within age group mean level comparisons were not significantly different; however, males aged 20-29 had
significantly higher levels than those aged 50-59,
P≤0.02, respectively. The standard deviations are
represented by the vertical lines.

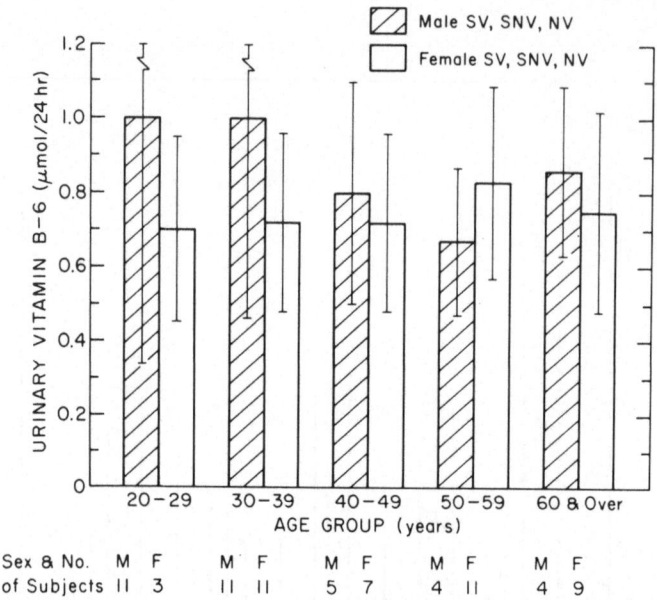

Fig. 3. Male and female non-vitamin user Seventh-day Adventist
        (SDA) vegetarians (SV), SDA non-vegetarians (SNV), and
        non-SDA non-vegetarians (NV) urinary vitamin B-6
        excretion levels for the respective age groups. Male
        and female within and between age group mean level
        comparisons were not significantly different. The
        standard deviations are represented by the vertical
        lines.

        In male subjects who were consuming more protein than females,
a threshold effect may be operating and as these subjects exceed a
certain level of protein intake, the relationship between vitamin
B-6 and protein intake and PLP levels may become more direct. This
is particularly true as long as dietary intake of either of these
is not modified by artificially altering the intake of vitamin B-6
or protein independently of one another. Although the human vitamin
B-6 requirement is related to the level of protein intake, investigators (4-6, 8) have reported that the urinary excretion of 4PA and
vitamin B-6 does not appear to be affected by protein intake. Conversely, Miller and Leklem (18) have found that as the amount of
protein increased in the diet the levels of 4PA and, to a lesser
extent, PLP decreased. These investigators kept the vitamin B-6
intake constant at 1.5 mg pyridoxine/day.

There was a significant correlation of both male and female 4PA, urinary vitamin B-6, and plasma PLP levels with dietary vitamin B-6 (P≤0.01; P≤0.001; P≤0.001, respectively). In controlled studies with adults, urinary excretion of free or total vitamin B-6, and 4PA, as well as PLP levels, have been found to be reflective of vitamin B-6 intake (5-8,12,16,40,42-45). Additionally, correlation between male and female 4PA and urinary vitamin B-6 levels with their respective B-6/protein ratios were significant (P≤0.001; P≤0.001); also, PLP levels were significantly related with their respective B-6/protein ratios (P≤0.02; P≤0.001). We have conclusively established that a significant relationship does exist between vitamin B-6 intake as well as B-6/protein ratios and 4PA, urinary vitamin B-6, and plasma PLP levels; therefore, 4PA, urinary vitamin B-6, and/or plasma PLP levels could possibly be used as an index for vitamin B-6 nutriture evaluation. Correlation coefficients were higher when male and female 4PA levels were correlated with B-6/protein ratios, rather than with vitamin B-6 intakes (Fig. 4, Fig. 5). However, no consistent preferential increase in correlation coefficients was noted when comparing male or female urinary vitamin B-6 and plasma PLP levels with either vitamin B-6 intakes or B-6/protein ratios. Regression analysis of male and female urinary 4PA, vitamin B-6, and plasma PLP levels revealed significant correlations between urinary 4PA and urinary vitamin B-6 (P≤0.001) and plasma PLP (P≤0.001), urinary vitamin B-6 and plasma PLP (P≤0.001), respectively.

Combining male and female non-vitamin users and vitamin users within each of their respective groups and comparing their urinary 4PA, vitamin B-6, and plasma PLP levels with dietary vitamin B-6 and dietary vitamin B-6 plus vitamin B-6 supplemental intake resulted in increasing of correlation coefficients in almost every instance, increasing an average of 22% for the six comparisons (r = 0.58 ± 0.10 vs r = 0.74 ± 0.07). Likewise, for these same groups, comparison between 4PA and urinary vitamin B-6, 4PA and PLP, urinary vitamin B-6, and PLP, revealed the correlation coefficients to be increased in every instance, increasing an average of 20% for these six comparisons (r = 0.69 ± 0.11 vs r = 0.86 ± 0.07).

From studies that have been conducted regarding the relationship between tryptophan and vitamin B-6 metabolism, it appears that 1.25 to 1.50 mg of pyridoxine is nutritionally adequate and corrects abnormal tryptophan metabolism. Using this range of vitamin B-6 intake and the protein intake associated with this range, we have calculated B-6/protein ratios from the aforementioned studies (4, 6,8,9-12,16; see Table 1). Consequently, we used the 1.25 to 1.50 mg vitamin B-6 intake and the B-6/protein ratio of 0.0125 to 0.015, and the fact that both vitamin B-6 intakes and B-6/protein ratios were significantly correlated with 4PA, urinary vitamin B-6, and

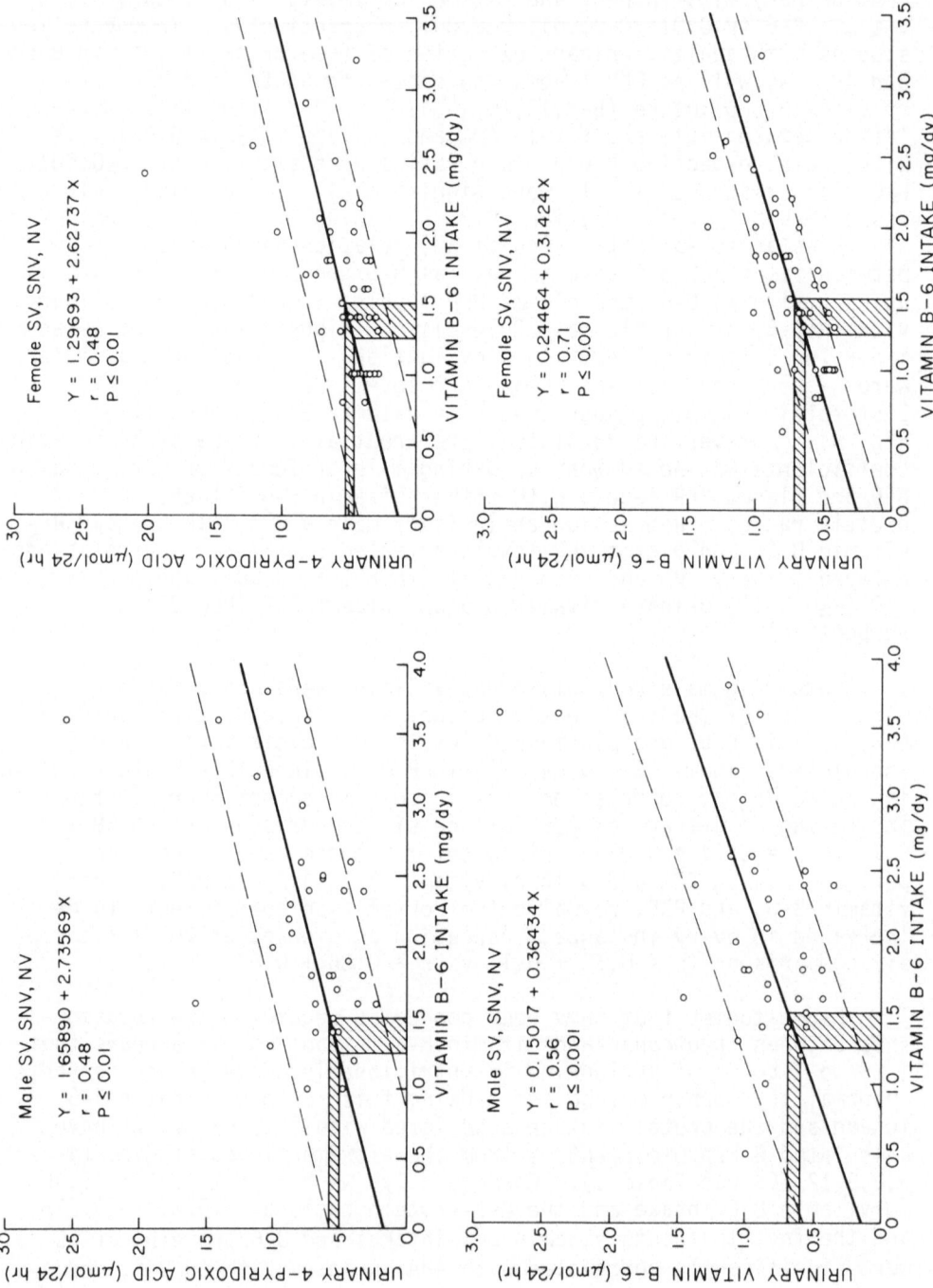

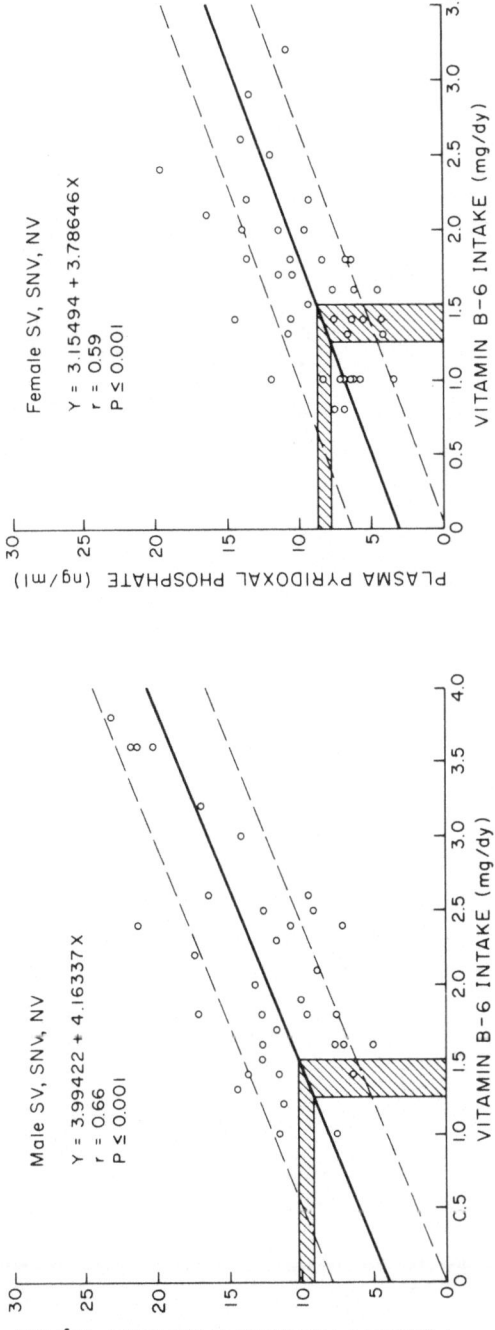

Fig. 4.   Male and female dietary vitamin B-6 intakes were correlated with urinary 4-pyridoxic acid and vitamin B-6 and plasma pyridoxal phosphate levels and extrapolations from regression lines were used to obtain marginal lower and upper range limits for 4PA, urinary vitamin B-6, and PLP using intakes of 1.25 and 1.50 mg of vitamin B-6/day, respectively. Each open circle represents an individual. The dashed lines indicate one standard deviation about the regression line.

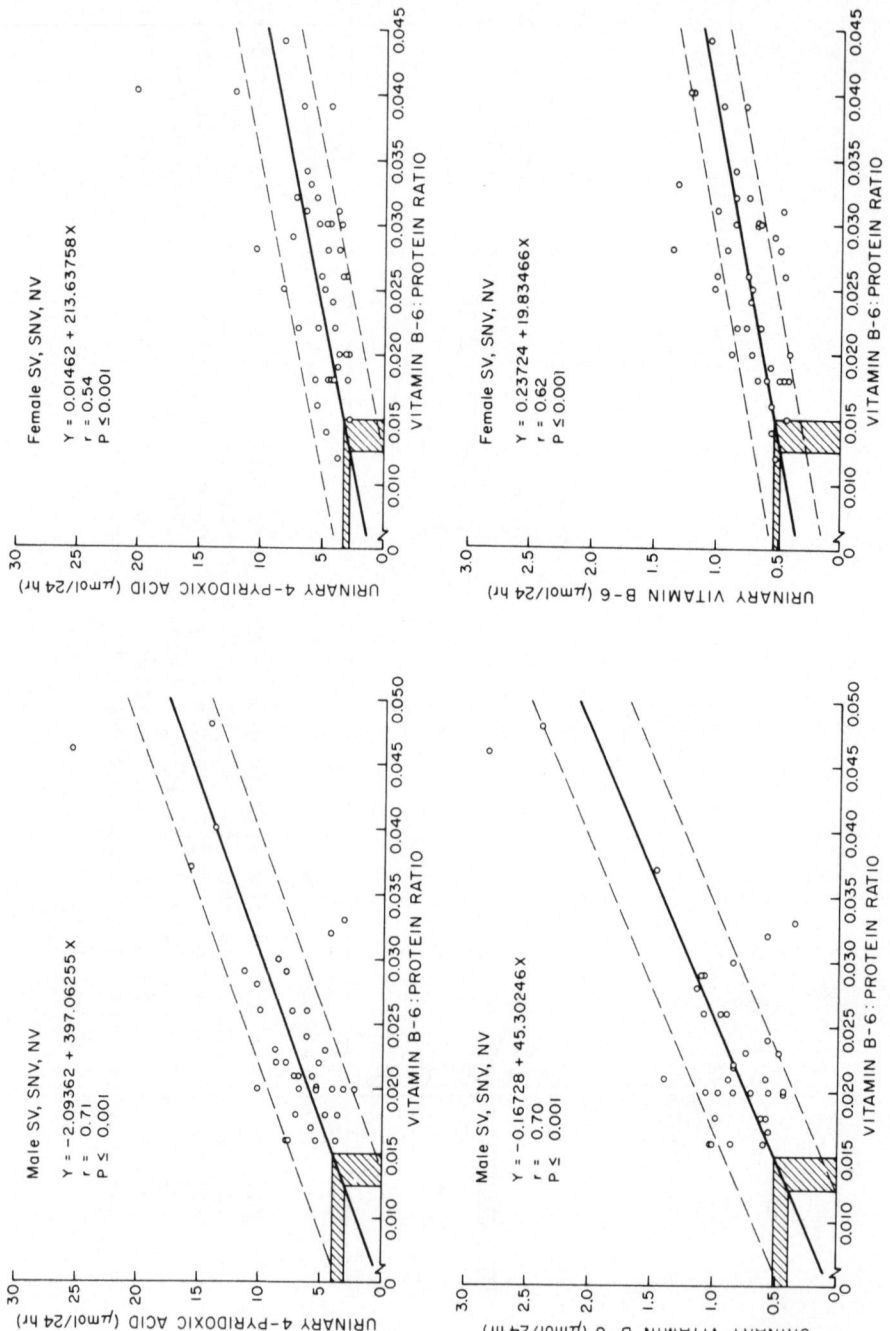

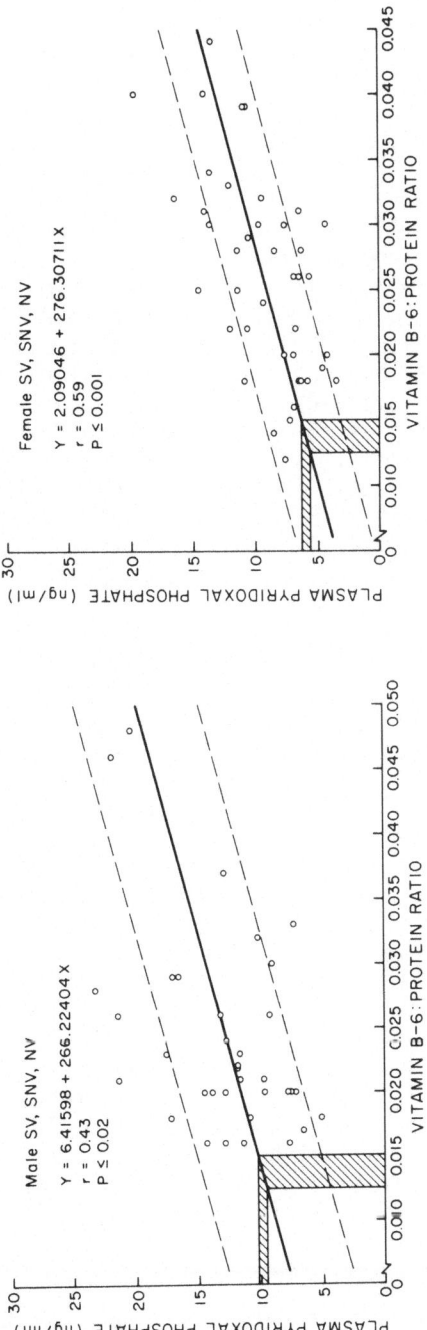

Fig. 5. Male and female dietary vitamin B-6/protein intake ratios were correlated with urinary 4-pyridoxic acid and vitamin B-6, and plasma pyridoxal phosphate levels and extrapolations from regresison lines were used to obtain marginal lower and upper range limits for urinary 4PA, vitamin B-6, and plasma PLP using B-6/protein ratios of 0.0125 and 0.015, respectively. Each open circle represents an individual. The dashed lines indicate one standard deviation about the regression line.

plasma PLP levels, to extrapolate lower and upper marginal range
limits for the aforementioned vitamin B-6 metabolites from appropriate regression lines. Thus, this procedure was used to provide
guidelines for use in assessing vitamin B-6 nutrition status in
adult males and females (Table 5). Lower and upper range limit
extrapolations from regression analysis between vitamin B-6 intakes
and 4PA, urinary vitamin B-6, and plasma PLP were 5.0 to 5.7 μmol/
24 hr, 4.6 to 5.2 μmol/24 hr; 0.6 to 0.7 μmol/24 hr, 0.6 to 0.7
μmol/24 hr; and 9.2 to 10.2 ng/ml, 7.8 to 8.8 ng/ml for males and
females, respectively (Fig. 4). Male and female lower and upper
range limit extrapolations from regression analysis between B-6/
protein ratios and 4PA, urinary vitamin B-6, and plasma PLP were
3.0 to 4.0 μmol/24 hr, 2.8 to 3.2 μmol/24 hr; 0.4 to 0.5 μmol/24 hr,
0.4 to 0.5 μmol/24 hr; and 9.5 to 10.2 ng/ml, 5.5 to 6.2 ng/ml,
respectively (Fig. 5). The lower and upper marginal range limits
were consistently lower for the B-6/protein ratios guideline than
the vitamin B-6 intake guideline for both males and females, except
for male PLP limits which were similar. According to Linkswiler
(5), adult men excreting less than 5.46 μmol/24 hr of 4PA or less
than 0.59 μmol/24 hr of vitamin B-6, may have an inadequate intake
of dietary vitamin B-6. Similarly, Sauberlich et al. (1) reported
that adult males and females excreting less than 2.72 to 4.36 μmol/
24 hr of 4PA or less than 0.33 to 0.53 μmol/24 hr of vitamin B-6[2],
may be consuming inadequate levels of dietary vitamin B-6. These
levels agree with our data derived from the vitamin B-6 intake and
B-6/protein ratio guidelines for marginal levels (Table 5).
Linkswiler (5) has also suggested that 4PA and vitamin B-6 excretions
of 0.54 to 1.08 μmol/24 hr and 0.18 to 0.30 μmol/24 hr, respectively,
indicate a state of vitamin B-6 deficiency. These values are well
below the marginal guidelines established in this study and provide
urinary estimations of severe vitamin B-6 deficiency. Using the
vitamin B-6 intake guideline, the percentage of males and females
with marginal 4PA (40%, 58%), urinary vitamin B-6 (34%, 48%), and
plasma PLP (37%, 51%) was higher than the percentage of males and
females with unacceptable levels of 4PA (14%, 12%), urinary vitamin
B-6 (11%, 24%), and plasma PLP (37%, 17%), according to the B-6/
protein ratios guideline (Table 4). No one particular group (SV,
SNV, NV) had a greater proportion of marginal vitamin B-6 deficient
subjects than another when employing either guideline. It appears
that the dietary vitamin B-6 guideline may have overestimated
inadequate vitamin B-6 urinary and plasma metabolite levels. This
discrepancy may be the result of not being able to take into account
the inherent interaction of dietary protein with vitamin B-6 intakes.

---

[2]Free (unhydrolyzed) urinary vitamin B-6 values were converted to
total urinary vitamin B-6 by assuming free urinary vitamin B-6
to equal approximately 60% of the total urinary vitamin B-6.

Table 5.   Urinary and Plasma Biochemical Evaluation of Vitamin B-6
            Nutritional Status in Adults--Tentative Guidelines

	Vitamin B-6 Status	
	B-6 Intake - 4PA, Urinary B-6, PLP[a]	B-6/Protein Ratio - 4PA, Urinary B-6, PLP[a]
	Marginal	Marginal
Urinary Metabolites		
4-pyridoxic acid μmol/24 hr		
Male	<.5.0 - 5.7	<3.0 - 4.0
Female	<4.6 - 5.2	<2.8 - 3.2
Vitamin B-6 μmol/24 hr[b]		
Male	<0.6 - 0.7	<0.4 - 0.5
Female	<0.6 - 0.7	<0.4 - 0.5
Plasma Metabolite		
Pyridoxal phosphate ng/ml		
Male	<9.2 - 10.2	<9.5 - 10.2
Female	<7.8 - 8.8	<5.5 - 6.2

[a] Dietary vitamin B-6 intakes of B-6/protein ratios were correlated
with urinary 4PA, vitamin B-6, and plasma PLP levels and extrapolations from these were used to obtain lower and upper range
limits using intakes of 1.25 and 1.50 mg of vitamin B-6/day,
respectively.
[b] Saccharomyces uvarum assay of hydrolyzed urine, as pyridoxine.

    Recognizing the importance of the relationship between dietary
vitamin B-6 and dietary protein, we wished to determine the extent
to which both the vitamin B-6 intake and B-6/protein ratio guidelines would assess marginal vitamin B-6 nutrition status under
controlled laboratory conditions. Miller and Leklem (18) studied
the effect of dietary protein intake on the metabolism of vitamin
B-6. In their study, eight men were fed diets containing 0.5 (low),
1.0 (medium), and 2.0 (high) g of protein/kg body weight. Each
level of protein was fed for 15 days. The total intake of pyridoxine
was 1.5 mg/day. The mean B-6/protein ratios for subjects on the
low, medium, and high protein diets were 0.044, 0.022, and 0.011,
respectively. The low, medium, and high protein intakes averaged
34 ± 4 g/day, 68 ± 7 g/day, and 136 ± 14 g/day, respectively. The

4PA and PLP levels decreased with increasing amounts of protein intake. On the medium protein intake diet, 4PA and PLP values averaged 3.64 $\pm$ 0.52 μmol/24 hr and 8.24 $\pm$ 2.16 ng/ml, respectively; while, on the high protein intake diet, 4PA and PLP levels averaged 2.77 $\pm$ 0.68 μmol/24 hr and 6.88 $\pm$ 2.84 ng/ml, respectively. Comparison of the analyzed 4PA and PLP individual values with both guidelines revealed the following: according to the dietary vitamin B-6 guideline, all individuals consuming the medium and high protein diets had marginal levels of 4PA, while 62% and 75% of the subjects ingesting the medium and high protein diets were considered to have inadequate PLP levels. Employing the B-6/protein ratio guideline revealed that only one of the subjects consuming the medium and 50% of the subjects ingesting the high protein diets had marginal levels of 4PA, while approximately 50% of the subjects consuming either the medium or high protein diets would be considered to have marginal PLP levels. Thus, data from the controlled metabolic study support the previous statement that the dietary vitamin B-6 guideline may tend to overestimate inadequate vitamin B-6 metabolite levels, especially 4PA, and this discrepancy may be the result of not being able to take into account the relationship between dietary vitamin B-6 and dietary protein.

Criteria used for nutritional assessment in this study have combined both indirect (tryptophan load test) and direct (urine, blood, and dietary measurements) vitamin B-6 assessment indices as detection variables in an attempt to determine with a greater degree of certainty when a state of marginal vitamin B-6 nutrition may exist. Because of the relationship between vitamin B-6 intake and the amount of protein consumed and recognizing vitamin B-6 and protein metabolic interrelationships, perhaps the most viable measurement of inadequate vitamin B-6 nutrition would be the B-6/protein ratios guideline. The guidelines described provide tentative lower and upper range limits for male and female 4PA, urinary vitamin B-6, and plasma PLP levels. They would also be reflective of the amount of dietary vitamin B-6 the body may need to correct metabolic-biochemical abnormalities caused by marginal dietary vitamin B-6 nutrition. Because of the significant interrelationships between 4PA, urinary vitamin B-6, plasma PLP, and vitamin B-6 intake, individual blood and urinary measurements may indeed be useful reflections of the subject's recent vitamin B-6 intake and vitamin B-6 status. It should be emphasized that these guidelines are based on 24-hr urine collections and fasting blood samples. Whether or not a shorter urine collection would be of value remains to be determined.

ACKNOWLEDGMENTS

Supported in part by NIH Biomedical Research Grant RR07079.

LITERATURE CITED

1. Sauberlich, H. E., Skala, J. H. & Dowdy, R. P. (1974)
   Laboratory test for assessment of nutritional status.
   pp. 37-49, CRC Press Inc., Cleveland, OH.
2. Shane, B. (1978) Vitamin B-6 and blood. In: Human Vitamin
   B-6 Requirements, pp. 111-128, Nat. Acad. Sci., Washington,
   DC.
3. Henderson, L. M. & Hulse, J. D. (1978) Vitamin B-6 relationship in tryptophan metabolism. In: Human Vitamin B-6
   Requirements, pp. 21-36, Nat. Acad. Sci., Washington, DC.
4. Sauberlich, H. E., Canham, J. E., Baker, E. M., Raica, N., Jr.
   & Herman, Y. F. (1970) Human vitamin B-6 nutriture. J. Sci.
   Ind. Res. 29, S28-S37.
5. Linkswiler, H. (1967) Biochemical and physiological changes
   in vitamin B-6 deficiency. Am. J. Clin. Nutr. 20, 547-557.
6. Canham, J. E., Baker, E. M., Harding, R. S., Sauberlich, H. E.
   & Plough, I. C. (1969) Dietary protein - its relationship
   to vitamin B-6 requirement and function. Ann. N.Y. Acad. Sci.
   166, 16-29.
7. Sauberlich, H. E., Canham, J. E., Baker, E. M., Raica, N., Jr.
   & Herman, Y. F. (1972) Biochemical assessment of the nutritional status of vitamin B-6 in the human. Am. J. Clin. Nutr.
   25, 629-642.
8. Baker, E. M., Canham, J. E., Nunes, W. T., Sauberlich, H. E.
   & McDowell, M. E. (1964) Vitamin B-6 requirement for adult
   men. Am. J. Clin. Nutr. 15, 59-66.
9. Miller, L. T. & Linkswiler, H. (1967) Effect of protein
   intake on the development of abnormal tryptophan metabolism
   by men during vitamin B-6 depletion. J. Nutr. 93, 53-59.
10. Yess, N., Price, J. M., Brown, R. R., Swan, P. B. & Linkswiler,
    H. (1964) Vitamin B-6 depletion in man: urinary excretion
    of tryptophan metabolites. J. Nutr. 84, 229-236.
11. Leklem, J. E., Brown, R. R., Rose, D. P., Linkswiler, H. &
    Arend, R. A. (1975) Metabolism of tryptophan and niacin in
    oral contraceptive users receiving controlled intakes of
    vitamin B-6. Am. J. Clin. Nutr. 28, 146-156.
12. Donald, E. A. & Bosse, T. R. (1979) The vitamin B-6 require-
    ment in oral contraceptive users. II. Assessment by tryptophan
    metabolites, vitamin B-6, and pyridoxic acid levels in urine.
    Am. J. Clin. Nutr. 32, 1024-1032.
13. Sauberlich, H. E. (1964) Human requirements for vitamin B-6.
    Vitam. Horm. 22, 807-854.
14. Cinnamon, A. D. & Beaton, J. R. (1970) Biochemical assess-
    ment of vitamin B-6 status in man. Am. J. Clin. Nutr. 23,
    696-702.

15. Brown, R. R., Miller, O. N., Coursin, D. B. & Rose, D. P.
    (1971) Biochemistry and pathology of tryptophan metabolism
    and its regulation by amino acids, vitamin B-6 and steroid
    hormones. Am. J. Clin. Nutr. 24, 653-746.
16. Donald, E. A., McBean, L. O., Simpson, M.H.W., Sun, M. F. &
    Aly. H. E. (1971) Vitamin B-6 requirement of young adult
    women. Am. J. Clin. Nutr. 24, 1028-1041.
17. Brown, R. R. (1972) Normal and pathological condition which
    may alter the human requirement for vitamin B-6. J. Agr. Food
    Chem. 20, 498-505.
18. Miller, L. T. & Leklem, J. E. (1978) Effect of dietary
    protein on metabolism of vitamin B-6. Fed. Proc. 37, 449
    (Abstract).
19. Basu, T. K. (1977) Interaction of drugs and nutrition. J.
    Human Nutr. 31, 449-458.
20. Pino, S., Benoth, J. & Gardyna, H. (1965) An automated method
    for urine creatinine which does not require a dialyzer module.
    Clin. Chem. 11, 664-666.
21. Reddy, S. K., Reynolds, M. S. & Price, J. M. (1958) The
    determination of 4-pyridoxic acid in urine. J. Biol. Chem.
    233, 691-696.
22. Storvick, C. A., Benson, E. M., Edwards, M. A. & Woodring, M. J.
    (1964) Clincal and microbiological determination of vitamin
    B-6. In: Methods of Biochemical Analysis (Glick, D., ed.),
    vol. 12, pp. 183-276, Wiley, New York, NY.
23. Chabner, B. & Livingston, D. (1970) A simple enzymic assay
    for pyridoxal phosphate. Anal. Biochem. 34, 413-423.
24. Schaum, K. D., Mason, M. & Sharp, J. L. (1973) Patient-
    oriented dietetic information system. J. Am. Dietet. Assoc.
    63, 39-41.
25. Orr, M. L. (1969) Pantothenic acid, vitamin B-6, and
    vitamin B-12 in foods. Home Economics Research Report No. 36,
    U.S. Dept. of Agriculture, Washington, DC.
26. Pennington, J. A. (1976) Dietary Nutrient Guide. The AVI
    Publishing Company, Inc., Westport, CT.
27. Posati, L. P. & Orr, M. L. (1976) Composition of Foods,
    Dairy and Egg Products. Agr. Handbook No. 8-1, U.S. Dept. of
    Agriculture, Washington, DC.
28. Campbell Soup Company. (1974) Nutritive Composition of
    Products, Camden, NJ.
29. Steel, R.G.D. & Torrie, J. H. (1960) Principles and Procedures
    of Statistics, pp. 57-66, 183-188. McGraw-Hill Book Company,
    Inc., New York, NY.
30. Contractor, S. F. & Shane, B. (1970) Blood and urine levels
    of vitamin B-6 in the mother and fetus before and after loading
    of the mother with vitamin B-6. Am. J. Obstet. Gynec. 107,
    635-740.

31. Chabner, B. A., DeVita, V. T., Livingston, D. M. & Oliverio, V. T. (1970) Abnormalities of tryptophan metabolism and plasma pyridoxal phosphate in Hodgkins disease. N. Eng. J. Med. 282, 838-843.
32. Hamfelt, A. (1964) Age variation of vitamin B-6 metabolism in man. Clin. Chim. Acta 10, 48-54.
33. Rose, C. S., György, P., Butler, M., Andres, R., Norris, A. H., Shock, N. W., Tobin, J., Brin, M. & Spiegel, H. (1976) Age differences in vitamin B-6 status of 617 men. Am. J. Clin. Nutr. 29, 847-853.
34. Lumeng, L. & Li, T.-K. (1974) Vitamin B-6 metabolism in chronic alcohol abuse. J. Clin. Invest. 53, 693-704.
35. Bureau of Nutritional Sciences. (1975) Dietary Standard for Canada, revised ed., Food Directorate, Health Protection Branch, Dept. of Natl. Hlth. & Welfare, pp. 110, Ottawa, Canada.
36. Harding, R. S., Plough, I. C. & Friedman, T. E. (1959) The effect of storage on the vitamin B-6 content of a packaged army ration, with a note on the human requirement for the vitamin. J. Nutr. 68, 323-331.
37. Swan, P., Wentworth, J. & Linkswiler, H. (1964) Vitamin B-6 depletion in man: urinary taurine and sulfate excretion and nitrogen balance. J. Nutr. 84, 220-228.
38. Food and Nutrition Board, National Research Council. (1980) Recommended Dietary Allowances, 7th ed., pp. 98, Nat. Acad. Sci., Washington, DC.
39. Johansson, S., Lindstedt, S., Register, U. & Wadstrom, L. (1966) Studies on the metabolism of labeled pyridoxine in man. Am. J. Clin. Nutr. 18, 185-196.
40. Baysal, A., Johnson, B. A. & Linkswiler, H. (1966) Vitamin B-6 depletion in man: blood vitamin B-6, plasma pyridoxal phosphate, serum cholesterol, serum transaminases and urinary vitamin B-6 and 4-pyridoxic acid. J. Nutr. 89, 19-23.
41. McCoy, E. E. & England, J. (1968) Excretion of 4-pyridoxic acid during deoxypyridoxine and pyridoxine administration to mongoloid and non-mongoloid subjects. J. Nutr. 96, 525-528.
42. Brown, R. R., Rose, D. P., Leklem, J. E., Linkswiler, H. & Anand, R. (1975) Urinary 4-pyridoxic acid, plasma pyridoxal phosphate, and erythrocyte aminotransferase levels in oral contraceptive users receiving controlled intakes of vitamin B-6. Am. J. Clin. Nutr. 28, 10-19.
43. Gailani, S. D., Holland, J. F., Nussbaum, A. & Olson, K. B. (1968) Clinical and biochemical studies of pyridoxine deficiency in patients with neoplastic diseases. Cancer 21, 975-988.

44. Snyderman, S. E., Holt, L. E., Jr., Carretero, R. & Jacobs, K.
     (1953) Pyridoxine deficiency in the human infant. Am. J.
     Clin. Nutr. 1, 200-207.
45. Bosse, T. R. & Donald, E. A. (1979) The vitamin B-6 require-
     ment in oral contraceptive users. I. Assessment by pyridoxal
     level and transferase activity in erythrocytes. Am. J. Clin.
     Nutr. 32, 1015-1023.

THE TRYPTOPHAN LOAD TEST AS AN INDEX OF VITAMIN B-6 NUTRITION

R. R. Brown

Department of Human Oncology
Wisconsin Clinical Cancer Center
University of Wisconsin Center for Health Sciences
Madison, WI   53706

The amino acid tryptophan was first isolated as the chromogenic substance in tryptic digests of proteins (1). Since that time, naturally occurring L-tryptophan has been shown to be one of the indispensable amino acids having a number of important biological functions.

The nutritional requirement for tryptophan in the diet, as determined by measurements of nitrogen balance, is about 160 mg/day for women and about 250 mg/day for men (2,3). The actual daily intake of tryptophan in the typical high protein diet of developed countries is about 800 to 1000 mg/day. Thus, the typical diet provides several times the minimal requirement. Although studies have not been well documented, it can be expected that the requirement for tryptophan by individuals may vary somewhat depending upon age, race, other nutrients, state of health, and other factors.

Some of the known metabolic pathways of tryptophan are summarized in Fig. 1. The enzyme tryptophan pyrrolase (L-tryptophan-2, 3-dioxygenase) which gives rise to kynurenine (via formylkynurenine, not shown) is an inducible enzyme which can increase many-fold in response to its substrate or in response to induction by cortisol or conditions which may increase cortisol. Since the action of tryptophan oxygenase is to initiate the first step of the irreversible kynurenine pathway of tryptophan metabolism, if substantial tryptophan passes via this pathway, the available tryptophan for other functions may well be reduced to limiting levels.

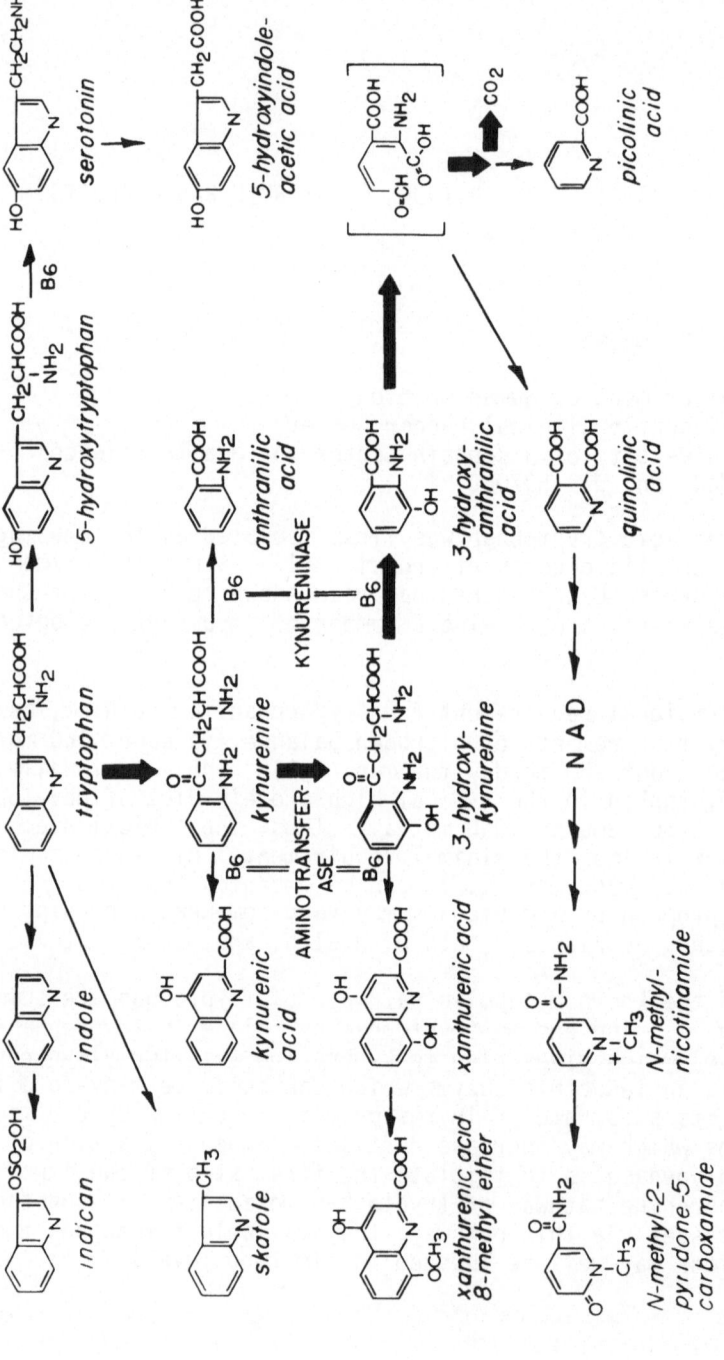

Fig. 1. Metabolic chart showing some of the metabolites of tryptophan. The large arrows indicate the pathway for degradation of the majority of ingested tryptophan. B-6 indicates the sites of action of enzymes requiring PLP as a cofactor.

Tryptophan is a nutritionally important precursor of the vitamin niacin, in addition to being a vital amino acid component of most proteins and enzymes. It is estimated that 60 mg of dietary tryptophan may give rise to about 1 mg of niacin (4,5) although this ratio may possibly vary with the amount of tryptophan ingested (6,7). With a diet containing 1000 mg of tryptophan (present in about 100 g protein), about 17 mg of niacin may be synthesized.

Another quantitatively minor, but functionally vital metabolite of tryptophan is serotonin (5-hydroxytryptamine), a biogenic amine having a variety of neuro-endocrine functions. Formation of this substance is initiated by the enzyme tryptophan-5-hydroxylase to form 5-hydroxytryptophan. Subsequent decarboxylation by a pyridoxal phosphate (PLP) dependent decarboxylase gives rise to serotonin.

Various types of experiments have led to the conclusion that when dietary intake of tryptophan is limited, it is preferentially used for maintenance of body protein, and serotonin production (8), and that metabolism via the kynurenine pathway is very limited. Only when excess tryptophan is ingested does the kynurenine pathway become quantitatively more important. This is borne out by human studies (8) and by animal studies (9,10) showing that the production of kynurenine pathway metabolites was more dependent upon the amount or concentration of tryptophan available rather than on the activity of tryptophan pyrrolase. At higher intakes of tryptophan, above the minimum required for maintenance of nitrogen balance and essential functions, increasingly greater amounts of tryptophan enter the kynurenine pathway. For example, we showed that at L-tryptophan loads from 2 to 8 grams, there was a non-linear excretion of kynurenine (Fig. 2) which suggests induction of the pyrrolase at doses somewhat above 2 g (11). A standardized loading dose of L-tryptophan of 50 mg/kg body weight has been suggested for men and women as providing the most reproducible results without overloading (12,13).

In addition to the above vital metabolites of tryptophan, more than 70 other metabolic intermediates or conjugates have been demonstrated arising either from tissue enzyme activity or from activity of microorganisms. These metabolites include a variety of indolic compounds, quinoline compounds, aromatic amines, aminophenols, and pyridines. With a few exceptions, the biological functions of these numerous metabolites, if indeed they have any, is not known. Picolinic acid is reported to be involved in zinc absorption (14). Xanthurenic acid is reported to complex with insulin to form a less active material (15). Indoles from tryptophan loads result in pulmonary edema in ruminants (16) while indole itself has been reported to cause leukemias (17,18). Hydroxykynurenine is a precursor of phenoxazone pigments in some crustaceans and insects (19), and cinnabarinic acid, a phenoxazone

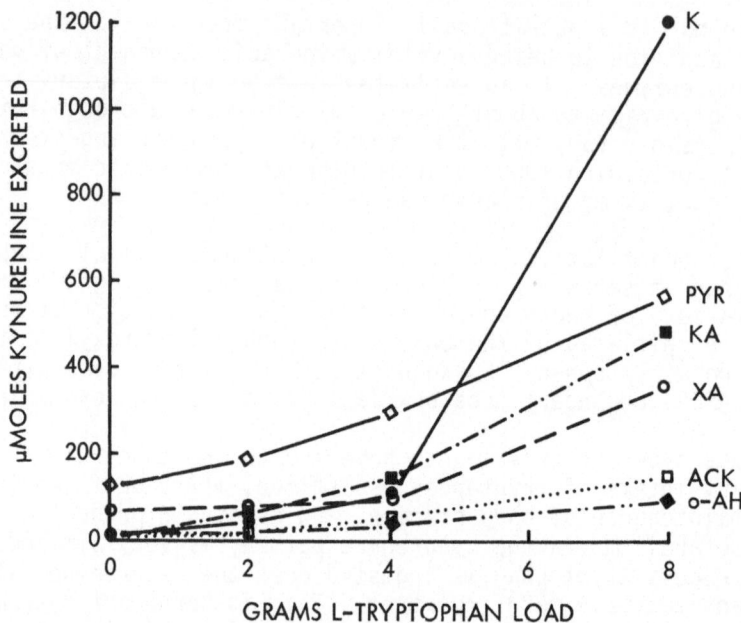

Fig. 2.   Chart showing urinary excretion of kynurenine by a single
          subject in the 24 hours after ingestion of 2, 4, or 8 g of
          L-tryptophan. Abbreviations are K, kynurenine; PYR, N'-
          methyl-2-pyridone-5-carboxamide; KA, kynurenic acid; XA,
          xanthurenic acid; ACK, N^{α}-acetyl-kynurenine; o-AH, o-
          aminohippuric acid. The curve for kynurenine shows a
          distinct change in slope at the 4 g loading point.

derived from 3-hydroxy-anthranilic acid, may result in induction
of several enzymes in rodents (20) although the occurrence of this
compound in mammalian species has not been demonstrated.

     Tryptophan occurs naturally as the "L" isomer. Synthetic
tryptophan is an equal mixture of the L and the unnatural D isomers.
These isomers may be resolved from each other by various means in
the laboratory. D-tryptophan may substitute nutritionally for the
L-isomer in rats, but is poorly utilized by the dog and by man (21).
Additionally, D-tryptophan is more slowly absorbed from the gut
resulting in bacterial production of a variety of unusual metabolites
For these reasons only L-tryptophan should be used in human studies.

ROLE OF VITAMIN B-6 IN TRYPTOPHAN METABOLISM

The metabolic map shown in Fig. 1 indicates several sites of action of PLP. The use of measurements of tryptophan metabolites for assessment of vitamin B-6 nutrition stems from the initial observations of a green urine collected from rats deficient in vitamin B-6 (22,23). This green color was shown to be the result of elevated urinary xanthurenic acid complexed with iron from metal cages and formed the basis of a simple colorimetric assay for urinary xanthurenic acid even though this assay is not very specific at low concentration (24). Thus, elevations of urinary xanthurenic acid, and subsequently of other tryptophan metabolites, were shown to occur in vitamin B-6 deficiency. Vitamin B-6, as PLP, is a required cofactor for kynureninase (kynurenine hydrolase) and kynurenine aminotransferase in the kynurenine pathway. These enzymes act on kynurenine and 3-hydroxykynurenine to form anthranilic and 3-hydroxy-anthranilic acids, and the quinoline derivatives, kynurenic and xanthurenic acids.

When metabolic blocks are present at kynureninase, a rather high percentage of the ingested tryptophan can be accounted for as metabolites of the kynurenine pathway. For example, Dalgliesh showed high levels of kynurenine metabolites in rats, accounting for much of the ingested tryptophan (25). In human subjects receiving vitamin B-6 deficient diets or with deficiencies induced by isoniazid or deoxypyridoxine (26,27) urinary excretion of metabolites preceding the kynureninase step can account for more than half of the tryptophan load. Additionally, a patient with a congenital defect in kynureninase was shown to excrete large amounts of kynurenine and hydroxykynurenine (28). These data lead us to conclude that the majority of excess tryptophan is metabolized via the kynurenine pathway and that the existence of an additional major pathway of quantitative significance is unlikely.

Since PLP is required for xanthurenic acid formation, the increased formation of xanthurenic acid in vitamin B-6 deficiency seems anomalous. Measurement of binding constants for kynureninase and kynurenine aminotransferase do not adequately explain this anomaly (29,30). Observations that mitochondrial kynurenine aminotransferase retains its PLP during vitamin B-6 deficiency while cytosolic aminotransferase and kynureninase do not (29), suggests an important role of mitochondrial membranes in retention of aminotransferase activity. Thus, intracellular distribution and probably organ distribution of these enzymes are important factors in determining the pattern of metabolite formation. This subject has been reviewed recently (31). In any case, with blockage of kynureninase activity by vitamin B-6 deficiency, 3-hydroxykynurenine

and kynurenine accumulate leading to increased formation and excretion of xanthurenic and kynurenic acids along with kynurenine and
hydroxykynurenine. In vitamin B-6 deficiency in rats there is a
corresponding decreased urinary excretion of products after kynur-
enase (32,33). However, in humans, quinolinic acid excretion is
actually increased (34). This suggests that vitamin B-6 may be
required at some point after quinolinic acid although we could not
find evidence for such a requirement (35).

        Increased production of metabolites of the kynurenine pathway
may also occur from an increased entry of tryptophan into the pathway. Tryptophan pyrrolase is an inducible enzyme. Its activity
can be increased by stabilization with increased tryptophan levels
and its rate of synthesis can be induced by cortisol or stresses
which stimulate steroid levels (36,37). This variability in tryptophan pyrrolase activity, which undoubtedly occurs in humans also,
must be taken into consideration in the interpretation of the
tryptophan load test used as an index of vitamin B-6 nutritional
status. Administration of adrenal steroids to humans indeed does
alter the tryptophan load test (38,39) and it has been suggested
that an abnormal tryptophan load test (i.e., urinary elevations of
kynurenine pathway metabolites) may be more a reflection of stress-
induced enzyme induction rather than a deficiency of vitamin B-6 (40).
Arguing against this are observations that supplements of vitamin B-6
can correct most abnormal tryptophan load tests (39). Additionally,
levels of tryptophan pyrrolase in liver biopsies from bladder cancer
patients did not correlate with urinary kynurenine levels, whereas
activity of kynureninase was better correlated (41). More recently,
data from use of a kynurenine load test, which presumably bypasses
the inducible pyrrolase step, has suggested a defect in kynureninase
activity in women receiving estrogens (42). Similarly, studies of
kynurenine metabolism using non-loading tracer doses of ^{14}C-kynur-
enine in patients having scleroderma, also suggest a defect at the
level of kynureninase (43,44).

METHODS OF ANALYSIS FOR URINARY TRYPTOPHAN METABOLITES

        A variety of analytical methods for tryptophan metabolites
has been developed in many laboratories. These methods include
paper or thin layer chromatographic systems, ion exchange chromatographic systems, high performance liquid chromatography, and
gas chromatography. It is not the purpose of this review to compare
or evaluate these methods, but advantages and disadvantages are
present in any method. In a given laboratory and for a given
experimental objective, one method may be more advantageous than
another. In general, results of different methods are comparable,
but lack of specificity with some systems results in interference
leading to erroneously high values. We have found ion-exchange

chromatographic separations, followed by spectrophotometric, colorimetric, or fluorometric detection to be adequate, sensitive, specific, and reproducible for many of the metabolites in human urine (45), and these methods have the advantage that many samples can be measured by operating multiple columns simultaneously and by automation of colorimetric methods (46).

COMPARISON OF THE TRYPTOPHAN LOAD TEST WITH OTHER INDICES OF VITAMIN B-6 NUTRITION

Studies of the effects of oral contraceptive use on requirements for vitamin B-6 provided the opportunity to compare several indices of vitamin B-6 nutrition in a control group of healthy young women not using oral contraceptives (47,48). Ten healthy women (ages 20-26 years) were fed a standardized diet deficient in vitamin B-6 for 4 weeks. This diet contained the equivalent of 0.19 mg of pyridoxine per day. For an additional 4 weeks, 6 of these subjects were supplemented with 0.8 mg/day of pyridoxine hydrochloride to give a total daily intake of 0.85 mg of vitamin B-6 as pyridoxine. At weekly intervals, several tests for vitamin B-6 status were done including a 2.0 g L-tryptophan load test, a 3.0 g L-methionine load test, plasma PLP levels, urinary 4-pyridoxic acid (4PA), and erythrocyte aminotransferase activities without and with PLP stimulation in vitro. These data are expressed as a percentage of initial non-depleted values in Fig. 3. There is almost a linear increase in excretion of tryptophan metabolites and cystathionine as deficiency progresses over the 4 weeks, with the greatest percentage change appearing in urinary 3-hydroxykynurenine. Marked decreases in urinary 4PA and plasma PLP also occurred with one week of feeding the deficient diet (Figs. 3 and 4). The shapes of the 4PA and plasma PLP curves suggest the occurrence of two or more body pools of vitamin B-6 with one pool depleting more rapidly than the other. Similarly, after starting repletion with 0.85 mg of PN, urinary 4PA and plasma PLP rose rapidly during the first week but then rose at a much slower rate throughout the remainder of the repletion period, suggesting an easily repleted pool and a second more slowly repleted pool. During depletion, the activity of erythrocyte aminotransferase decreased (48) but the percent stimulation by PLP in our hands was not as rapid or reliable an index of vitamin B-6 nutritional status as were the other indices measured. A similar conclusion regarding the usefulness of the erythrocyte aminotransferases was recently expressed (49). It should be noted that there is a plotting error in Fig. 2 of reference 48; the numerical data of Table 6, reference 48 are correct.

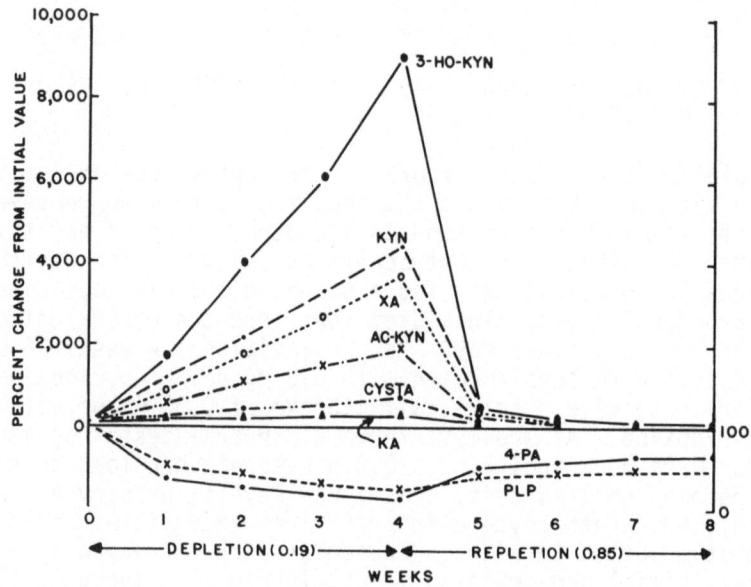

Fig. 3.   Chart showing percentage change from pre-depletion values
          of various indices of vitamin B-6 nutritional status. Ten
          healthy young women, not using oral contraceptives, were
          depleted of vitamin B-6 by ingestion of diet containing
          the equivalent of 0.19 mg of pyridoxine/day for 4 weeks
          at which time they were repleted with 0.85 mg pyridoxine/
          day (47,48). Oral loading doses of 2 g L-tryptophan or
          3 g L-methionine were given at intervals. Urinary tryp-
          tophan metabolites, methionine metabolites, 4-pyridoxic
          acid, and plasma PLP were measured and expressed as a
          percentage of the pre-depletion level. Abbreviations
          are 3-OH-KYN, 3-hydroxykynurenine; KYN, kynurenine; XA,
          xanthurenic acid; AC-KYN, acetylkynurenine; CYSTA,
          cystathionine; KA, kynurenic acid; 4PA, 4-pyridoxic acid;
          PLP, pyridoxal phosphate.

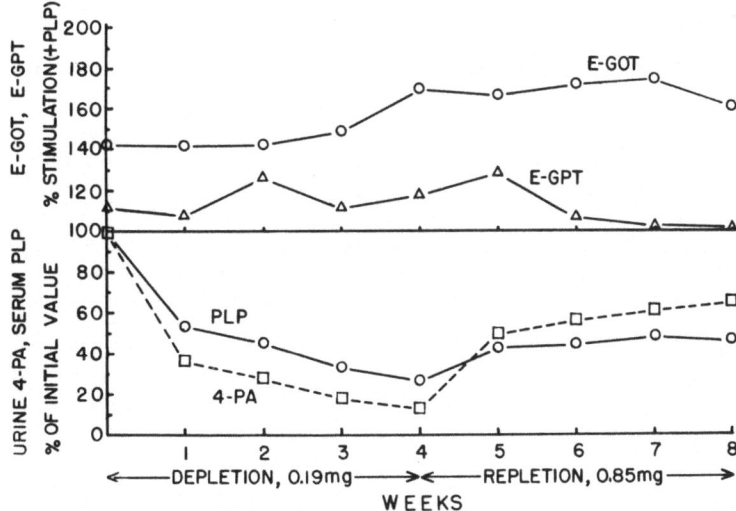

Fig. 4.   Chart showing urinary 4PA, plasma PLP, and percent stimu-
          lation by in vitro PLP saturation of erythrocyte glutamate-
          oxaloacetate aminotransferase (E-GOT) and erythrocyte
          glutamate-pyruvate aminotransferase (E-GPT) in the same
          healthy young women described in Fig. 3.   Changes in PLP
          stimulation of E-GOT and E-GPT were not as responsive to
          pyridoxine intake as were other indices.

It is my opinion that the most sensitive and responsive
indices of the functional adequacy of vitamin B-6 nutrition in
healthy subjects are the tryptophan load test with measurement of
urinary kynurenine, 3-hydroxykynurenine and/or xanthurenic acid,
and the methionine load test with the measurement of urinary
cystathionine. Furthermore, it has been pointed out that the
measurement of urinary 4PA and plasma PLP reflect intake of the
vitamin (50,51) and may reflect tissue levels of the vitamin,
whereas the tryptophan and methionine load tests more nearly indicate the functional adequacy of coenzyme levels. As an example of
this problem, we observed that one of the control women in our
depletion study had very high plasma levels of PLP, approximately
28 ng/ml. She confessed to regularly taking supplemental pyridoxine
because it made her feel better. Though she was not included in
the study, we continued making measurements on her through 4 weeks
of vitamin B-6 depletion and 4 additional weeks of supplementation.
After one week of vitamin depletion, her plasma PLP levels were
still very high, yet her tryptophan load test was abnormal. Even
after 4 weeks of depletion, her plasma PLP levels were in the
normal range, yet her functional tests were as abnormal as other
subjects whose plasma PLP levels were 2-3 ng/ml. Clearly for this

woman normal levels of plasma PLP were not adequate to maintain
normal tryptophan metabolism, and there may be a very good biochemical
reason why she felt better when taking extra vitamin B-6. Thus,
changes in plasma PLP and urinary 4PA, while reliable and responsive
to dietary intake of vitamin B-6, do not give as great a change as
do the functional tests. In our hands, as well as in others, the
erythrocyte aminotransferases and the PLP stimulation of these
enzymes in vitro were not as sensitive or as helpful as the other
tests. In subjects with serious disease or complicated medical or
endocrine problems, the tryptophan load test may be difficult to
interpret and other indices should be considered including the
kynurenine load test described below.

THE KYNURENINE LOAD TEST

     In subjects having disease or stress, there is greater diffi-
culty in interpreting the tryptophan load test because of the
inducible nature of tryptophan pyrrolase. Therefore, we have
attempted to develop a load test using kynurenine to by-pass tryptophan pyrrolase. At the same time, this test might be able to
help us better interpret the tryptophan load test. For example,
if the tryptophan load test is abnormal in a given subject, but the
kynurenine test is normal, we might reasonably conclude that the
abnormal tryptophan load test is due to an induced pyrrolase. On
the other hand, if both tests are abnormal, it would suggest that
the defect is located after kynurenine in the pathway.

     Using gradually increasing loads of L-kynurenine sulfate mono-
hydrate, we determined that an oral load of 200 mg gave an increase
in urine metabolites comparable to that of our standard 2.0 g load
of L-tryptophan in normal control subjects. We have compared this
load of L-kynurenine with a 2.0 g load of L-tryptophan in 12 control
women and in 18 women using oral contraceptives (Fig. 5) (52).
Basal excretions of metabolites measured do not differ appreciably
between the two groups. However, as we and others have observed,
after a tryptophan load, several metabolites are excreted in
elevated amounts by the oral contraceptive users. These metabolites
include kynurenine (K), acetylkynurenine (ACK), 3-hydroxykynurenine
(HK), 3-hydroxyanthranilic acid (HA), and most strikingly, xanthurenic
acid (XA). The ratio of HK/HA has been suggested as an index of
kynureninase activity (55). In this study it was about 1.0 in
basal urines of both groups. After tryptophan loading, this ratio
was elevated to about 1.5 in oral contraceptive users, but was less
than 1.0 in control subjects. After the kynurenine load, excretions
of K, ACK, HK, and the HK/HA ratio were significantly elevated in
the oral contraceptive users. These data strongly suggest that
kynureninase activity is impaired in oral contraceptive users and
that it is this impairment of kynureninase, possibly in conjunction

with an estrogen induced tryptophan pyrrolase (54), which is responsible for the altered tryptophan metabolism in oral contraceptive users. It is interesting to note that the pattern of metabolites after kynurenine load is not identical to that after

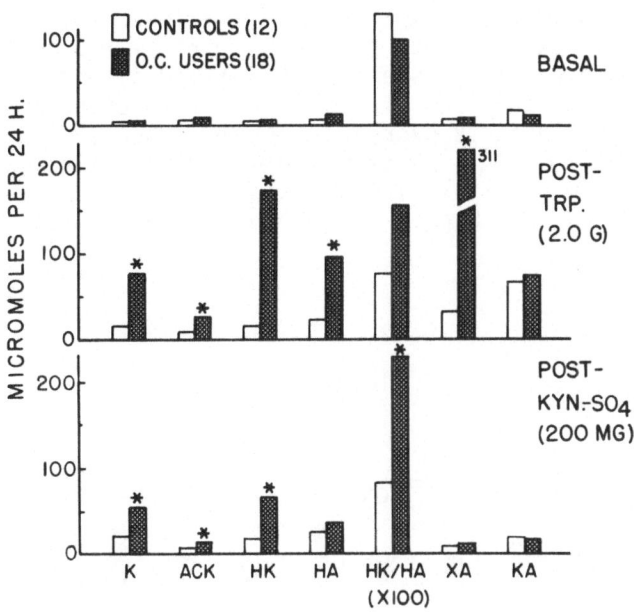

Fig. 5.   Excretion of tryptophan metabolites by 12 control women and 18 women using oral contraceptives (OC) before (basal) and after loading with either 2.0 g L-tryptophan (post-TRP) or 200 mg L-kynurenine sulfate (KYN-SO$_4$) (52). Abbreviations are K, kynurenine; ACK, acetylkynurenine; HK, 3-hydroxykynurenine; HA, 3-hydroxyanthranilic acid; HK/HA, ratio of HK to HA; XA, xanthurenic acid; KA, kynurenic acid. Asterisks indicate values significantly different (P< 0.05) from control values (Student's t test).

tryptophan load in that XA is remarkably low both in controls and in oral contraceptive users, even though levels of its precursor, HK, were responsive to the kynurenine load. Rates of absorption, renal clearance, as well as organ and intracellular distributions may influence these in vivo tests.

We have also compared tryptophan and kynurenine load tests in post-menopausal women without and with estrogen replacement therapy (42,55). In this study, 15 control women were compared with 12 age-matched women who received orally, 2 mg of β-estradiol and 1 mg of estriol per day for 20 days followed by 8 days without hormones. Metabolic studies were done in the last 5 days of hormone adminis-tration of the fourth 20-day cycle. The results are summarized in Fig. 6. They show that basal levels of metabolites are comparable between groups with the exception of a lower mean excretion of 4PA in the hormone-treated group. After 2.0 g of L-tryptophan, the subjects receiving estrogens excreted elevated amounts of K, HK, HA, and XA. After the load of 200 mg of L-kynurenine sulfate, estrogen-treated subjects excreted elevated amounts of K and HK, and lower levels of 4PA. As in the oral contraceptive users, the excretion of XA was not elevated after kynurenine load, even though its precursor, HK, was higher than after tryptophan loading.

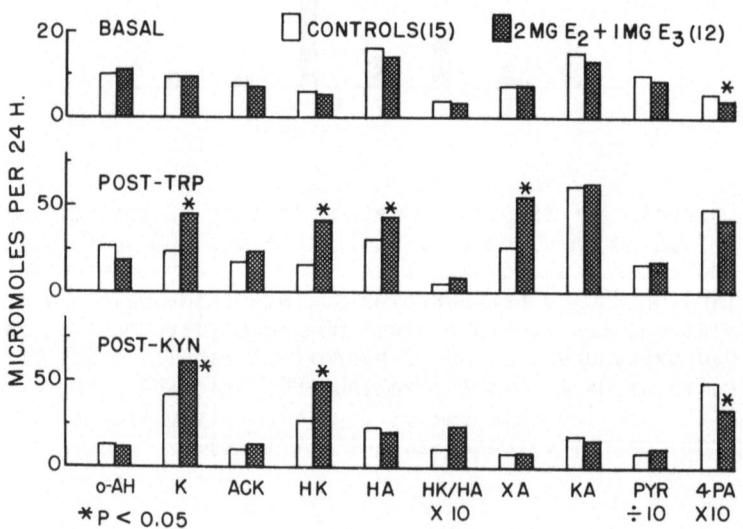

Fig. 6.   Excretion of tryptophan metabolites by 12 post-menopausal subjects given a combination of β-estradiol (E2) and estriol (E3) and 15 age-matched control women not taking estrogens (42). Abbreviations are o-AH, o-amino-hippuric acid; PYR, N'-methyl-2-pyridone-5-carboxamide. Other abbreviations are as in Fig. 5.

TRYPTOPHAN METABOLISM IN HUMAN DISEASE

Many laboratories have examined tryptophan metabolism in various human diseases (56,57), and have found abnormal metabolism in a number of conditions. In our laboratory, using a constant 2.0 g loading dose of L-tryptophan we have shown that a large percentage of patients with a variety of diseases or clinical conditions have abnormal tryptophan load tests (Fig. 7). These include tuberculosis patients given deoxypyridoxine or isonizaid and patients having disseminated lupus erythematosis, scleroderma, cancer, and pregnancy. Of interest is the different pattern of metabolites found in these various conditions. For example, in pregnancy, as in women using oral contraceptives, XA is excreted in largest amounts followed by HK. However, in patients treated with the vitamin B-6 antagonist deoxypyridoxine, HK excretion is greater than XA. This suggests that isoniazid is able to deplete not only cytosolic vitamin B-6 but also the mitochondrial component.

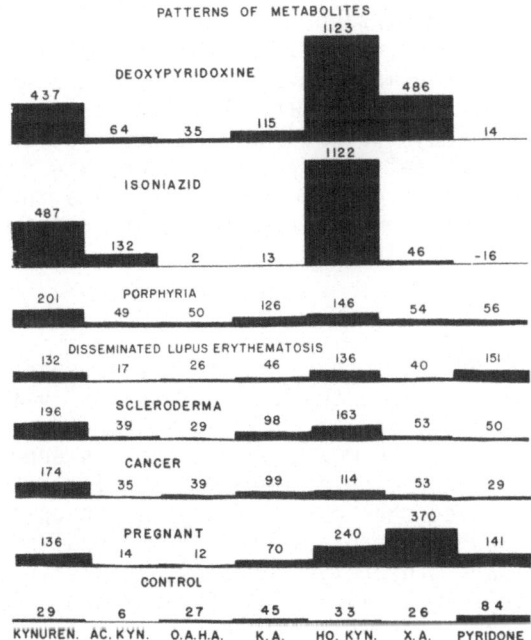

Fig. 7.   Patterns of excretion of tryptophan metabolites. Values
           shown by numbers over each bar are the yield of metabolite
           (post-tryptophan excretion minus basal excretion) in
           μmol/day in response to a 2.0 g load of L-tryptophan.

An interesting study of disease/tryptophan/vitamin B-6 interactions was done in Hodgkin's disease patients (58,59). Patients
with active Hodgkin's disease generally had abnormal tryptophan
metabolism, lower plasma pyridoxal phosphate levels and impaired
immune functions. When patients received chemotherapy and entered
remission, tryptophan metabolism was usually corrected, serum pyridoxal phosphate levels were increased, and immune functions were
improved. We have shown that tryptophan metabolism is abnormal in
a large percentage of patients with breast cancer (60,61) and
associated with this abnormality are low plasma pyridoxal phosphate
levels and elevated levels of a pyridoxal phosphate phosphatase
associated with erythrocyte membranes. Thus, in these patients
there is a good inverse correlation between the activity of the
erythrocyte phosphatase and plasma pyridoxal phosphate levels. The
importance of an alkaline phosphatase activity in the levels of
pyridoxal phosphate has been well studied and recently reviewed (62).
This phosphatase is induced by acetaldehyde, and we have observed
increased activity in subjects given ACTH (Potera, C., Rose, D. P.
& Brown, R. R., unpublished data). Associated with ACTH-induced
phosphatase elevations were decreased plasma levels of pyridoxal
phosphate.

In view of the role of zinc in immune lymphocyte functions
(63,64) and the importance of vitamin B-6 through its role in the
production of picolinic acid from tryptophan in the uptake of zinc
(14), it is interesting to speculate that immunosuppression seen
in vitamin B-6 deficiency (65,66) and in cancer patients may really
be the result of a zinc deficiency and to speculate further on the
role of these interactions of zinc/tryptophan/vitamin B-6 in a
variety of disease conditions including cancer, autoimmune diseases,
transplantation problems, and the like.

SUMMARY

The metabolism of tryptophan in humans was reviewed and the
usefulness of tryptophan load tests as an index of vitamin B-6
nutrition was discussed. For an adult, a loading dose of 2.0 g of
L-tryptophan or a dose of 50 mg/kg body weight is enough to cause
an increased urinary excretion of metabolites of the kynurenine
pathway. It is believed that doses of tryptophan up to this level
do not induce tryptophan pyrrolase. In normal healthy subjects,
measurement of urinary 3-hydroxykynurenine, kynurenine, or
xanthurenic acid is a sensitive index of functional vitamin B-6
deficiency which correlates well with other indices of vitamin B-6
status such as urinary 4-pyridoxic acid, plasma pyridoxal phosphate,
or methionine load tests at all degrees of deficiency. In subjects
having serious diseases, interpretation of the tryptophan load test
is difficult because of the possibility that tryptophan pyrrolase
may be induced by the stress of the disease and that the levels of

metabolite measured may be the result of this induction rather than the result of vitamin B-6 deficiency. The pattern of tryptophan metabolites in the urine in a variety of disease conditions was shown to vary considerably, suggesting that the tryptophan load test, by itself, is not an unambiguous test of vitamin B-6 nutritional status. We describe preliminary studies with a kynurenine load test which by-passes tryptophan pyrrolase. An oral loading dose of 200 mg of L-kynurenine sulfate in normal subjects results in modest and reproducible increases in several urinary metabolites, comparable in amount to the levels seen after a 2.0 g tryptophan load. However, xanthurenic acid excretion is not altered by kynurenine loads. Premenopausal women using oral contraceptives and post-menopausal women receiving small doses of estradiol had abnormal kynurenine load tests as well as abnormal tryptophan load tests. These data are interpreted as indicating that estrogens alter the activity of kynureninase and in this manner simulate a functional deficiency of vitamin B-6.

LITERATURE CITED

1. Hopkins, F. G. & Cole, S. W. (1901) A contribution to the chemistry of proteids. Part I. A preliminary study of a hitherto undescribed product of tryptic digestion. J. Physiol. 27, 418-428.
2. Reynolds, M. S. (1957) Amino acid requirements of adults. J. Am. Dietet. Assoc. 33, 1015-1018.
3. Rose, W. C., Lambert, G. F. & Coon, M. J. (1954) The amino acid requirements of man. VII. General procedures; the tryptophan requirement. J. Biol. Chem. 211, 815-827.
4. Horwitt, M. K., Harvey, C. C., Rothwell, W. S., Cutler, J. L. & Haffron, D. (1956) Tryptophan-niacin relationships in man. Studies with diets deficient in riboflavin and niacin, together with observations on the excretion of nitrogen and niacin metabolites. J. Nutr., Suppl. 1, 60, 1-43.
5. Goldsmith, G. A., Miller, O. N. & Unglaub, W. G. (1961) Efficiency of tryptophan as a niacin precursor in man. J. Nutr. 73, 172-176.
6. Nakagawa, I., Takahashi, T., Suzuki, T. & Masana, Y. (1969) Effect in man of the addition of tryptophan or niacin to the diet on the excretion of their metabolites. J. Nutr. 99, 325-330.
7. Patterson, J. I. (1979) Conversion of tryptophan to nicotinamide in the human and the rat. Ph.D. Thesis. University of Wisconsin, Madison.
8. Vivian, V. M., Brown, R. R., Price, J. M. & Reynolds, M. S. (1966) Some aspects of tryptophan and niacin metabolism in young women consuming a low tryptophan diet supplemented with niacin. J. Nutr. 88, 93-99.

9. Kim, J. H. & Miller, L. L. (1969) The functional significance
    of changes in activity of the enzymes, tryptophan pyrrolase
    and tyrosine transaminase, after induction in intact rats and
    in isolated perfused rat liver. J. Biol. Chem. 244, 1410-1416.
10. Milholland, R. J. & Rosen, F. (1971) The role of tryptophan
    pyrrolase adaptation in the excretion of xanthurenic acid by
    rats deficient in vitamin B-6. Am. J. Clin. Nutr. 24, 740-746.
11. Brown, R. R. & Price, J. M. (1956) Quantitative studies on
    metabolites of tryptophan in the urine of the dog, cat, rat,
    and man. J. Biol. Chem. 219, 985-997.
12. Allegri, G., Costa, C. & De Antoni, A. (1978) A further
    contribution to the choice of the dose for L-tryptophan load
    test. Acta Vitamin. Enzymol. 32, 163-166.
13. Costa, C., De Antoni, A., Allegri, G. & Vanzan, S. (1979)
    Studies on the tryptophan load test in man. La Ricerca Clin.
    Lab. 9, 165-175.
14. Evans, G. W. & Johnson, E. C. (1979) Zinc absorption in rats
    fed varying levels of vitamin B-6 and a vitamin B-6 antagonist.
    Clin. Res. 27, 682A.
15. Kotake, Y. & Murakami, E. (1971) A possible diabetogenic role
    for trypotphan metabolites and effects of xanthurenic acid on
    insulin. Am. J. Clin. Nutr. 24, 826-829.
16. Carlson, J. R., Yokoyama, M. T. & Dickinson, E. O. (1972)
    Induction of pulmonary edema and emphysema in cattle and goats
    with 3-methylindole. Science 176, 298-299.
17. Bungeler, W. (1932) Die experimentalle erzengung von leukamie
    und lymphosarcom durch chronische indolvergifting der maus.
    Frankfurter A. Pathol. 44, 202-271.
18. Ehrhart, H. & Stitch, W. (1957) Untersuchungen über experi-
    mentalleukamien. II. Die indol-leukamie bei der weissen
    maus. Klin. Wochschr. 35, 504-511.
19. Butenandt, A., Weidel, W. & Schlossberger, H. (1949)
    3-Oxykynurenine als cn^+-gen-abhangiges glied im intermediaren
    tryptophan-stoffwechsel. Z. Naturforsch. 4B, 242-244.
20. Kido, R., Nishino, M. & Tsuda, H. (1971) Studies on the
    mechanism of tryptophan induction of certain hepatic enzymes.
    Am. J. Clin. Nutr. 24, 766-769.
21. Triebwasser, K. C., Swan, P. B., Henderson, L. M. & Budny, J. A.
    (1976) Metabolism of D- and L-tryptophan in dogs. J. Nutr.
    106, 642-652.
22. Lepkovsky, S., Roboz, E. & Haagen-Smit, A. J. (1943) Xanthu-
    renic acid and its role in the tryptophan metabolism of pyri-
    doxine-deficient rats. J. Biol. Chem. 149, 195-201.
23. Miller, E. C. & Baumann, C. A. (1945) Relative effects of
    casein and tryptophan on the health and xanthurenic acid
    excretion of pyridoxine-deficient mice. J. Biol. Chem. 157,
    551-562.

24. Satoh, K. & Price, J. M. (1958) Fluorometric determination of kynurenic acid and xanthurenic acid in human urine. J. Biol. Chem. 230, 781-789.

25. Dalgliesh, C. E. (1952) The relation between pyridoxine and tryptophan metabolism, studied in the rat. Biochem. J. 52, 3-14.

26. Yess, N., Price, J. M., Brown, R. R., Swan, P. B. & Linkswiler, H. (1964) Vitamin B-6 depletion in man: Urinary excretion of tryptophan metabolites. J. Nutr. 84, 229-236.

27. Price, J. M., Brown, R. R. & Larson, F. C. (1957) Quantitative studies on human urinary metabolites of tryptophan as affected by isoniazid and deoxypyridoxine. J. Clin. Invest. 36, 1600-1607.

28. Komrower, G. M., Wilson, V., Clamp, J. R. & Westall, R. G. (1964) Hydroxykynureninuria. A case of abnormal tryptophan metabolism probably due to a deficiency of kynureninase. Arch. Disease Childhood 39, 250-256.

29. Ogasawara, N., Hagino, Y. & Kotake, Y. (1962) Kynurenine-transaminase, kynureninase and the increase in xanthurenic acid excretion. J. Biochem. (Tokyo) 52, 162-166.

30. Ueno, Y., Hayaishi, K. & Shukuya, R. (1963) Kynurenine transaminase from horse kidney. J. Biochem. (Tokyo) 54, 75-80.

31. Henderson, L. M. & Hulse, J. D. (1978) Vitamin B-6 relationship in tryptophan metabolism. In: Human Vitamin B-6 Requirements, pp. 21-36. Nat. Acad. Sci., Washington, DC.

32. Rosen, F., Huff, J. W. & Perlzweig, A. (1947) The role of B-6 deficiency in the tryptophane-niacin relationships in rats. J. Nutr. 33, 561-567.

33. Henderson, L. M., Weinstock, I. M. & Ramasarma, G. B. (1951) Effect of deficiency of B vitamins on the metabolism of tryptophan by the rat. J. Biol. Chem. 189, 19-29.

34. Brown, R. R., Yess, N., Price, J. M., Linkswiler, H., Swan, P. & Hankes, L. V. (1965) Vitamin B-6 depletion in man: Urinary excretion of quinolinic acid and niacin metabolites. J. Nutr. 87, 419-423.

35. Yeh, J. K-J. (1974) Nutritional factors affecting the conversion of tryptophan to niacin. Ph.D. Thesis. University of Wisconsin, Madison.

36. Knox, W. E. (1951) Two mechanisms which increase in vivo the liver tryptophan peroxidase activity: Specific enzyme adaptation and stimulation of the pituitary-adrenal system. Brit. J. Exptl. Pathol. 32, 462-469.

37. Schimke, R. T., Sweeny, E. W. & Berlin, C. M. (1964) An analysis of the kinetics of rat liver tryptophan pyrrolase induction. The significance of both enzyme synthesis and degradation. Biochem. Biophys. Res. Commun. 15, 214-219.

38. Rose, D. P. & McGinty, F. (1968) The influence of adreno-cortical hormones and vitamins upon tryptophan metabolism in man. Clin. Sci. 35, 1-9.

39. Wolf, H. (1973) The effect of hydrocortisone and tryptophan load on the metabolism of tryptophan along the kynurenine pathway. Scand. J. Clin. Lab. Invest. Suppl. 36, 77-87.

40. Altman, K. & Greengard, O. (1966) Correlation of kynurenine excretion with liver tryptophan pyrrolase levels in disease and after hydrocortisone induction. J. Clin. Invest. 45, 1527-1534.

41. Gailani, S., Murphy, G., Kenny, G., Nussabaum, A. & Silvernail, P. (1973) Studies on tryptophan metabolism in patients with bladder cancer. Cancer Res. 33, 1071-1077.

42. Wolf, H., Walter, S., Brown, R. R. & Arend, R. A. (1980) Effect of natural oestrogens on tryptophan metabolism: Evidence for interference of oestrogens with kynureninase. Scand. J. Clin. Lab. Invest. 40, 15-21.

43. Hankes, L. V., Brown, R. R., Leklem, J., Schmaeler, M. & Jesseph, J. (1972) Metabolism of C^{14} labeled enantiomers of tryptophan, kynurenine and hydroxykynurenine in humans with scleroderma. J. Invest. Derm. 58, 85-95.

44. Brown, R. R. (1975) Twenty years of tryptophan studies in humans. Acta Vitamin. Enzymol. 29, 12-16.

45. Price, J. M., Brown, R. R. & Yess, N. (1965) Testing the functional capacity of the tryptophan niacin pathway in man by analysis of urinary metabolites. Advan. Metab. Disor. 2, 159-225.

46. Arend, R. A., Leklem, J. E. & Brown, R. R. (1970) Direct and steam distillation autoanalyzer methods for assay of diazo-tizable aromatic amine metabolites of tryptophan in urine and in serum. Biochem. Med. 4, 457-468.

47. Leklem, J. E., Brown, R. R., Rose, D. P., Linkswiler, H. & Arend, R. A. (1975) Metabolism of tryptophan and niacin in oral contraceptive users receiving controlled intakes of vitamin B-6. Am. J. Clin. Nutr. 28, 146-156.

48. Brown, R. R., Rose, D. P., Leklem, J. E., Linkswiler, H. & Anand, R. (1975) Urinary 4-pyridoxic acid, plasma pyridoxal phosphate, and erythrocyte aminotransferase levels in oral contraceptive users receiving controlled intakes of vitamin B-6. Am. J. Clin. Nutr. 28, 10-19.

49. Shane, B. (1978) Vitamin B-6 and blood. In: Human Vitamin B-6 Requirements, pp. 111-128, Nat. Acad. Sci., Washington, DC.

50. Shane, B. & Contractor, S. F. (1980) Vitamin B-6 status and metabolism in pregnancy. In: Vitamin B-6 Metabolism and Role in Growth (Tryfiates, G. P., ed.), pp. 137-171, Food and Nutrition Press, Inc., Westport, Connecticut.

51. Linkswiler, H. M. (1978) Vitamin B-6 requirements of men.
     In: Human Vitamin B-6 Requirements, pp. 279-290, Nat. Acad.
     Sci., Washington, DC.
52. Leklem, J. E., Rose, D. P. & Brown, R. R. (1973) Effects of
     oral contraceptives on urinary metabolite excretions after
     administration of L-tryptophan or L-kynurenine sulfate.
     Metabolism 22, 1499-1505.
53. Hansson, O. (1969) Tryptophan loading and pyridoxine treat-
     ment in children with epilepsy. Ann. N.Y. Acad. Sci. 166,
     306-309.
54. Braidman, I. P. & Rose, D. P. (1971) Effects of sex hormones
     on three glucocorticoid-inducible enzymes concerned with amino
     acid metabolism in rat liver. Endocrinology 89, 1250-1255.
55. Wolf, H., Brown, R. R. & Arend, R. A. (1980) The kynurenine
     load test, an adjunct to the tryptophan load test. Scand. J.
     Clin. Lab. Invest. 40, 9-14.
56. Musajo, L. & Benassi, C. A. (1964) Aspects of disorders of
     the kynurenine pathway of tryptophan metabolism in man. Adv.
     Clin. Chem. 7, 63-135.
57. Price, J. M. (1958) Disorders of tryptophan metabolism.
     Univ. Mich. Med. Bull. 24, 461-485.
58. Chabner, B. A., DeVita, V. T., Livingston, D. M. & Oliverio,
     V. T. (1970) Abnormalities of tryptophan metabolism and
     plasma pyridoxal phosphate in Hodgkin's disease. New Eng. J.
     Med. 282, 838-843.
59. DeVita, V. T., Chabner, B. A., Livingston, D. M. & Oliverio,
     V. T. (1971) Anergy and tryptophan metabolism in Hodgkin's
     disease. Am. J. Clin. Nutr. 24, 835-840.
60. Potera, C., Brown, R. R. & Rose, D. P. (1977) Role of pyri-
     doxal phosphate (PLP) phosphatase activity in regulation of
     plasma PLP in cancer patients. Fed. Proc. 36, 1137.
61. Potera, C., Rose, D. P. & Brown, R. R. (1977) Vitamin B-6
     deficiency in cancer patients. Am. J. Clin. Nutr. 30, 1677-
     1679.
62. Lumeng, L. & Li, T.-K. (1980) Mammalian vitamin B-6 metab-
     olism: regulatory role of protein-binding and the hydrolysis
     of pyridoxal-5'-phosphate in storage and transport. In:
     Vitamin B-6 Metabolism and Role in Growth (Tryfiates, G. P.,
     ed.), pp. 27-51. Food and Nutrition Press, Westport,
     Connecticut.
63. Gross, L. R. & Newburne, P. M. (1980) Role of nutrition in
     immunologic function. Physiolog. Rev. 60, 265-269.
64. Schloen, L. H., Fernandes, G., Garofalo, J. A. & Good, R. A.
     (1979) Nutrition, immunity and cancer--a review. Part II:
     Zinc, immune function and cancer. Clin. Bull. 9, 63-75.

65. Axelrod, A. E. & Trakatellis, A. C. (1964) Relationship of
     pyridoxine to immunological phenomena. Vitamins and Hormones
     <u>22</u>, 591-607.
66. Robson, L. C. & Schwarz, M. R. (1975) Vitamin B-6 deficiency
     and the lymphoid system. II. Effects of vitamin B-6 deficiency
     in utero on the immunological competence of the offspring.
     Cell. Immunol. <u>16</u>, 145-152.

VITAMIN B-6 AND SULFUR AMINO ACID METABOLISM

John A. Sturman

Developmental Neurochemistry Laboratory
Department of Pathological Neurobiology
Institute for Basic Research in Mental Retardation
Staten Island, NY   10314

Vitamin B-6, in the form of pyridoxal 5'-phosphate, is the coenzyme required by many of the enzymes involved in the metabolism of sulfur-containing amino acids (Fig. 1). Methionine, cyst(e)ine, and taurine, of the chemicals listed in this scheme, are generally available in the diet. Methionine is an essential amino acid for mammals, although the requirement can be spared to some extent by cystine. Cyst(e)ine is not generally an essential amino acid for mammals, since adequate amounts may be produced from methionine via the transsulfuration pathway, although it may be essential for a period after birth in some species as a result of the postnatal development of cystathionase. Taurine is an aminosulfonic acid whose role in development and nutrition has been the subject of much recent research and debate. It is an essential nutrient for the cat and kitten, and may be for some primates, including man. These species have low activities of cysteinesulfinic acid decarboxylase, the enzyme considered to be responsible for taurine biosynthesis in mammals. Methionine and cysteine are utilized for protein synthesis, taurine is not.

Those enzymes requiring pyridoxal 5'-phosphate as coenzyme are affected by a dietary deficiency of vitamin B-6, although not to the same extent. In addition, there are a number of human conditions, in which there is a greater dependency on vitamin B-6, which are alleviated somewhat by an increased dietary intake of the vitamin. Inborn errors of amino acid metabolism in man have been described involving two of the enzymes in Fig. 1 which require pyridoxal 5'-phosphate as coenzyme, and, for each of these enzymes, conditions occur in which enzymatic activity is reduced or absent. These conditions, and their response to dietary vitamin B-6 will be discussed in more detail.

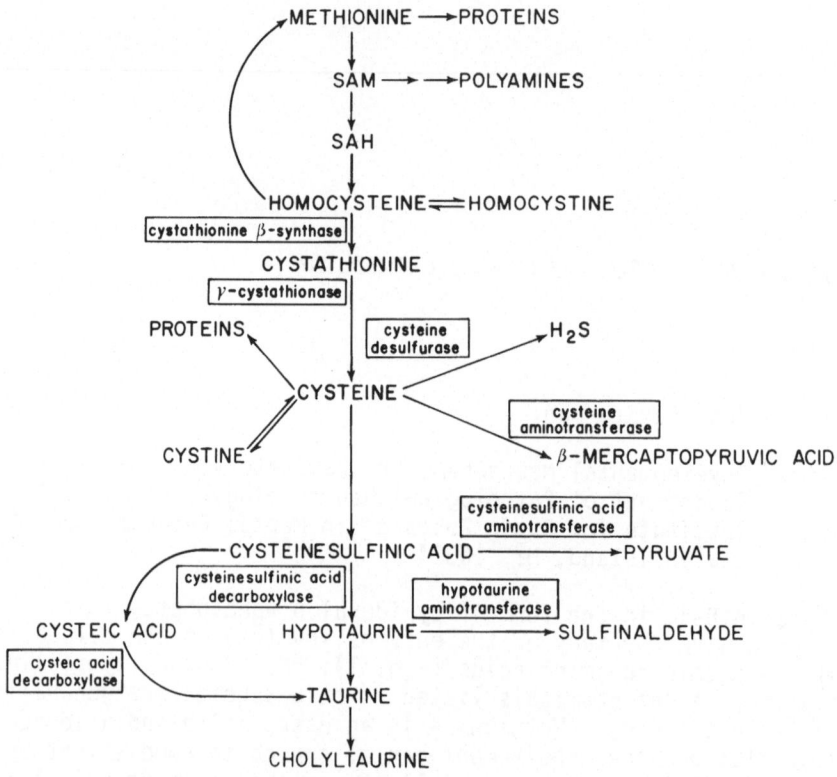

Fig. 1. Methionine metabolism in mammals. The enzymes listed
        utilize pyridoxal 5'-phosphate as coenzyme.

CYSTATHIONINE β-SYNTHASE (EC 4.2.1.22)

     In mammals, this enzyme is responsible for the formation of
cystathionine via the transsulfuration pathway of methionine metabolism (1). The reaction proceeds by the β-activation of serine and
the addition of homocysteine (Fig. 2). Cystathionine β-synthase is
also capable of carrying out the β-activation of cysteine and the
addition of homocysteine to form cystathionine (Fig. 3) (2,3). The
sulfur atom of cystathionine is derived from homocysteine in both
reactions. The sulfur atom of cysteine can be incorporated into
cystathionine by γ-activation of homocysteine or of homoserine,
mediated by γ-cystathionase (4-8).

     Cystathionine β-synthase activity is widespread among tissues
(brain, liver, kidney, pancreas) and among species--it has been
measured in liver of every species examined (9,10). In addition,
the enzymatic activity is present in fibroblasts derived from human
skin (11) and, to a lesser extent, in long-term lymphoid cell lines
established from human peripheral blood leucocytes after stimulation
of the lymphocytes with phytohemagglutinin (12,13).

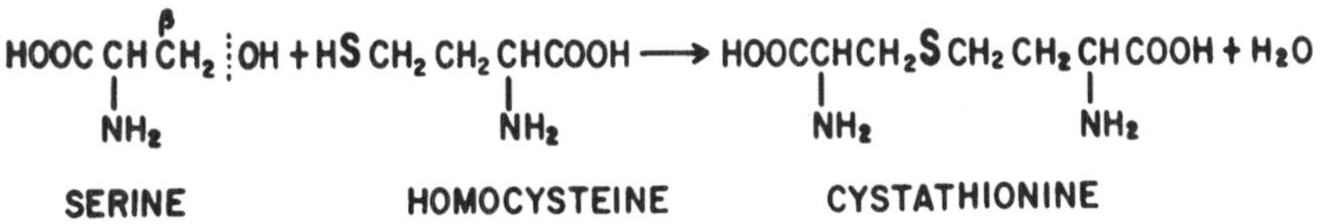

$$\underset{\substack{|\\ NH_2}}{HOOC\ CH}\ \overset{\beta}{CH_2}\ |\ OH + HS\ CH_2\ CH_2\ \underset{\substack{|\\ NH_2}}{CHCOOH} \longrightarrow HOOCCHCH_2\underset{\substack{|\\ NH_2}}{S}CH_2\ CH_2\ \underset{\substack{|\\ NH_2}}{CHCOOH} + H_2O$$

SERINE HOMOCYSTEINE CYSTATHIONINE

Fig. 2. The reaction catalyzed by cystathionine β-synthase in the transsulfuration pathway of methionine metabolism.

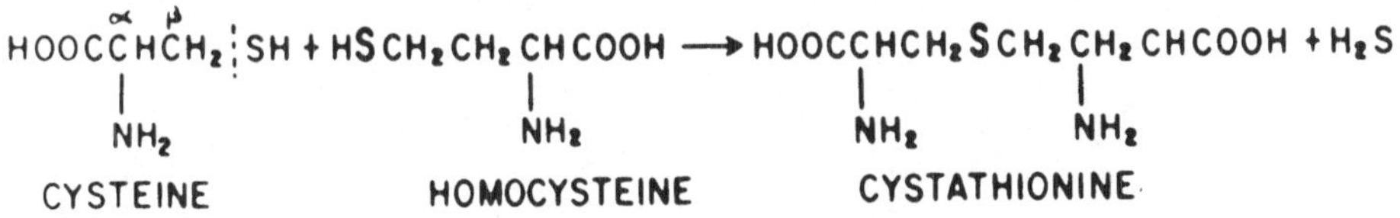

$$HOOC\overset{\alpha}{C}\overset{\beta}{CH}_2\ |\ SH + HS\ CH_2\ CH_2\ \underset{\substack{|\\ NH_2}}{CHCOOH} \longrightarrow HOOCCHCH_2\ \underset{\substack{|\\ NH_2}}{S}CH_2\ CH_2\ \underset{\substack{|\\ NH_2}}{CHCOOH} + H_2S$$

CYSTEINE HOMOCYSTEINE CYSTATHIONINE

Fig. 3. Synthesis of cystathionine from cysteine and homocysteine catalyzed by cystathionine β-synthase (also known as serine sulfhydrase).

Cystathionine β-synthase activity is present in fetal (2nd trimester) human liver (14,15), although lower than in adult human liver, whereas in fetal rhesus monkey liver during the third trimester its activity is greater than that in postnatal and adult rhesus monkey liver (Fig. 4) (16). Activity in fetal human and fetal rhesus monkey brain is lower than found in mature brain, and in the monkey, at least, increases slowly during development (Fig. 5). The concentration of cystathionine in rhesus monkey tissues parallels the activity of cystathionine β-synthase (Fig. 6), although the activity of γ-cystathionase, the cystathionine cleaving enzyme, is also partly responsible for these results (16,17).

The enzyme is almost entirely located in the soluble fraction of liver homogenates whereas it is chiefly located in the particulate fraction of brain homogenates (18-20). It has been extensively purified from rat liver and from human liver, and from cultured human fibroblasts (21-27). The enzyme from these sources consists of subunits (27-29).' Purification of the enzyme from brain has not been reported to date.

Homocystinuria due to cystathionine β-synthase deficiency is a disease in man inherited in an autosomal recessive manner (30). It may be accompanied by several clinical signs and symptoms, including mental retardation, thromboembolic disease, dislocated lenses and skeletal abnormalities (31). It is usually characterized biochemically by abnormally high concentrations of homocystine and methionine and abnormally low concentrations of cystine in plasma and urine. In such patients the activity of cystathionine β-synthase

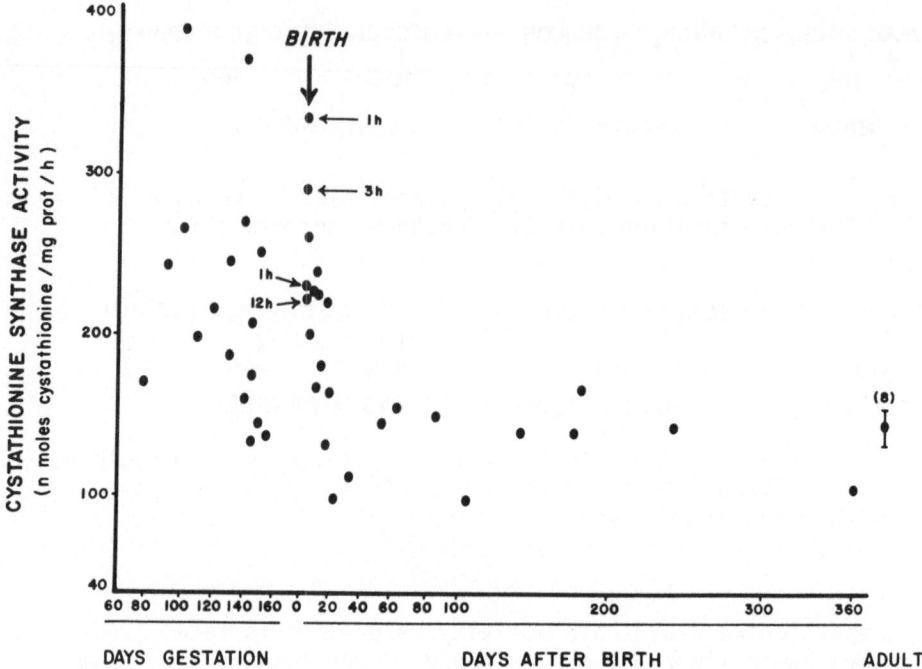

Fig. 4.   Specific activity of cystathionine β-synthase in rhesus
          monkey liver during development. From reference 16 with
          permission.

has been demonstrated to be abnormally low or absent in liver, brain,
cultured skin fibroblasts, and in long-term lymphoid lines (11,12,
32-39). The biochemical consequences of this deficiency of enzymatic
activity include a virtual absence of cystathionine in the brain
(40,41), which normally contains a high concentration of cystathionine. Whether or not this has any important consequences is
not known, although it has been suggested that cystathionine has a
neurochemical function (42,43). In addition, elevated concentrations
of methionine are present in liver, which may contribute to the
ultrastructural abnormalities that have been observed in the liver
of these patients (38,44). Although the presence of homocystine
was reported in liver from one patient at autopsy (45), it was not
identified in tissues from two other patients at autopsy (41), or
in liver biopsies obtained from two other patients (44). It is of
note that the livers from the last two patients contained apparently
normal concentrations of cystine. The explanation of the failure
to detect homocystine in tissues of patients was recently provided
by a report which demonstrated that homocysteine bound to proteins
with disulfide bonds was not released by conventional extraction

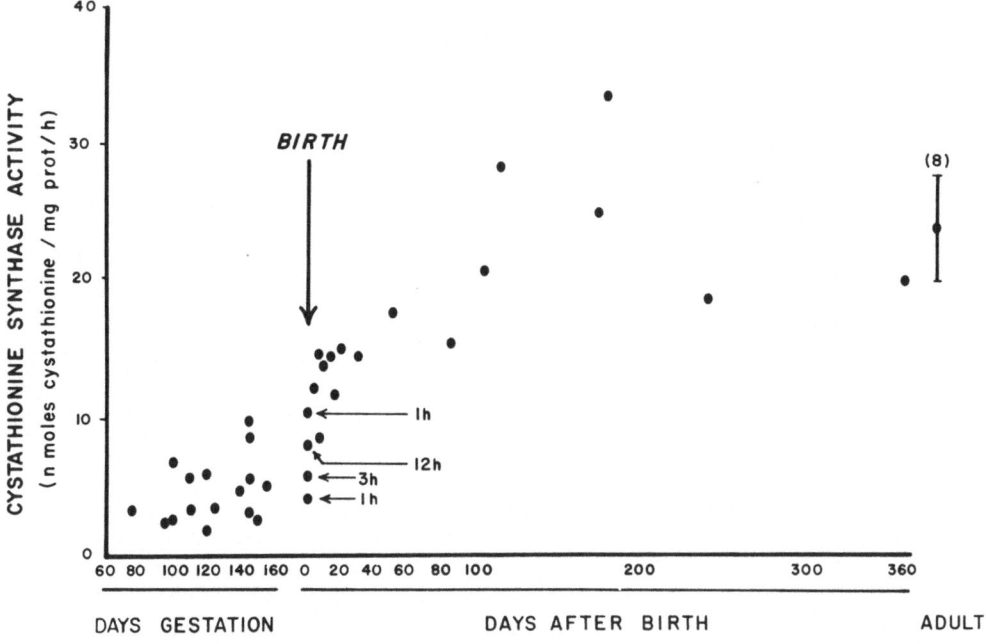

Fig. 5. Specific activity of cystathionine β-synthase in rhesus
         monkey brain (occipital lobe) during development. From
         reference 16 with permission.

procedures (46). When such tissues were incubated with 2-mercapto-
ethanol, large amounts of homocysteine were released from brain,
liver, and kidney obtained at autopsy from a patient.

     Dietary treatment with large doses of vitamin B-6, in the form
of pyridoxine hydrochloride, ameliorates or eliminates the biochemical abnormalities of some patients with homocystinuria due to
cystathionine β-synthase deficiency (47-51). Such treatment, which
may require 25 to 1500 mg of pyridoxine hydrochloride daily, when
successful will eliminate homocystine from plasma and urine, reduce
the concentrations of methionine in plasma and urine, and result in
the appearance of normal cystine concentrations in plasma and urine
within a few days (Fig. 7). Treatment with vitamin B-6 reduces the
concentration of methionine in the livers of such responsive patients
(44), but it is not known if the concentration of cystathionine in
their brains is altered. In some patients with this disease, these
biochemical abnormalities in plasma and urine are unaffected by
vitamin B-6 therapy, and are termed unresponsive (52).

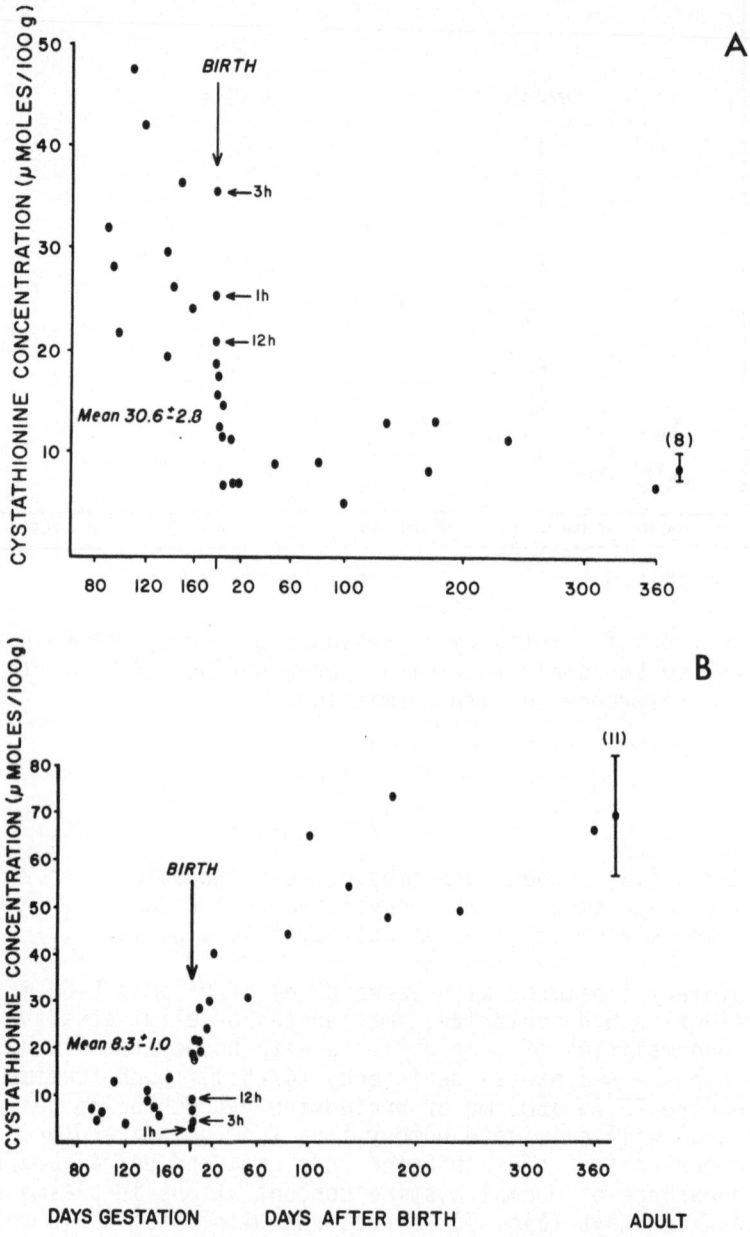

Fig. 6. Concentration of cystathionine during development of the
rhesus monkey (A) in liver (B) in brain (occipital lobe).
From reference 16 with permission.

The mechanism of action of vitamin B-6 in homocystinuria due to cystathionine β-synthase deficiency has been the subject of much study and speculation in recent years (24,33,35,53-56). In general, unresponsive patients do not have any measurable hepatic activity, whereas responsive patients usually do. Furthermore, from the limited studies performed to date, the hepatic activity in responsive patients is generally increased by vitamin B-6 therapy, whereas the

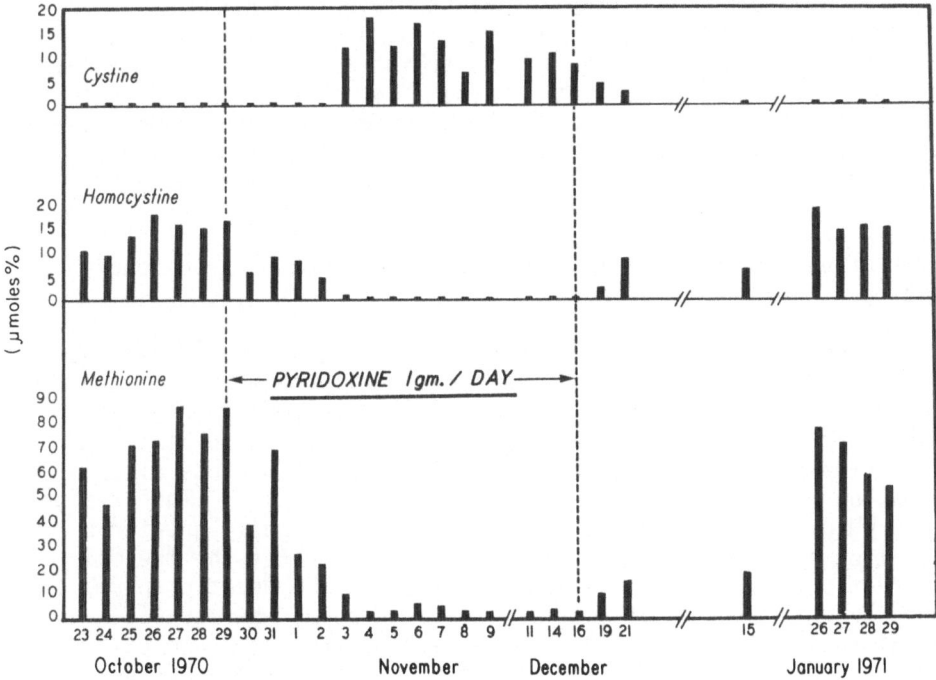

Fig. 7.   Effect of oral pyridoxine treatment on the concentration of methionine, homocystine, and cystine in plasma of a typical vitamin B-6-responsive, cystathionine β-synthase-deficient individual.

unresponsive patients still have no measurable activity (38). Because of the ethical and practical problems of studying the hepatic enzyme, most studies have been carried out with the enzyme contained in cultured skin fibroblasts. One study observed that skin fibroblasts cultured from responsive patients contained some measurable activity of the enzyme, whereas skin fibroblasts cultured from unresponsive patients contained no measurable activity. This suggested that there was a simple genetic heterogeneity in such patients that could easily be explained by a mutant enzyme with a reduced affinity for the coenzyme, which had sufficient activity in vivo during vitamin B-6 therapy to normalize the sulfur amino acid metabolite profile,

and by a mutant so greatly altered that it has lost all catalytic
activity (or complete absence of the enzyme protein). Further
studies indicated that the situation was more complex, since skin
fibroblasts cultured from responsive and unresponsive patients were
reported with no measurable activity, with measurable activity which
was greatly increased by pyridoxal 5'-phosphate in vitro, and, only
in skin fibroblasts cultured from responsive patients, measurable
activity which was increased only modestly by pyridoxal 5-phosphate
in vitro, as found with skin fibroblasts cultured from unaffected
individuals (11,24,32,57). These results made it necessary to
invoke three distinct classes of cystathionine β-synthase mutants:
those with no residual activity; those with reduced activity and
normal affinity for the pyridoxal 5'-phosphate coenzyme; and those
with reduced activity and a reduced affinity for the pyridoxal
5'-phosphate coenzyme. Moreover, the responsiveness or unrespon-
siveness of a patient could not be correlated simply with the
presence or absence of residual activity in vitro, or with stimulation of enzyme activity in vitro by the pyridoxal 5'-phosphate
coenzyme.

Another aspect of cystathionine β-synthase which has received
much attention is the stability of the activity to heat, and the
role of vitamin B-6 in this phenomenon. The enzyme from normal
human liver is activated more than 2-fold by incubation at 55⁰ for
3-4 minutes prior to assay (Fig. 8) (55). Longer periods of preincubation result in progressive thermal inactivation. The presence
of 1.3 mM pyridoxal 5'-phosphate results in a slightly greater
activation during the first 3-4 minutes and prevents the thermal
inactivation. Activation was not observed in the hepatic enzyme of
responsive patients prior to vitamin B-6 therapy, whereas after
several weeks of therapy, the hepatic enzyme from the same patients
was activated by preincubation at 55⁰. This result may be taken to
indicate that the enzyme from these responsive patients has an
abnormal structure, since activation is an expression of the ability
of the normal enzyme to undergo heat-induced coformational changes.
Apparently vitamin B-6 therapy allows the mutant enzyme to maintain
a more normal conformation in vivo, since it did undergo heat-induced
activation.

For the reasons previously listed, this research has been pur-
sued in cultured skin fibroblasts (57,58). The heat-induced activation of the enzyme is retained by normal skin fibroblasts,
although pyridoxal 5'-phosphate does not have such a complete
protective effect on the subsequent inactivation of the enzyme from
this source as it did on the normal liver enzyme (Fig. 9(. The
enzyme in cultured skin fibroblasts from all patients but one shows
no heat-induced activation and a variety of rates of inactivation.
The effect of pyridoxal 5'-phosphate on this phenomenon revealed

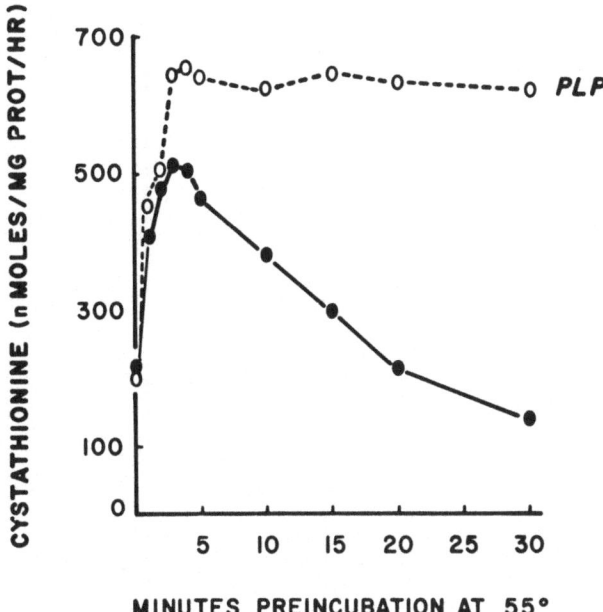

Fig. 8.   Effect of preincubation at 55° on the specific activity of
cystathionine β-synthase in an extract of normal human
liver, and the effect of 1.3 mM pyridoxal 5'-phosphate.
From reference 55 with permission.

two distinct variations (Fig. 9). The first of these, designated
type 1, is characterized by some protection against inactivation,
similar to that observed in normal skin fibroblasts. The second
variant, designated type 2, is relatively resistant to heat inactivation, unless pyridoxal 5'-phosphate is present, when the enzyme
is quickly inactivated. This effect of the coenzyme, while reducing
the ability of the enzyme to withstand heat-induced inactivation,
may, nevertheless, be considered as a normalizing effect.

Reexamination of some previously puzzling results obtained from
responsive patients in vivo suggests that a similar phenomenon may
occur in the intact patient (56). Oral loads of homocysteine (free-
base) administered to untreated responsive patients produced two
distinct types of results (Figs. 10 and 11). The first, designated
type 1, produced the predicted effect; i.e., it caused whatever
cystine was present in plasma to be removed, presumably by formation
of the mixed disulfide of cysteine and homocysteine, and no change
in the minimal amount of cystine excreted in urine. The second type
of result, designated type 2, was the appearance in plasma of large
concentrations of cystine, which previously was low or absent, and

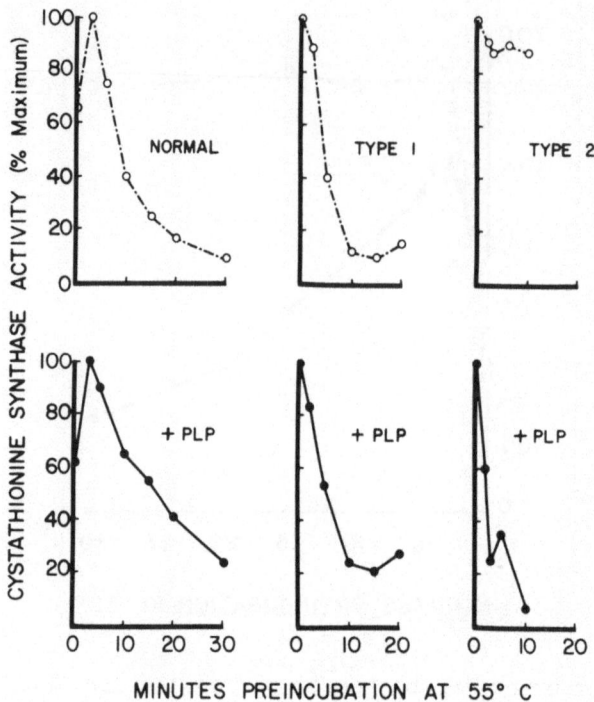

Fig. 9.   Effect of preincubation at 55° on the specific activity
           of cystathionine β-synthase in extracts of cultured skin
           fibroblasts from a normal individual and from vitamin B-6-
           responsive, cystathionine β-synthase-deficient individuals,
           illustrating the different effects of 0.4 mM pyridoxal
           5'-phosphate. Adapted from reference 58.

the excretion of large amounts of cystine in the urine. After a few
weeks of oral therapy with vitamin B-6, the loads of homocysteine
were repeated. Under these conditions, the responses were similar;
i.e., the cystine present in plasma (now in much greater concentrations than in the untreated condition) is largely or completely
removed, again, presumably, by formation of the mixed disulfide of
cysteine and homocysteine, and there is a small reduction or no
change in the cystine excreted in the urine. It should be noted
that the results of oral homocysteine loads in a normal individual
were similar to those obtained in the type 1 response.

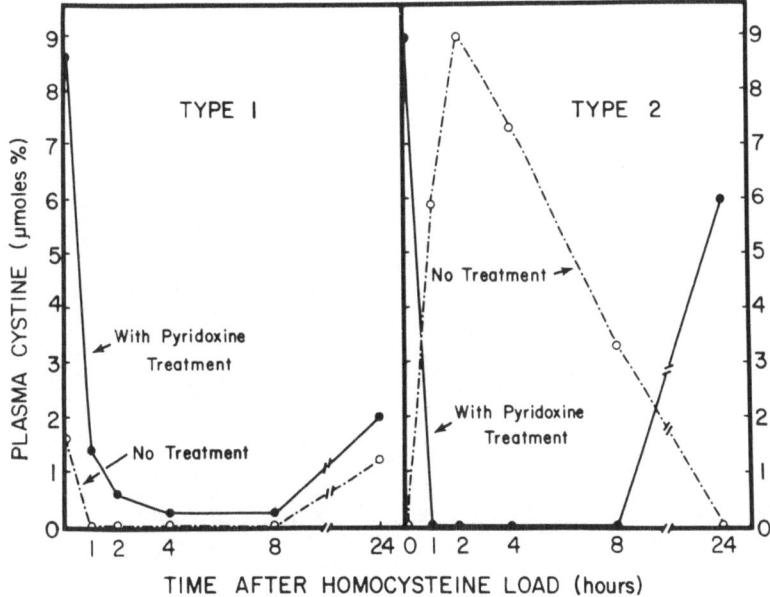

Fig. 10.   Different types of results obtained after an oral load of
homocysteine on the concentration of cystine in plasma of
vitamin B-6-responsive, cystathionine β-synthase-deficient
individuals with and without oral pyridoxine treatment.
Adapted from reference 56.

These results suggest that normal individuals and type 1 responsive patients do not have large amounts of cysteine bound to proteins
within the body by disulfide bonds, or, if they do, the homocysteine
free base is not a strong enough reducing agent to release it.   Type
2 responsive patients clearly have a large pool of cysteine bound
to proteins within the body by disulfide bonds which is released by
homocysteine.   Oral vitamin B-6 therapy normalizes this response in
a similar fashion to the type 2 response observed in vitro with the
enzyme from cultured skin fibroblasts.   One must conclude that the
mechanism involves some conformational change in vivo of a protein
or proteins within the body that alters the accessibility of the
thiol groups.   The implications of the result in vivo, however, are
greater than those in vitro for the following reason.   Proteins
other than cystathionine β-synthase may be involved because of the
large number of protein sulfhydryl sites required to bind the amount
of cystine released.   Changes in the conformation of these proteins
may contribute to some of the structural abnormalities which result
in the clinical signs and symptoms observed in these patients.

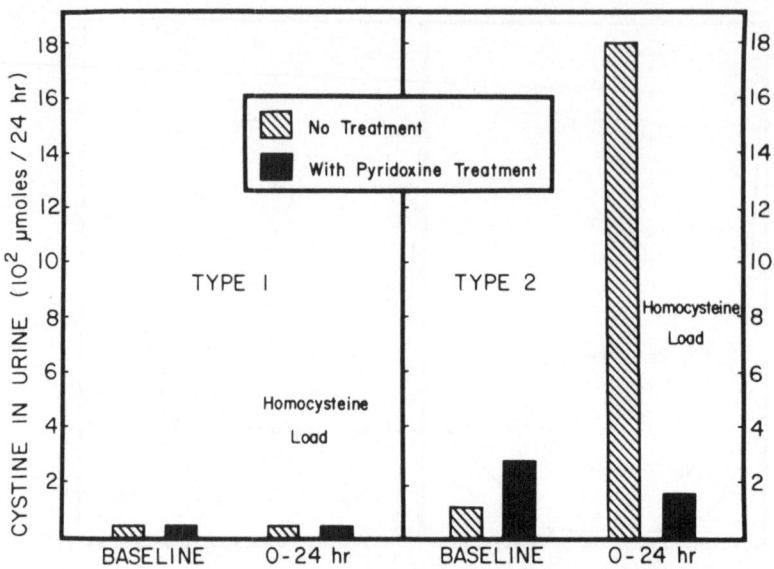

Fig. 11.   Different types of results obtained after an oral load of
           homocysteine on the excretion of cystine in urine of
           vitamin B-6-responsive, cystathionine β-synthase-deficient
           individuals with and without oral pyridoxine treatment.
           Adapted from reference 56.

γ-CYSTATHIONASE (EC 4.4.1.1)

     This enzyme in mammals completes the transsulfuration process
by cleaving cystathionine in the γ-position to form cysteine (Fig.
12). The mammalian enzyme is also capable of synthesizing cystathionine from cysteine and homoserine or homocysteine, and of
synthesizing the symmetrical homologue of cystathionine, homolanthionine, from homocysteine and homoserine (Fig. 13). γ-Cystathionase
also catalyzes the degradation of homoserine to α-oxobutyrate, NH_3
and H_2S (homoserine dehydratase) and of cysteine to pyruvate, NH_3
and H_2S (cysteine desulfurase). The degradation of cysteine involves
activation at the γ-carbon atom, whereas all of the other reactions
involve activation at the β-carbon atom, and involves a separate
active site on the enzyme.

     γ-Cystathionase activity is widespread among tissues (brain,
liver, kidney, pancreas) and among species--it is present at high
levels in the liver of every species examined (9,10,59). In brain,
the activity of this enzyme is low, and is a contributing factor,
at least, to the high concentration of cystathionine found in this
organ. The enzymatic activity is present in long-term lymphoid

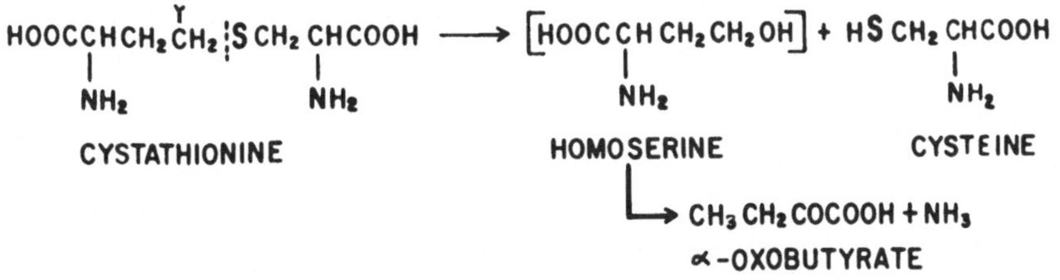
HOOCCHCH2CH2 S CH2 CHCOOH
NH2
NH2
CYSTATHIONINE
HOOCCHCH2CH2OH
NH2
HOMOSERINE
HS CH2 CHCOOH
NH2
CYSTEINE
CH3CH2COCOOH + NH3
α-OXOBUTYRATE

Fig. 12. The reaction catalyzed by γ-cystathionase in the transsulfuration pathway. No direct evidence exists for the production of homoserine as an intermediate, although it is required along with cysteine for the reverse reaction.

cell lines established from human peripheral blood leucocytes after stimulation of the leucocytes with phytohemagglutinin (60) and, to a lesser extent, in fibroblasts derived from human skin (61).

In contrast to cystathionine β-synthase, activity of γ-cystathionase is virtually absent from fetal (2nd trimester) human liver or brain (14,15,62). Cysteine, therefore, is an essential amino acid for the human fetus and must be supplied by the mother. It is probable that cysteine is an essential amino acid also for the prematurely born and full term human infant since the data available indicate that development of γ-cystathionase activity is a postnatal phenomenon. Rhesus monkey liver (16) and rat liver (63) have an increasing activity of γ-cystathionase after birth, but, in contrast to fetal human liver, do have measurable activity in liver prior to birth (Fig. 14).

The enzyme is almost entirely located in the soluble fraction of liver homogenates whereas a considerable proportion is located in the particulate fraction of brain homogenates (20). It has been extensively purified from rat liver, mouse liver, and from human liver (4,64-68). The enzymes from these sources have somewhat different properties, although all require pyridoxal 5'-phosphate as coenzyme. The amino acid composition of rat liver γ-cystathionase has been reported (69), and it has been shown to have two separate active sites (65,70).

Primary cystathioninuria is an inborn error resulting from an inherited deficiency of γ-cystathionase. Although this was first described in a patient with severe mental deficiency (71), and many cases with a variety of clinical signs and symptoms have subsequently been reported (72-74), several cases have also been reported in healthy individuals (75-77). The prevalent view is that clinical manifestations are not causally related to a deficiency of γ-cystathionase. The activity of γ-cystathionase has been demonstrated to

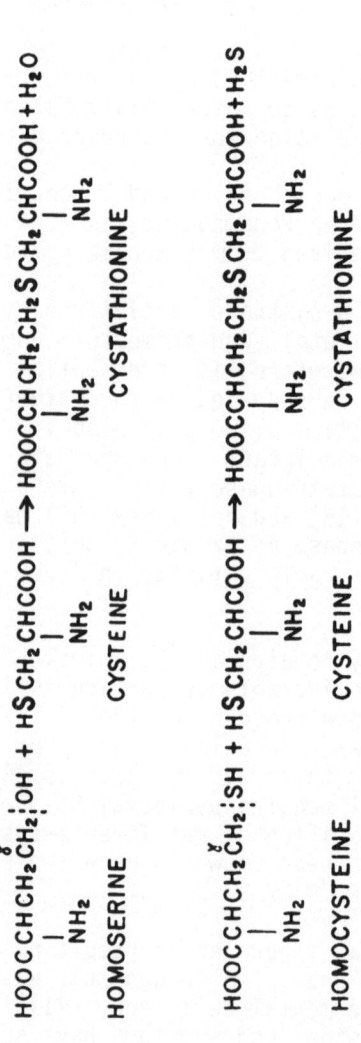

Fig. 13.   Other reactions mediated by γ-cystathionase.

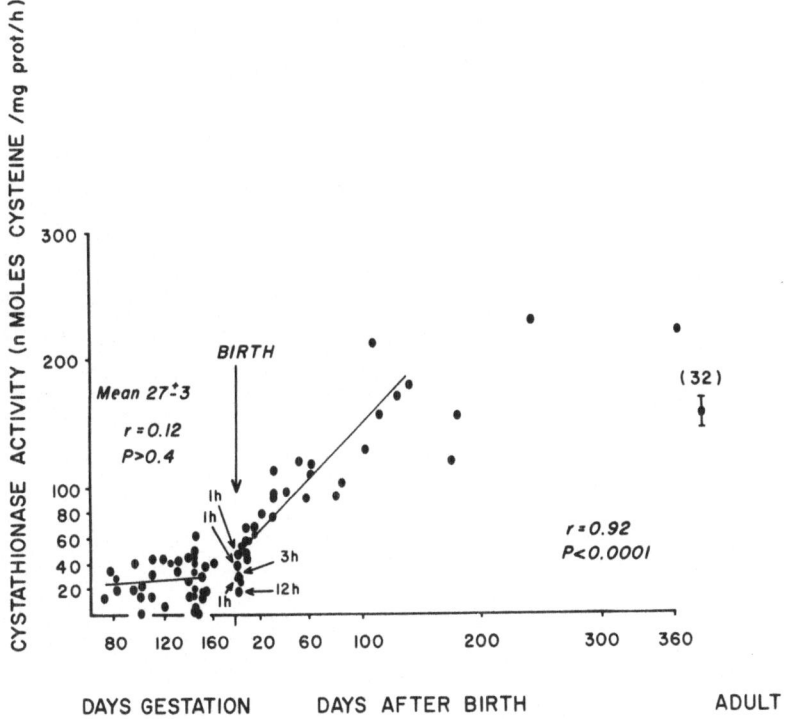

Fig. 14.   Specific activity of γ-cystathionase in rhesus monkey
           liver during development. From reference 16 with
           permission.

be abnormally low or absent in liver (72,78), cultured skin fibroblasts (61), and in long-term lymphoid lines (60). The biochemical
consequences of this enzymatic deficiency include the presence of
cystathionine in plasma, the excretion of large quantities of
cystathionine in urine, and the accumulation of cystathionine in
body organs, such as liver and kidney. It is not certain whether
cystathionine accumulates in brain because the minimal data available are not distinguishable from normal brain, which has a high
concentration of cystathionine.

Dietary treatment with large doses of vitamin B-6, in the form
of pyridoxine hydrochloride, ameliorates or eliminates the cystathioninemia and cystathioninuria in the majority of patients (72,
75,79), although two unresponsive cases have been reported (80,81).
The mechanism of action of vitamin B-6 in γ-cystathionase deficiency
could not be determined from the two reports of studies with limited
amounts of liver, but has been considerably clarified by extensive
studies using long-term lymphoid lines. The results to date suggest

that primary cystathioninuria is caused by two different mutations
affecting the γ-cystathionase molecule, the vitamin B-6-responsive
and -unresponsive forms (60,82). The unresponsive form appears to
result from a failure to synthesize the enzyme protein, for no
enzymatic activity can be detected nor can any protein with antigenic
identity to the γ-cystathionase protein be detected. The responsive
form appears to result from the synthesis of a mutant enzyme with
reduced affinity for the coenzyme. This form has some residual
activity (Fig. 15) but needs much greater concentrations of pyridoxal
5'-phosphate than does the normal enzyme to exhibit maximum activity
(Fig. 16). This mutant enzyme retains antigenic identity with the
normal enzyme, although the antigenic binding capacity may be reduced.

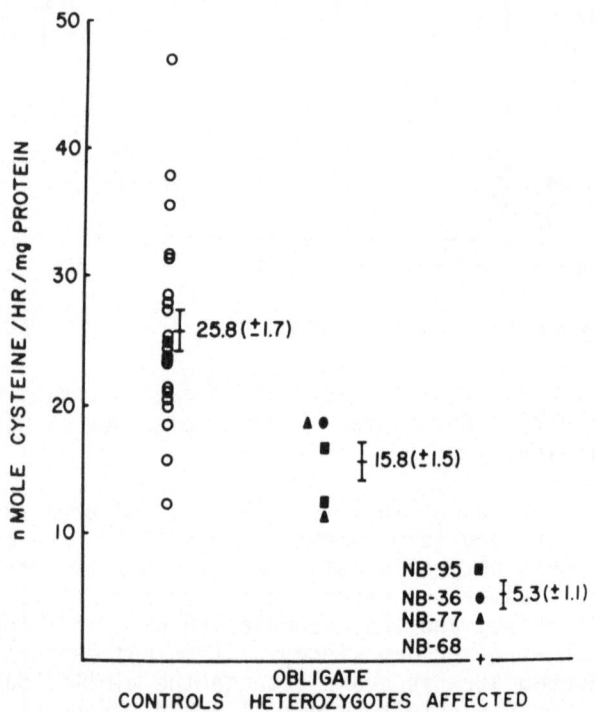

Fig. 15.   Specific activity of γ-cystathionase in extracts of long-
           term lymphoid cell lines established from 21 normal indi-
           viduals, from 5 obligate heterozygotes for vitamin B-6-
           responsive cystathioninuria, from 3 patients with vitamin
           B-6-responsive cystathioninuria (NB 36, NB 77, NB 95),
           and from one patient with vitamin B-6-unresponsive
           cystathioninuria (NB 68). From reference 82 with
           permission.

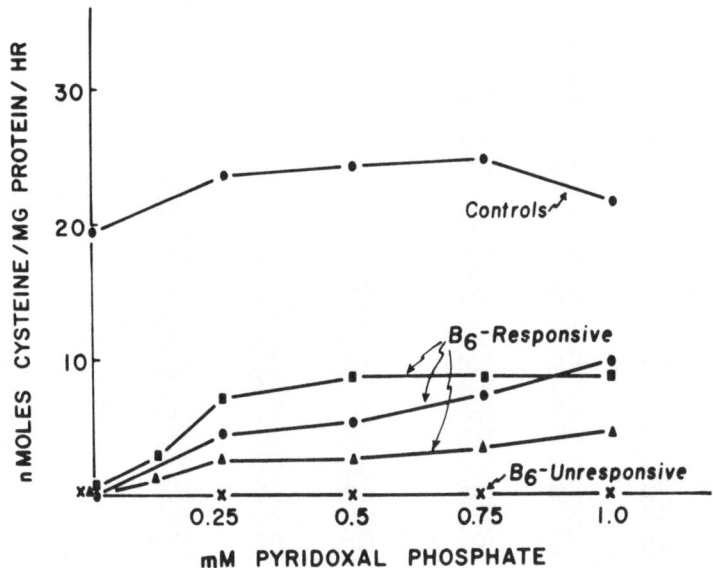

Fig. 16. The effects of increasing concentrations of pyridoxal 5'-phosphate on the specific activity of γ-cystathionase in extracts of lymphoid cell lines from a normal individual, from three patients with vitamin B-6-responsive cystathioninuria, and from one patient with vitamin B-6-unresponsive cystathioninuria. From reference 82 with permission.

Another interesting demonstration of an altered structure of the mutant enzyme resulted from the measurement of the thermostability of the enzymatic activity, and the effect of pyridoxal 5'-phosphate on this parameter (83). Extracts of cells from normal individuals were inactivated to varying degrees by heating at 70° for 90 minutes prior to measurement of cystathionase activity. The presence of 0.5 mM pyridoxal 5'-phosphate afforded complete protection against heat inactivation (Fig. 17). Extracts of cells from heterozygotes behaved similarly. In contrast, extracts of cells from responsive γ-cystathionase-deficient patients, although inactivated to a similar extent by heating alone, were inactivated to an even greater extent in the presence of 0.5 mM pyridoxal 5'-phosphate. In this respect, the mutant γ-cystathionase resembles the type 2 mutant cystathionine β-synthase discussed earlier.

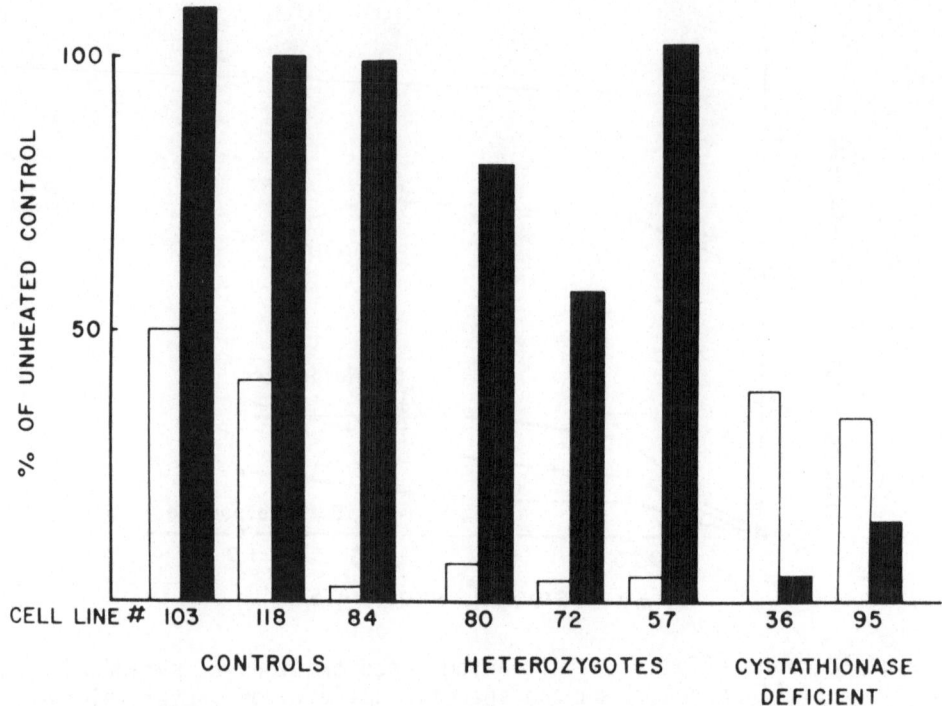

Fig. 17. The effect of preincubation at 70° for 90 minutes on the
specific activity of γ-cystathionase in extracts of long-
term lymphoid cells (open bars) and the effect of 0.5 mM
pyridoxal 5'-phosphate (solid bars). From reference 83
with permission.

CYSTEINESULFINIC ACID DECARBOXYLASE (EC 4.1.1.19)

This enzyme is considered to be responsible for the bulk, if
not all, of the taurine biosynthesized by mammals. The immediate
product of the reaction is hypotaurine (Fig. 18), which is then
converted rapidly to taurine by either or both chemical oxidation
and enzymatic oxidation. Hypotaurine is rarely found in mammalian
tissues in measurable amounts (84-86). Taurine has been the subject
of much recent research and its role in nutrition and development
has been extensively examined (87).

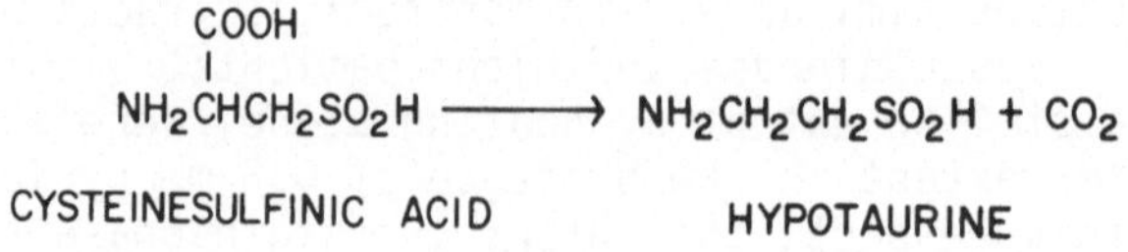

$$\underset{\text{CYSTEINESULFINIC ACID}}{NH_2CHCH_2SO_2H} \overset{\text{COOH}}{\underset{}{|}} \longrightarrow \underset{\text{HYPOTAURINE}}{NH_2CH_2CH_2SO_2H} + CO_2$$

Fig. 18. The reaction catalyzed by cysteinesulfinic acid
decarboxylase.

Cysteinesulfinic acid decarboxylase activity has been measured in various tissues (brain, liver, kidney) from a variety of species (87,88). Its activity in liver, especially, varies greatly from species to species. The activity in liver, brain, and retina increases during development (89-92). The enzyme is almost entirely located in the soluble fraction of liver homogenates whereas it is chiefly located in the particulate fraction of brain homogenates (20,89,90). During development, the activity of the soluble enzyme in rat brain increases approximately 2-fold, whereas the activity of the particulate enzyme increases approximately 20-fold (Fig. 19) (90). In addition, the soluble enzyme apparently has a lower requirement for the pyridoxal 5'-phosphate coenzyme. The enzyme has been purified from rat liver and from horse kidney (93-98). The present consensus is that the same enzyme catalyzes the decarboxylation of cysteinesulfinic acid and of cysteic acid.

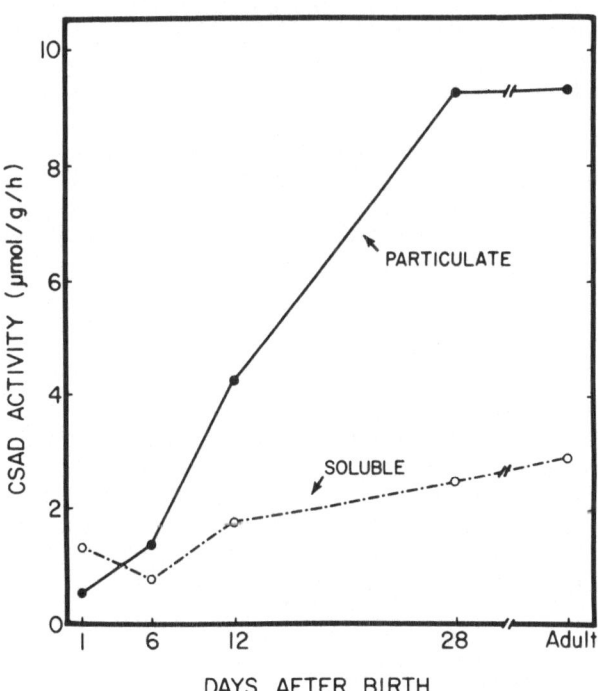

Fig. 19. Distribution of the activity of cysteinesulfinic acid decarboxylase between the soluble and particulate fractions of a rat brain homogenate during development. Adapted from reference 90.

There have been no reports to date of a disease in man involving cysteinesulfinic acid decarboxylase, nor have there been any reported attempts to purify and characterize the enzyme from human tissue, probably because the activity is so small.

CYSTEINE DESULFURASE

This enzyme degrades cysteine to form H_2S, NH_3, and pyruvate. The enzyme has been highly purified from rat liver and has been demonstrated unequivocally to be the same enzyme as cystathionase (99,100). It is worth noting that the cysteine desulfurase of bacteria is not identical with cystathionase (101). The active site for cysteine desulfurase activity on the enzyme from rat liver has been shown by kinetic studies and by immunochemical studies to be different from the active site for cystathionase activity (and the several other activities exhibited by this enzyme) (65,70). No reports on cysteine desulfurase activity of human liver have been published, although some preliminary studies suggest that it is present, but at lower activity than found in rat liver (Pascal, unpublished data). This is of interest because of the considerable differences between the cystathionase enzymes of rat liver and of human liver. It is also not known whether cysteine desulfurase activity is reduced in patients with primary cystathioninuria due to γ-cystathionase deficiency. It has been shown that other activities of the cystathionase active site, such as homoserine dehydratase, are reduced in this condition (78,102). Presumably the activity is absent in unresponsive cystathioninuria where the enzyme protein is apparently absent, but the activity may or may not be deficient in responsive cystathioninuria since it is mediated by a different part of the protein molecule.

CYSTEINE AMINOTRANSFERASE

Cysteine can be transaminated with α-oxobutyrate or with pyruvate by extracts of rat liver to form β-mercaptopyruvate. These two reactions are catalyzed by separate enzymes, both located in the mitochondrial fraction of a rat liver homogenate (103). An enzyme catalyzing cysteine-glutamate transamination has been purified from rat liver (104). All of these transamination reactions require pyridoxal 5'-phosphate as coenzyme.

CYSTEINESULFINIC ACID AMINOTRANSFERASE

Cysteinesulfinic acid is transaminated by extracts of rat liver to pyruvate, via β-sulfinylpyruvate (105,106). This enzyme is different from aspartate aminotransferase (EC 2.6.1.1) which catalyzes the transamination between aspartate and α-oxobutyrate and between glutamate and oxaloacetate in rat liver and rat brain

and in chick retina, in contrast to the bacterial enzyme (107-110).
Although the subcellular location of the two enzymes in mammalian
tissue is similar, the developmental pattern and requirement for
the pyridoxal 5'-phosphate coenzyme are distinct.

HYPOTAURINE AMINOTRANSFERASE

It has been reported that sonicated mitochondria from rat liver
and rat kidney will transaminate selenohypotaurine with α-oxobutyrate,
but will not transaminate hypotaurine (111). More recent investigations have revealed the presence of an enzyme in rat liver and
rat kidney which will transaminate hypotaurine which apparently
requires pyridoxal 5'-phosphate as coenzyme (Fellman, unpublished
data).

CYSTEIC ACID DECARBOXYLASE

Extracts of several mammalian tissues (brain, liver, kidney)
will decarboxylate cysteic acid to form taurine, and sensitive
methods for such measurements are available (88,112,113). The
enzyme is generally considered to be the same as cysteinesulfinic
acid decarboxylase. It has been considered that since little or no
in vitro oxidation of hypotaurine to taurine can be demonstrated in
brain, then the pathway of taurine biosynthesis may proceed via
cysteic acid in this tissue (114). However, there has been no
demonstration to date of oxidation of cysteinesulfinic acid to
cysteic acid, so the role of this enzymatic activity is still
uncertain.

NUTRITIONAL DEFICIENCY OF VITAMIN B-6

The enzymes discussed above all require pyridoxal 5'-phosphate
as coenzyme, and, therefore, would be expected to be sensitive to
any nutritional deprivation of vitamin B-6. Such an effect may be
expressed in several ways: there may be little or no change in the
activity of the holoenzyme if the binding between coenzyme and apoenzyme is relatively strong; e.g., as observed for cystathionine
β-synthase (115-117), there may be a relatively large decrease in
activity of the holoenzyme if the binding between coenzyme and apoenzyme is relatively weak; e.g., as observed for γ-cystathionase
and aminotransferases (115,116,118), and there may even be a loss
of apoenzyme protein if it is unstable in the absence of coenzyme;
e.g., as observed for cysteinesulfinic acid decarboxylase (119,120).
The metabolic consequences of a nutritional deficiency of vitamin
B-6 can thus be related in most instances to the effect on individual
enzymes. Because cystathionine β-synthase is little affected, there
is no homocystinuria or homocystinemia observed in this condition.
Under the same conditions, holo γ-cystathionase is reduced rapidly,

even though the apoenzyme is not substantially decreased, resulting
in cystathioninemia and cystathioninuria (121,122). This also
occurs in man when the nutritional intake of vitamin B-6 is curtailed,
and cystathioninuria is the most sensitive index afforded by sulfur
amino acids of the adequacy of dietary vitamin B-6.

Other consequences include the reduced synthesis of cysteine,
an important amino acid constituent of proteins, but this would
only cause adverse effects if the diet were also deficient in this
amino acid. Excretion of taurine is also severly reduced because
biosynthesis is decreased. In rats, this results in a decreased
turnover of taurine, rather than a decreased concentration (123).
In species that are known to suffer from taurine depletion, cats
and primates, adverse effects would only be possible in the unlikely
event that the diet was also deficient in taurine. In general,
protein synthesis does not seem to be affected by a deficiency of
vitamin B-6, although hair is a dramatic exception. There is a
severely reduced incorporation of cystine, the major amino acid
constituent of hair, into the hair of vitamin B-6-deficient rats
(124). This is not the result of a deficiency of cyst(e)ine, and
probably is the cause of the alopecia observed in these animals.

SUMMARY

Vitamin B-6 clearly plays an important role in the metabolism
of sulfur amino acids, and an inadequate nutritional supply will
clearly result in alterations in the performance of a number of
important enzymes. These alterations can contribute to a variety
of clinical signs and symptoms, such as seizures. In addition, there
exist a number of human conditions in which there is a greater
dependency on vitamin B-6. These certainly include the two enzymes
involved in sulfur amino acid metabolism which have a decreased
affinity for their coenzyme pyridoxal 5'-phosphate, cystathionine
β-synthase and γ-cystathionase, discussed in detail earlier. They
may also include other conditions if one includes the possibility
of modification of protein conformation which may alter the accessibility of various portions of protein molecules, since the bulk of
pyridoxal 5'-phosphate is protein bound in normal nutritional
conditions (125).

LITERATURE CITED

1. Brinkley, F. (1950) Synthesis of cystathionine by prepara-
    tions from rat liver. J. Biol. Chem. 191, 531-534.
2. Braunstein, A. E., Goryachenkova, E. V. & Lac, N. D. (1969)
    Reactions catalyzed by serine sulfhydrase from chicken liver.
    Biochim. Biophys. Acta 171, 366-368.

3. Braunstein, A. E., Goryachenkova, E. V., Tolosa, E. A., Willhardt, I. H. & Yefremova, L. L. (1971) Specificity and some other properties of liver serine sulphhydrase: Evidence for its identity with cystathionine β-synthase. Biochim. Biophys. Acta 242, 247-260.

4. Matsua, Y & Greenberg, D. M. (1959) A crystalline enzyme that cleaves homoserine and cystathionine. IV. Mechanism of action, reversibility, and substrate specificity. J. Biol. Chem. 234, 516-519.

5. Wong, P.W.K., Schwarz, V. & Komrower, G. M. (1968) The biosynthesis of cystathionine in patients with homocystinuria. Pediat. Res. 2, 149-160.

6. Chatagner, F., Tixier, M. & Portemer, C. (1969) Biosynthesis of cystathionine from homoserine and cysteine by rat liver cystathionase. FEBS Letters 4, 231-233.

7. Gaull, G. E., Wada, Y., Schneidman, K., Rassin, D. K., Tallan, H. H. & Sturman, J. A. (1971) Homocystinuria: Observations on the biosynthesis of cystathionine and homolanthionine. Pediat. Res. 5, 265-273.

8. Tallan, H. H., Sturman, J. A., Pascal, T. A. & Gaull, G. E. (1974) Cystathionine γ-synthesis from homocysteine and cysteine by mammalian tissue. Biochem. Med. 9, 90-101.

9. Mudd, S. H., Finkelstein, J. D., Irreverre, F. & Laster, L. (1965) Transsulfuration in mammals: Microassays and tissue distributions of three enzymes of the pathway. J. Biol. Chem. 240, 4382-4392.

10. Sturman, J. A., Rassin, D. K. & Gaull, G. E. (1970) Distribution of transsulfuration enzymes in various organs and species. Int. J. Biochem. 1, 251-253.

11. Uhlendorf, B. W. & Mudd, S. H. (1968) Cystathionine synthase in tissue culture derived from human skin: Enzyme defect in homocystinuria. Science 160, 1007-1009.

12. Goldstein, J. L., Campbell, B. K. & Gartler, S. M. (1972) Cystathionine synthase activity in human lymphocytes: Induction by phytohemagglutinin. J. Clin. Invest. 51, 1034-1037.

13. Fleisher, L. D., Beratis, N. C., Hirschorn, K. & Gaull, G. E. (1972) Detection of cystathionine synthase in long-term lymphoid-cell lines. Lancet 2, 482.

14. Sturman, J. A., Gaull, G. E. & Raiha, N. (1970) Absence of cystathionase in human fetal liver: Is cystine essential? Science 169, 74-76.

15. Gaull, G. E., Sturman, J. A. & Raiha, N.C.R. (1972) Development of mammalian sulfur metabolism: Absence of cystathionase in human fetal tissues. Pediat. Res. 6, 538-547.

16. Sturman, J. A., Gaull, G. E. & Niemann, W. H. (1976) Cystathionine synthesis and degradation in brain, liver and kidney of the developing monkey. J. Neurochem. 26, 457-463.

17. Sturman, J. A. & Gaull, G. E. (1978) Methionine and poly-
     amine metabolism in the brain and liver of the developing
     human and rhesus monkey. Adv. Polyamine Res. 2, 213-240.
18. Kashiwamata, S. (1971) Subcellular localization of cysta-
     thionine synthase in rat brain. FEBS Letter 19, 69-71.
19. Kashiwamata, S. (1971) Brain cystathionine synthase:
     Vitamin B-6 requirement for its enzymic reaction and changes
     in enzymic activity during early development of rats. Brain
     Res. 30, 185-192.
20. Rassin, D. K. & Gaull, G. E. (1975) Subcellular distribution
     of enzymes of transmethylation and transsulphuration in rat
     brain. J. Neurochem. 24, 969-978.
21. Brown, F. C. & Gordon, P. H. (1970) Cystathionine synthase
     from rat liver: partial purification and properties. Can.
     J. Biochem. 49, 484-491.
22. Kashiwamata, S. & Greenberg, D. M. (1970) Studies on cysta-
     thionine synthase of rat liver: Properties of the highly
     purified enzyme. Biochim. Biophys. Acta 212, 488-500.
23. Kimura, H. & Nakagawa, H. (1970) Studies on cystathionine
     synthetase: Characteristics of purified rat liver enzyme.
     J. Biochem. 69, 711-723.
24. Kim. Y. J. & Rosenberg, L. E. (1974) On the mechanism of
     pyridoxine responsive homocystinuria. II. Properties of
     normal and mutant cystathionine β-synthase from cultured
     fibroblasts. Proc. Nat. Acad. Sci. 71, 4821-4825.
25. Porter, P. N., Grishaver, M. S. & Jones, O. W. (1974)
     Characterization of human cystathionine β-synthase: Evidence
     for the identity of human L-serine dehydratase and cysta-
     thionine β-synthase. Biochim. Biophys. Acta 364, 128-139.
26. Tudball, N. & Reed, M. A. (1975) Purification and properties
     of cystathionine synthase from human liver. Biochem. Biophys.
     Res. Comm. 67, 550-555.
27. Kraus, J., Packman, S., Fowler, B. & Rosenberg, L. E. (1978)
     Purification and properties of cystathionine β-synthase from
     human liver: Evidence for identical subunits. J. Biol.
     Chem. 253, 6523-6528.
28. Kashiwamata, S. & Kotake, Y. (1970) Studies of cystathionine
     synthase of rat liver: Dissociation into two components by
     sodium dodecyl sulfate electrophoresis. Biochim. Biophys.
     Acta 212, 501-503.
29. Ansell, P.R.J. & Tudball, N. (1977) The existence of human
     liver cystathionine β-synthase in multiple molecular forms.
     Biochim. Biophys. Acta 483, 443-451.
30. Finkelstein, J. D., Mudd, S. H., Irreverre, F. & Laster, L.
     (1964) Homocystinuria due to cystathionine synthetase
     deficiency: The mode of inheritance. Science 146, 785-787.

31. Gaull, G.E., Tallan, H.H., Lajtha, A. & Rassin, D.K. (1975) Pathogenesis of brain dysfunction in inborn errors of amino acid metabolism. In: Biology of Brain Dysfunction (Gaull, G. E., ed.), vol. 3, pp. 47-143, Plenum Press, NY.

32. Mudd, S. H., Finkelstein, J. D., Irreverre, F. & Laster, L. (1964) Homocystinuria: An enzymatic defect. Science 143, 1443-1445.

33. Gaull, G. E., Rassin, D. K. & Sturman, J. A. (1969) Enzymatic and metabolic studies of homocystinuria: Effects of pyridoxine. Neuropadiatrie 1, 199-226.

34. Griffiths, R. & Tudball, N. (1976) Studies on the use of skin fibroblasts for the measurement of cystathionine synthase activity with respect to homocystinuria. Clin. Chim. Acta 83, 157-162.

35. Mudd, S. H., Edwards, W. A., Loeb, P. M., Brown, M. S. & Laster, L. (1970) Homocystinuria due to cystathionine synthase deficiency: The effect of pyridoxine. J. Clin. Invest. 49, 1762-1773.

36. Griffiths, R. & Tudball, N. (1977) The molecular defect in a case of (Cystathionine β-synthase)-deficient homocystinuria. Eur. J. Biochem. 74, 269-273.

37. Gaull, G. E. & Sturman, J. A. (1971) Vitamin B-6 dependency in homocystinuria. Brit. Med. J. 3, 532-533.

38. Gaull, G., Sturman, J. A. & Schaffner, F. (1974) Homocystinuria due to cystathionine synthase deficiency: Enzymatic and ultrastructural studies. J. Pediat. 84, 381-390.

39. Fleisher, L. D., Tallan, H. H., Beratis, N. G., Hirschhorn, K. & Gaull, G. E. (1973) Cystathionine synthase deficiency: Heterozygote detection using cultured skin fibroblasts. Biochem. Biophys. Res. Comm. 55, 38-44.

40. Gerritsen, T. & Waisman, H. A. (1964) Homocystinuria: Absence of cystathionine in the brain. Science 145, 588.

41. Brenton, D. P., Cusworth, D. C. & Gaull, G. E. (1965) Homocystinuria: Biochemical studies of tissues including a comparison with cystathioninuria. Pediatrics 35, 50-56.

42. Griffiths, R. & Tudball, N. (1976) Observations on the fate of cystathionine in rat brain. Life Sci. 19, 1217-1223.

43. Tudball, N. & Beaumone, A. (1979) Studies on the neurochemical properties of cystathionine. Biochim. Biophys. Acta 588, 285-293.

44. Rassin, D. K., Longhi, R. C. & Gaull, G. E. (1977) Free amino acids in liver of patients with homocystinuria due to cystathionine synthase deficiency: Effects of vitamin B-6. J. Pediat. 91, 574-577.

45. Tada, K., Yoshida, T. & Arakawa, T. (1970) Free amino acid pattern in the liver from the patients with amino acid disorders: Postmortem diagnosis of inborn errors of amino acid metabolism. Tohoku J. Exp. Med. 101, 223-226.

46. Kang, S.-S., Wong, P.W.K. & Becker, N. (1979) Protein-bound
     homocyst(e)ine in normal subjects and in patients with homo-
     cystinuria. Pediat. Res. 13, 1141-1143.
47. Barber, G. W. & Spaeth, G. L. (1967) Pyridoxine therapy in
     homocystinuria. Lancet 1, 337.
48. Yoshida, T., Tada, K., Yokoyama, Y. & Arakawa, T. (1968)
     Homocystinuria of vitamin B-6 dependent type. Tohoku J. Exp.
     Med. 96, 235-242.
49. Barber, G. W. & Spaeth, G. L. (1969) The successful treat-
     ment of homocystinuria with pyridoxine. J. Pediat. 75,
     463-478.
50. Carson, N.A.J. & Carre, I. J. (1969) Treatment of homo-
     cystinuria with pyridoxine: A preliminary study. Arch. Dis.
     Child. 44, 387-392.
51. Hagberg, B., Hambraeus, L. & Hamfelt, A. (1969) Pyridoxine
     in homocystinuria. Lancet 2, 271.
52. Shih, V. E. & Efron, M. (1970) Pyridoxine-unresponsive
     homocystinuria. New Eng. J. Med. 283, 1206-1208.
53. Kelly, S. & Copeland, W. (1968) A hypothesis on the homo-
     cystinuric's response to pyridoxine. Metabolism 17, 794-795.
54. Seashore, M. R., Durant, J. L. & Rosenberg, L. E. (1972)
     Studies of the mechanism of pyridoxine-responsive homo-
     cystinuria. Pediat. Res. 6, 187-196.
55. Longhi, R. C., Fleisher, L. D., Tallan, H. H. & Gaull, G. E.
     (1977) Cystathionine β-synthase deficiency: a qualitative
     abnormality of the deficient enzyme modified by vitamin B-6
     therapy. Pediat. Res. 11, 100-103.
56. Rassin, D. K., Longhi, R. C., Sternowsky, H. J., Sturman, J.
     A. & Gaull, G. E. (1977) Homocysteine and cysteine loads in
     patients with homocystinuria due to cystathionine synthase
     deficiency: Effects of vitamin B-6. Clin. Chim. Acta 79,
     197-210.
57. Fowler, B., Kraus, J., Packman, S. & Rosenberg, L. E. (1978)
     Homocystinuria: Evidence for three distinct classes of
     cystathionine β-synthase mutants in cultured fibroblasts.
     J. Clin. Invest. 61, 645-653.
58. Fleisher, L. D., Longhi, R., Tallan, H. H. & Gaull, G. E.
     (1978) Cystathionine β-synthase deficiency: Differences in
     thermostability between normal and abnormal enzyme from
     cultured human cells. Pediat. Res. 12, 293-296.
59. Radcliffe, B. C. & Egan, A. R. (1974) A survey of methionine
     adenosyltransferase and cystathionine γ-lyase activities in
     ruminant tissues. Austr. J. Biol. Sci. 27, 465-471.
60. Pascal, T. A., Gaull, G. E., Beratis, N. G., Gillam, B. M.,
     Tallan, H. H. & Hirschhorn, H. (1975) Vitamin B-6-responsive
     and -unresponsive cystathioninuria: Two variant molecular
     forms. Science 190, 1209-1211.

61. Bittles, A. H. & Carson, N. A. (1974) Cystathionase deficiency in fibroblast cultures from a patient with primary cystathioninuria. J. Med. Genet. 11, 121-122.

62. Pascal, T. A., Gillam, B. M. & Gaull, G. E. (1972) Cystathionase: Immunochemical evidence for absence from human fetal liver. Pediat. Res. 6, 773-778.

63. Heinonen, K. (1973) Studies on cystathionase activity in rat liver and brain during development. Biochem. J. 136, 1011-1015.

64. Deme, D., Durieu-Trautmann, O. & Chatagner, F. (1971) The thiol groups of rat liver cystathionase. Eur. J. Biochem. 20, 269-275.

65. Pascal, T. A., Tallan, H. H. & Gillam, B. M. (1972) Hepatic cystathionase: Immunochemical and electrophoretic studies of the human and rat forms. Biochim. Biophys. Acta 285, 48-59.

66. Brown, F. C. & DeFoor, M. C. (1974) γ-Cystathionase of rat liver: The role of sulfhydryl groups in the catalytic function. Eur. J. Biochem. 46, 317-322.

67. Brown, F. C. (1975) γ-Cystathionase of rat liver: Effects of pyridoxal phosphate and other compounds on reaction rates. Arch. Biochem. Biophys. 171, 378-384.

68. Bikel, I., Pavlatos, T. N. & Livingston, D. M. (1978) Purification and subunit structure of mouse liver cystathionase. Arch. Biochem. Biophys. 186, 168-174.

69. Loiselet, J. & Chatagner, F. (1966) Amino acid composition of "ethionine-induced" cystathionase of rat liver. Biochim. Biophys. Acta 130, 180-183.

70. Deme, D. & Chatagner, F. (1972) Etude du centre actif de l'homoserine dehydratase du foie de rat. Biochim. Biophys. Acta 258, 643-654.

71. Harris, H., Penrose, L. S. & Thomas, D.H.H. (1959) Cystathioninuria. Ann. Human Gen. 23, 442-453.

72. Frimpter, G. W. (1965) Cystathioninuria: Nature of the defect. Science 149, 1095-1096.

73. Perry, T. L., Robinson, G. C., Teasdale, J. M. & Hansen, S. (1967) Concurrence of cystathioninuria, nephrogenic diabetes insipidus and severe anemia. New Eng. J. Med. 276, 721-725.

74. AvRuskin, T. W. & Kang, E. S. (1974) Cystathioninuria, mental retardation and juvenile diabetes mellitus. Am. J. Dis. Child. 127, 250-253.

75. Scott, R. C., Dassell, S. W., Clark, S. H., Chiang-Teng, C. & Swedberg, K. R. (1970) Cystathioninemia: A benign genetic condition. J. Pediat. 76, 571-577.

76. Lyon, I.C.T., Procopis, P. G. & Turner, B. (1971) Cystathioninuria in a well baby population. Acta Paediat. Scand. 60, 324-328.

77. Perry, T. L., Hardwick, D. F., Hansen, S., Love, D. L. &
     Isreals, S. (1968) Cystathioninuria in two healthy siblings.
     New Eng. J. Med. 278, 590-592.
78. Finkelstein, J. D., Mudd, S. H., Irreverre, F. & Laster, L.
     (1966) Deficiencies of cystathionase and homoserine dehy-
     dratase activities in cystathioninuria. Biochemistry 55,
     865-872.
79. Shaw, K.N.F., Lieberman, E., Koch, R. & Donnell, G. N. (1967)
     Cystathioninuria. Am. J. Dis. Child. 113, 119-127.
80. Tada, K., Yoshida, T., Yokoyama, Y., Sato, T., Nakagawa, H.
     & Arakawa, T. (1968) Cystathioninuria not associated with
     vitamin B-6 dependency: A probable new type of cystathi-
     oninuria. Tohoku J. Exp. Med. 95, 235-242.
81. Levy, H. L., Mudd, S. H. & Madigan, P. M. (1973) Pyridoxine-
     unresponsive cystathioninemia. Pediat. Res. 7, 390.
82. Pascal, T. A., Gaull, G. E., Beratis, N. G., Gillam, B. M. &
     Tallan, H. H. (1978) Cystathionase deficiency: Evidence
     for genetic heterogeneity in primary cystathioninuria.
     Pediat. Res. 12, 125-133.
83. Pascal, T. A., Beratis, N. G., Tallan, H. H. & Gaull, G. E.
     (1979) Cystathionase deficiency: The effect of cofactor on
     the stability of normal and abnormal enzyme from lymphoid
     cell lines. Enzyme 24, 265-268.
84. Van der Horst, C.J.G. & Kuiper, C. J. (1972) Investigation
     into the occurrence of some steroids, amino acids and carbo-
     hydrates on specific days of the oestrus cycle of the pig.
     Neth. J. Vet. Sci. 5, 35-46.
85. Amende, L. M. & Pierce, S. K. (1978) Hypotaurine: The
     identity of an unknown ninhydrin-positive compound co-eluting
     with urea in amino acid extracts of bivalve tissue. Comp.
     Biochem. Physiol. 59B, 257-261.
86. Sturman, J. A. (1980) Formation and accumulation of hypo-
     taurine in rat liver regenerating after partial hepatectomy.
     Life Sci. 26, 267-272.
87. Sturman, J. A. & Hayes, K. C. (1980) The biology of taurine
     in nutrition and development. Adv. Nutr. Res. 3, 231-299.
88. Jacobsen, J. G., Thomas, L. L. & Smith, L. H., Jr. (1964)
     Properties and distribution of mammalian L-cysteine sulfinate
     carboxylyases. Biochim. Biophys. Acta 85, 103-116.
89. Agrawal, H. C., Davison, A. N. & Kaczmarek, L. K. (1971)
     Subcellular distribution of taurine and cysteinesulphinate
     decarboxylase in developing rat brain. Biochem. J. 122,
     759-763.
90. Pasantes-Morales, H., Mapes, C., Tapia, M. R. & Mandel, P.
     (1976) Properties of soluble and particulate cysteine sul-
     finate decarboxylase of the adult and the developing rat
     brain. Brain Res. 107, 575-589.

91. Loriette, C. & Chatagner, F. (1978) Cysteine oxidase and
     cysteine sulfinic acid decarboxylase in developing rat liver.
     Experientia 34, 981-982.
92. Pasantes-Morales, H., Lopez-Colome, A. M., Salceda, R. &
     Mandel, P. (1976) Cysteine sulphinate decarboxylase in
     chick and rat retina during development. J. Neurochem. 27,
     1103-1106.
93. Sorbo, B. & Heyman, T. (1957) On the purification of
     cysteinesulfinic acid decarboxylase and its substrate
     specificity. Biochim. Biophys. Acta 23, 624-627.
94. Chatagner, F., Durieu-Trautmann, O. & Rain, M. C. (1968)
     Influence du phosphate de pyridoxal et de quelques autres
     derives de la pyridoxine sur la stabilite in vitro de la
     cystathionase et de la decarboxylase de l'acide cysteine
     sulfinique. Bull. Soc. Chim. Biol. 50, 129-141.
95. Lin, Y.-C., Demeio, R. H. & Metrione, R. M. (1971) Purifi-
     cation and properties of rat liver cysteine sulfinate decar-
     boxylase. Biochim. Biophys. Acta 250, 558-567.
96. Guion-Rain, M. C. & Chatagner, F. (1972) Rat liver cysteine
     sulfinate decarboxylase: Some observations about substrate
     specificity. Biochim. Biophys. Acta 276, 272-276.
97. Federici, G., Santoro, L., Tomati, U. & Cannella, C. (1973)
     Purificazione e proprieta della L-cisteinsolfinico decar-
     bossilasi dal rene di cavallo. Boll. Soc. Ital. Biol. Sper.
     49, 679-685.
98. Guion-Rain, M. C., Portemer, C. & Chatagner, F. (1975) Rat
     liver cysteine sulfinate decarboxylase: Purification, new
     appraisal of the molecular weight and determination of
     catalytic properties. Biochim. Biophys. Acta 384, 265-276.
99. Cavallini, B., Mondovi, B. & De Marco, C. (1963) The identity
     of cysteine desulfhydrase with cystathionase and mechanism of
     cysteine-cystine desulfhydration. Proc. Sympos. Chem. Biol.
     Aspects of Pyridoxal Catalysis, pp. 361-376.
100. Jolles-Bergeret, B., Brun, D., Labouesse, J. & Chatagner, F.
     (1963) Etude de la degradation de la l-cysteine par un enzyme
     purifie isole du foie de rat (Cysteine desulfurase "soluble"
     ou cystathionase). Bull. Soc. Chim. Biol. 45, 397-411.
101. Kredich, N. M., Keenan, B. S. & Foote, L. J. (1972) The
     purification and subunit structure of cysteine desulfhydrase
     from Salmonella typhimurium. J. Biol. Chem. 247, 7157-7162.
102. Kint, J. A. & Carton, D. (1971) New evidence for the identity
     of homoserine deaminase and cystathionase in human liver.
     Arch. Int. Physiol. Biochim. 79, 202.
103. Ubuka, T., Umemura, S., Ishimoto, Y & Shimomura, M. (1977)
     Transaminase of L-cysteine in rat liver mitochondria. Physiol.
     Chem. Phys. 9, 91-96.

104. Ip, M.P.C., Thibert, R. J. & Schmidt, D. E. (1977) Purifi-
      cation and partial characterization of cysteine-glutamate
      transaminase from rat liver. Canad. J. Biochem. 55, 958-964.
105. Chatagner, F., Bergeret, B., Sejourne, T. & Fromageot, C.
      (1952) Transamination et desulfination de l'acide L-cysteine-
      sulfinique. Biochim. Biophys. Acta 9, 340-341.
106. Singer, T. P. & Kearney, E. B. (1954) Pathways of L-cysteine-
      sulfinate metabolism in animal tissues. Biochim. Biophys.
      Acta 14, 570-571.
107. Recasens, M., Gabellec, M. M., Austin, L. & Mandel, A. (1978)
      Regional and subcellular distribution of cysteine sulfinate
      transaminase in rat nervous system. Biochem. Biophys. Res.
      Comm. 83, 449-456.
108. Recasens, M., Gabellec, M. M., Mack, G. & Mandel, P. (1978)
      Comparative study of miscellaneous properties of cysteine
      sulfinate transaminase and glutamate oxaloacetate transaminase
      in chick retina homogenate. Neurochem. Res. 3, 27-35.
109. Recasens, M., Benezra, R., Gabellec, M. M., Delaunoy, J. P. &
      Mandel, P. (1979) Purification and some properties of cys-
      teine sulfinate transaminase. FEBS Letter 99, 51-54.
110. Yagi, T., Kagamiyama, H. & Nozaki, M. (1979) Cysteine sul-
      finate transamination activity of aspartate aminotransferases.
      Biochem. Biophys. Res. Comm. 90, 447-452.
111. Rinaldi, A., Floris, G., Cossu, P. & DeMarco, C. (1978)
      Transamination of selenohypotaurine. Bull. Molec. Biol. Med.
      3, 234-242.
112. Yam, C. F., Tunnicliff, G., Ngo, T. T. & Barbeau, A. (1977)
      A sensitive radiometric assay for cysteic acid decarboxylase
      activity in crude enzyme preparations of rat liver and brain.
      Comp. Biochem. Physiol. 58, 115-117.
113. Wu, J.-Y., Moss, L. G. & Chen, M.-S. (1979) Tissue and
      regional distribution of cysteic acid decarboxylase: A new
      assay method. Neurochem. Res. 4, 201-212.
114. Kontro, P. & Oja, S. S. (1980) Hypotaurine oxidation by
      mouse tissues. In: Natural Sulfur Compounds: Novel Bio-
      chemical and Structural Aspects (Cavallini, D., Gaull, G. E.
      & Zappia, V., eds.), pp. 201-212, Plenum Press, New York.
115. Sturman, J. A., Cohen, P. A. & Gaull, G. E. (1969) Effects
      of deficiency of vitamin B-6 on transsulfuration. Biochem.
      Med. 3, 244-251.
116. Pan, F. & Pai, S. (1970) Dietary vitamin B-6 and enzymes of
      methionine metabolism in rat liver. J. Chinese Chem. Soc.
      17, 46-53.
117. Finkelstein, J. D. & Chalmers, F. T. (1970) Pyridoxine
      effects on cystathionine synthase in rat liver. J. Nutr.
      100, 467-469.

118. Meister, A., Morris, H. P. & Tice, S. V. (1953) Effect of vitamin B-6 deficiency on hepatic transaminase and cysteine desulfhydrase systems. Proc. Soc. Exp. Biol. Med. 82, 301-304.

119. Hope, D. B. (1955) Pyridoxal phosphate as the coenzyme of the mammalian decarboxylase for L-cysteine sulphinic and L-cysteic acids. Biochem. J. 59, 497-500.

120. Rassin, D. K. & Sturman, J. A. (1975) Cysteine sulfinic acid decarboxylase in rat brain: Effect of vitamin B-6 deficiency on soluble and particulate components. Life Sci. 16, 875-882.

121. Sturman, J. A., Cohen, P. A. & Gaull, G. E. (1970) Metabolism of L-^{35}S-methionine in vitamin B-6 deficiency: Observations on cystathioninuria. Biochem. Med. 3, 510-523.

122. Sturman, J. A. & Rivlin, R. S. (1975) Pathogenesis of brain dysfunction in deficiency of thiamine, riboflavin, pantothenic acid, or vitamin B-6. In: Biology of Brain Dysfunction (Gaull, G. E., ed.), vol 3, pp. 425-475, Plenum Press, NY.

123. Sturman, J. A. (1973) Taurine pool sizes in the rat: Effects of vitamin B-6 deficiency and high taurine diet. J. Nutr. 102, 1566-1580.

124. Sturman, J. A. & Cohen, P. A. (1971) Cystine metabolism in vitamin B-6 deficiency: Evidence of multiple taurine pools. Biochem. Med. 5, 245-268.

125. Bosron, W. F., Veitch, R. L., Lumeng, L. & Li, T.-K. (1978) Subcellular localization and identification of pyridoxal 5'-phosphate-binding proteins in rat liver. J. Biol. Chem. 253, 1488-1492.

METHIONINE METABOLITE EXCRETION AS AFFECTED BY A VITAMIN B-6

DEFICIENCY

Hellen M. Linkswiler

Department of Nutritional Sciences
College of Agricultural & Life Sciences
University of Wisconsin
Madison, WI   53706

The effect of a vitamin B-6 deficiency on the metabolism of methionine was investigated in three different studies conducted at the University of Wisconsin. In the first study, 49 days in length, six young men were subjects (1), and in the second study, 35 days in length, five young women participated (2). The purpose of these two studies was to determine the effect of a vitamin B-6 deficiency on the urinary excretion of homocystine, cystathionine, cysteine sulfinic acid and taurine, all metabolites of methionine whose formation and/or degradation are dependent upon the presence of vitamin B-6. The third study, 60 days in length, dealt with the effect of a vitamin B-6 deficiency on the metabolism of methionine by 14 oral contraceptive users and 10 nonusers as determined by the urinary excretion of the same five metabolites mentioned earlier (3). Since there was no significant difference between the oral contraceptive users and the nonusers in the excretion of any of the compounds, the two groups were combined for the purpose of this discussion.

Information concerning the subjects, certain details of the diet including the vitamin B-6 intake and the lengths of the pre-depletion, deficient and repletion periods are given in Table 1. Except for the level of protein intake and the daily supplements of methionine to the first two groups, the diet for all subjects was similar in composition. Casein and gelatin provided from 83 to 96% of the total protein; the remainder came from rice and a few low-protein fruits and vegetables. Sugar and fat additions raised the calorie intake to the desired levels. Supplements of vitamins and minerals were given, and except for vitamin B-6, the diets were adequate in all nutrients known to be essential for man.

Table 1. Description of the Three Studies

Study	1970[a]	1974[b]	1977[c]
Subjects			
Number	6	5	24[d]
Sex	male	female	female
Age, Years	19-25	19-29	20-31
Weight, kg	64-71	40-54	46-72
Diet			
Protein Intake, g	150	109	78
Methionine Supply, g	2.50	2.50	none
Vitamin B-6 Intake, mg			
Predepletion	2.16	2.16	0.99
Deficient	0.16	0.16	0.19
Repletion	2.16	2.16	0.99
Length of Study, Days			
Predepletion	14	7	4
Deficient	21	14	28
Repletion	14	14	28[e]

[a]Park and Linkswiler (1970).
[b]Shin and Linkswiler (1974).
[c]Leklem et al. (1977).
[d]The 24 subjects were both the controls and the oral contraceptive users; the two groups were combined since there
  was no significant difference between the two groups.
[e]Only 10 subjects were repleted with 2.0 mg vitamin B-6.

The 24-hour urinary excretion of homocystine, cystathionine,
L-cysteine sulfinic acid, and taurine (Fig. 1) was measured before
methionine loading (basal) on specified days and after loading with
3 g L-methionine on the day after the basal sample was collected.
These measurements were made during the predepletion, deficient,
and repletion periods.

HOMOCYSTEINE

None of the 35 subjects studied excreted any homocysteine in
either the basal or the post methionine urines during the predepletion periods when they consumed the experimental diets supplemented
with 2.0 (the 6 men fed 150 g protein and the 5 women fed 109 g
protein) or 0.8 mg of pyridoxine (24 women fed 78 g protein).

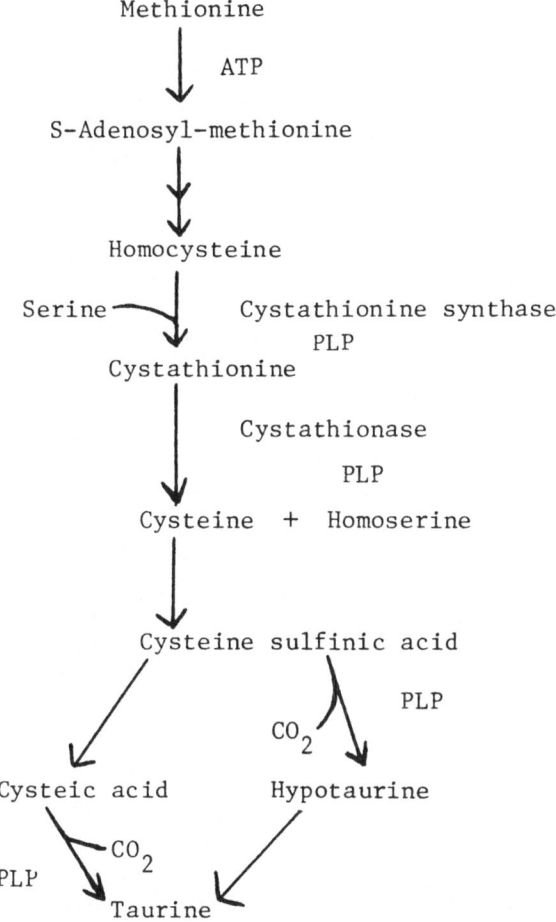

Fig. 1. An abbreviated pathway of methionine metabolism showing
the pyridoxal phosphate (PLP) dependent steps.

Trace amounts of homocystine were found in the basal urines
of two of the male subjects ingesting 150 g of protein daily after
14 and 21 days of vitamin B-6 deficiency. The post methionine urines
of the males had trace amounts of homocystine after 14 days of
deficiency and after 21 days they excreted substantial amounts of
homocystine (30 to 124 μmol/24 hours).

The women given 109 g of protein daily did not excrete any
homocystine in the basal urines, but two of the subjects excreted
54 and 111 µmol of homocystine following loading with 3 g L-
methionine after 14 days of vitamin B-6 deprivation. Even after
four weeks of vitamin B-6 deficiency, none of the 24 women given
the 78 g protein diet excreted any homocysteine either in the basal
or post methionine urines.

CYSTATIONINE

Cystathionine was the only methionine metabolite which increased
to any significant degree in the urine during vitamin B-6 deficiency.
Greatly increased amounts were excreted without the stress of the
methionine load, but oral ingestion of 3 g L-methionine increased
the excretion of cystathionine to a much greater extent. The
amount of cystathionine excreted by the three groups of subjects
before and during vitamin B-6 deficiency and following repletion
with 2.0 mg of the vitamin is given in Table 2. During the 14-day
predepletion period when the males fed the experimental diet containing 150 g protein were supplemented with 2.0 mg vitamin B-6,
the mean basal excretion of cystathionine was 128 µmol; the mean
post methionine value for the same period was 163 µmol/24 hours.
The mean basal and post methionine values for the women given the
109 g protein diet and the 2.0 mg supplement of vitamin B-6 were
122 and 226 µmol, respectively, whereas those for the women consuming the 78 g protein diet and 0.8 mg of the vitamin were 55
and 115 µmol.

When the vitamin B-6 supplement was withheld from the subjects,
abnormal methionine metabolism, as evidenced by the increase in
urinary cystathionine, developed within one week in all three groups
of subjects. After 14 days of deficiency, the basal excretion of
cystathionine had increased 4- to 5-fold in the men consuming 150 g
protein and in the women consuming 109 g whereas the post methionine
excretion had increased 8- to 9-fold in the same two groups. After
being deprived of vitamin B-6 for 21 days, the men had a 5-fold
increase in basal urinary cystathionine but a 23-fold increase in
the post methionine excretion.

The women given the diet containing 78 g of protein developed
abnormal methionine metabolism much more slowly than the other two
groups. After 28 days of vitamin B-6 deficiency, the basal and
post methionine excretion of cystathionine had increased only 3-fold
and 7-fold, respectively. The slower response of these women to
the vitamin deficiency than the other two groups may have been the
result of the lower protein intake. It is important to remember,

Table 2. Basal and Post Methionine Excretion of
Cystathionine by Men and Women During
Vitamin B-6 Adequacy and Deficiency

Sex	Males[a]		Females[b]		Females[c]	
Protein Intake, g/day	150		109		78	
Diet Period[d]	Cystathionine Extraction					
	B[e]	PM[e]	B	PM	B	PM
	μmol/24 hours					
Predepletion	112	161				
	144	165	122	226	55	115
Deficient	195	397	176	527	63	239
	500	1466	517	1877	112	511
	508	3719			165	809
					152	856
Repletion	163	244	140	201	50	160
	139	178	109	171	53	133
					44	130
					50	83

[a]Adapted from Park and Linkswiler (1970).
[b]Adapted from Shin and Linkswiler (1974).
[c]Adapted from Leklem et al. (1977).
[d]The length of the predepletion periods varied among the
studies (see Table 1). The basal and post methionine
excretion was measured once during each 7 days during
the deficient and the repletion periods.
[e]B = premethionine (basal); PM = post methionine.

however, that the two groups with the higher protein intakes also
had daily supplements of 2.5 g L-methionine, and it is possible
that these supplements contributed to the rate and extent of
abnormal methionine metabolism.

It has been reported that the rate and extent of abnormal tryptophan metabolism development in men during vitamin B-6 deficiency is related to the protein intake (4). After 40 days, men fed a diet containing 54 g protein and 0.16 mg vitamin B-6 daily excreted from zero to 29% of a 2.0 g loading dose of L-tryptophan as kynurenine, hydroxykynurenine, xanthurenic acid, kynurenic acid, and acetylkynurenine while men given 150 g protein excreted 29% of the dose as the five metabolites after 14 days of vitamin deficiency.

CYSTEINE SULFINIC ACID

The effect of a vitamin B-6 deficiency on the urinary excretion of cysteine sulfinic acid is so slight that the measurement of this compound is of no importance in assessing vitamin B-6 adequacy or deficiency (Table 3). The males given the 150 g protein diet showed a small but significant increase in cysteine sulfinic acid excretion after 14 days of vitamin B-6 deficiency in both the basal and post methionine urines. The basal urinary cysteine sulfinic acid of the women given the 109 g protein diet was not affected during the deficiency period of 14 days, but the post methionine excretion was slightly but significantly increased. Neither the basal nor the post methionine excretion of cysteine sulfinic acid was affected by the vitamin B-6 deficiency in the women consuming the 78 g protein diet.

TAURINE

The basal and post methionine excretion of taurine by the subjects of the three studies is given in Table 4. The basal taurine values did not differ significantly from the post methionine values in either the predepletion, the deficient, or the repletion periods. The state of vitamin B-6 nutriture had no effect on the amount of taurine excreted. In all three groups of subjects, both basal and post methionine values decreased during the period of vitamin B-6 deficiency, but they continued to decrease after the vitamin was reinstated in the diets. At the end of 28 days of vitamin B-6 repletion, the urinary taurine of the women given the 78 g protein diet was about one-third the amount found at the beginning of the study.

The taurine contents of the diets are not known, and the decrease in urinary taurine may simply be a reflection of low taurine intake. Sturman stated that studies from his laboratory suggest that the human infant, and probably the adult as well, is dependent upon a dietary source of taurine (5). The cat clearly requires a dietary source of taurine (6).

Table 3. Basal and Post Methionine Excretion of Cysteine Sulfinic Acid by Men and Women During Vitamin B-6 Adequacy and Deficiency

Sex	Males[a]		Females[b]		Females[c]	
Protein Intake, g/day	150		109		78	
Diet Period[d]	Cysteine Sulfinic Acid Excretion					
	B[e]	PM[e]	B	PM	B	PM
			μmol/24 hours			
Predepletion	92	87				
	96	101	70	72	66	77
Deficient	101	107	66	81	64	71
	117	128	73	117	64	93
	117	153			78	73
					73	90
Repletion	91	95	79	73	55	85
	91	85	77	70	67	92
					76	60
					62	63

[a]Adapted from Park and Linkswiler (1970).
[b]Adapted from Shin and Linkswiler (1974).
[c]Adapted from Leklem et al. (1977).
[d]The length of the predepletion periods varied among the studies (see Table 1). The basal and post methionine excretion was measured once during each 7 days during the deficient and the repletion periods.
[e]B = premethionine (basal); PM = post methionine.

Table 4. Basal and Post Methionine Excretion of Taurine by Men and Women During Vitamin B-6 Adequacy and Deficiency

Sex	Males[a]		Females[b]		Females[c]	
Protein Intake, g/day	150		109		78	
Diet Period[d]	Taurine Excretion					
	B[e]	PM[e]	B	PM	B	PM
	μmol/24 hours					
Predepletion	641	489				
	568	617	299	421	215	278
Deficient	560	572	144	204	215	227
	653	560	145	192	125	175
	473	455			121	96
					95	96
Repletion	343	295	141	175	87	93
	290	339	120	156	94	74
					58	96
					78	80

[a] Adapted from Park and Linkswiler (1970).
[b] Adapted from Shin and Linkswiler (1974).
[c] Adapted from Leklem et al. (1977).
[d] The length of the predepletion periods varied among the studies (see Table 1). The basal and post methionine excretion was measured once during each 7 days during the deficient and the repletion periods.
[e] B = premethionine (basal); PM = post methionine.

CONCLUSION

Cystathionine was the only methionine metabolite which was elevated substantially by the withdrawal of vitamin B-6 from the diet. Men and women deprived of vitamin B-6 for only 7 days excreted elevated quantities of cystathionine in both basal and post methionine urines. The amount excreted continued to increase as the periods of deficiency were prolonged. The level of dietary protein and/or methionine affected the rate and extent of abnormal methionine metabolism. After three weeks of vitamin B-6 deficiency, the basal excretion of cystathionine of men given 150 g protein had increased 5-fold whereas the post methionine excretion had increased 23-fold. In contrast, the basal and post methionine excretion of cystathionine of women consuming a 78 g protein diet increased only 3- and 7-fold, respectively, after 28 days of deficiency.

LITERATURE CITED

1. Park, Y. K. & Linkswiler, H. (1970) Effect of vitamin B-6 depletion in adult man on the excretion of cystathionine and other methionine metabolites. J. Nutr. 100, 110-116.
2. Shin, H. K. & Linkswiler, H. M. (1974) Tryptophan and methionine metabolism of adult females as affected by vitamin B-6 deficiency. J. Nutr. 104, 1348-1355.
3. Leklem, J. E., Linkswiler, H. M., Brown, R. R., Rose, D. P. & Anand, C. R. (1977) Metabolism of methionine in oral contraceptive users and control women receiving controlled intakes of vitamin B-6. Am. J. Clin. Nutr. 30, 1122-1127.
4. Miller, L. T. & Linkswiler, H. (1967) Effect of protein intake on the development of abnormal tryptophan metabolism by men during vitamin B-6 depletion. J. Nutr. 93, 53-59.
5. Sturman, J. A. (1978) Vitamin B-6 and the metabolism of sulfur amino acids. In: Human Vitamin B-6 Requirements, pp. 37-60. Nat. Acad. Sci., Washington, DC.
6. Hayes, K. C., Carey, R. E. & Schmidt, S. Y. (1975) Retinol degeneration associated with taurine deficiency in the cat. Science 188, 949-951.

RECOMMENDED METHODS FOR VITAMIN B-6 ANALYSIS

Robert D. Reynolds and James E. Leklem

Beltsville Human Nutrition Research Center
United States Department of Agriculture
Beltsville, MD 20705

and

Department of Foods and Nutrition
Oregon State University
Corvallis, OR 97331

This and the following paper are summaries of the recommendations formulated during open discussions on the final day of the Workshop. All the recommendations are based on current state-of-the-art methodologies and are subject to change as the analytical precision develops and new assessment criteria are validated.

TERMINOLOGY

Vitamin B-6 exists as six predominant physiologically significant forms: pyridoxine, pyridoxal, pyridoxamine, and their respective 5'-phosphate esters. When reporting about these compounds, the full chemical name, as recommended by the International Union of Pure and Applied Chemistry (IUPAC) and the International Union of Biochemistry (IUB) (1), should be given, i.e., pyridoxal 5'-phosphate rather than pyridoxal phosphate, etc. The predominant urinary form, 4-pyridoxic acid, should also be written so as to identify the position of the carboxyl group on the pyridine ring. The above recommendations are in accordance with previously published recommendations (1,2).

Where appropriate, the names of the above seven compounds may be abbreviated in accordance with the IUPAC-IUB recommendations (1,2), i.e., PN for pyridoxine, PL for pyridoxal, PM for pyridoxamine, and PNP, PLP, and PMP for the respective 5'-phosphate esters.

Not covered by the IUPAC-IUB recommendations is the abbreviation
for 4-pyridoxic acid, which, it was agreed, should be abbreviated
as 4PA (no hyphen between the 4 and PA). Nonstandard abbreviations
for the above compounds, such as PALP, PIN, PAMP, PIC, etc., should
no longer be used in any subsequent writings. Finally, in keeping
with the policy of many journals which use computerized typesetting,
the generic term should be written as vitamin B-6 instead of the
historical form, vitamin B_6.

CONCENTRATION OF VITAMERS

   Since the concentration of several of the B-6 vitamers relative
to others seems to be of importance in certain metabolic conditions,
a uniform expression of concentration of all forms is highly
desirable. This would also facilitate comparison of results obtained
in different laboratories. The consensus reached during the Workshop
was to express all as pmol/ml, nmol/ml, etc., when dealing with
liquid samples such as plasma, saliva, etc., and to similarly
express all as nmol/g or μmol/g, etc., when discussing content in
solid tissues such as liver or muscle. Previously used expressions
such as ng/ml, nmol/dl, etc., should no longer be used.

   Due to the nonhomogenous distribution of compounds within solid
tissues as a result of compartmentalization and binding to specific
proteins, reference should be made to the "tissue content" of the
vitamer rather than to the "concentration" of the vitamer in these
tissues. Although less of a problem, consideration should also be
given along these lines towards using the same expression for
liquid samples due to the binding of many of the vitamers to specific
proteins in the samples.

EVALUATION OF ESTABLISHED METHODOLOGIES

   There are at present three major approaches for determining
the concentration of B-6 vitamers: microbiological, enzymatic, and
chemical assays. The microbiological assays, as presently developed,
are cumbersome in the extraction step, are time-consuming in the
column separation of the vitamers (when used), and are not equally
sensitive to all the vitamers when assayed in various laboratories.
This discussion brought out this problem very prominantly.
Saccharomyces uvarum is less responsive to pyridoxamine than to
pyridoxine or pyridoxal in some laboratories but the organism is
equally responsive to all three forms in other laboratories. The
reason(s) for this important discrepancy was not resolved at the
Workshop. Other microorganisms have been reported to respond
equally to pyridoxine, pyridoxal, and pyridoxamine, but these data
have not been substantiated in other laboratories (see article by
Polansky). The harsh extraction conditions may result in changes

in the relative vitamer concentrations as well as produce conjugates to which the assay microorganism is only weakly responsive or totally non-responsive. In spite of these problems, the microbiological assay appears to be the method of choice for analyses of foods. Large numbers of samples can be assayed in one run for "total vitamin B-6 content", which appears to be the most appropriate measurement when considering dietary intake. The problems of differential response must be accounted for when expressing these data.

Enzymatic assays, especially the stimulation assay of apo-tyrosine decarboxylase, appear to be very reliable and, at present, are the most sensitive widely-used assays for pyridoxal 5'-phosphate. But that very point is one of the major shortcomings of this partic-ular method in that it measures only pyridoxal 5'-phosphate and none of the other vitamers. In metabolic studies, knowledge of the concentration of some of the other vitamers is becoming more important, such as when determining flux of the various vitamers from the non-phosphorylated to the phosphorylated form and then to 4-pyridoxic acid. An additional problem with the apotyrosine decarboxylase assay is that it is relatively difficult for techni-cians to obtain accurate and reproducible results for several months after setting up the assay. There has been an informal "round robin" of sending new technicians to different laboratories to learn the procedure. This should not be necessary if the method were as simple as it appears on paper. For reasons not yet known, use of the apotyrosine decarboxylase assay does not yield repro-ducible results when analyzing whole blood. The problems may be largely due to small variations in sample handling or extraction conditions on a day-to-day basis. The papers by Vanderslice and by Yang very poignantly address the problems with present sample extraction procedures and how markedly different values can be obtained when using only slightly different extraction conditions. Which extraction condition is the right one; i.e., the one which yields a complete extraction of the sample without changing either the concentration or form of the pyridoxal 5'-phosphate? With all the problems discussed above, the apotyrosine decarboxylase assay still appears to be the method of choice for determining the content of pyridoxal 5'-phosphate in many tissues.

Chemical assays predominantly require the fluorometric determination of the compounds of interest. The fluorometric determinations are made regardless whether the samples are in solution or on thin layer chromatography or electrophoretic supports. Inherent in any fluorometric determination is the pre-sence of interfering compounds generated from the sample, from the sample derivatization (if used) or from minute contamination of the glassware or plasticware used. Thus, the present chemical assay of biological samples is very prone to overestimation of concentra-tion due to the contaminating substances. Additionally, most of

the vitamers, especially pyridoxal 5'-phosphate, are sensitive to
white light. The resulting photolysis may produce compounds which
have markedly different fluorescent properties from the compound of
interest, yielding gross over or underestimations of the actual
concentrations. Rigorous attention must be given to protecting all
relevant compounds from light of destructive wavelengths. The
destructive wavelengths may also vary in an unpredictable manner
for the various derivatives. The problem of photolysis is not
unique to chemical assays and equal care must be given when assaying
any of the vitamers by any of the methods discussed.

RECOMMENDATIONS FOR FUTURE METHODOLOGICAL DEVELOPMENT

        There is much room for improvement in all the existing analyt-
ical methodological approaches. Development of new strains of
microorganisms which are equally responsive to PN, PL, and PM under
a wide range of growth conditions is needed. Equivalent growth
response of cells to the nonphosphorylated and the phosphorylated
forms would be a major contribution to the field of food composition
analysis. Finding a microorganism which readily transports the
phosphorylated forms across the cell membrane may be a Herculean
task, but the eventual scientific rewards would be worth the effort.
The cell lines used do not need to be restricted to bacteria or
yeast. Cell fusion techniques have opened up the possibility of
using hybridomas of two different mammalian cells to produce a
perpetually growing culture as the cell line of choice.

        Enzymatic assays which are responsive to more than just pyri-
doxal 5'-phosphate are needed. The beginnings of this procedure
have been presented in the paper by Yang and future advances along
these lines should be encouraged. Concomitant with enzymatic
assays of broader specificity is, however, the increased uncertainty
of the concentration of each individual vitamer in question. In
the development of appropriate enzymatic assays, one must not
restrict their search only to those enzymes which use the vitamers
as a cofactor. Perhaps enzymes exist which recognize specific
regions of the pyridine ring and for which the resulting reaction
is ammenable to development of high sensitivity and as much vitamer
specificity as desired. Should these enzymes not exist, then
thought should be given to their development using genetic engi-
neering techniques when such procedures become available in that
field.

        Development of any assay which could be used for mass screening
or for routine clinical analyses must be capable of being adapted
to as much automation as possible. Procedures which eliminate or
simplify sample extraction are especially desirable. While high
performance liquid chromatography can easily be adapted to automation,

problems of sample extraction persist and a relatively small number
of samples at present can be analyzed per 24-hour cycle. Improvement in column selection and optimum operating conditions should
enhance the applicability of high performance liquid chromatography.
Perhaps the most promising method which needs to be developed is
the utilization of radioimmunoassay (RIA) or enzyme-linked immuno-
sorbent assay (ELISA) procedures for all the metabolically important
forms of vitamin B-6. The production of antibodies is possible, as
demonstrated by Thanassi and Cidlowski (3), and further development
should lead to a near-ideal assay in which large numbers of samples
may be analyzed for any of the desired vitamers. It should be
theoretically possible to develop antibodies against the bound
forms of the vitamers, thus simplifying or eliminating the need
for sample extraction.

In developing any analytical method to be used for assessing
nutritional status in humans, limitations on the type of sample to
be used, the sample size, and the metabolite concentration in the
sample must always be considered. Thus, it is impossible for the
fields of methodology and of status assessment to progress
independently of each other.

The above discussion mentions only a few of the possible
avenues open to great strides in analytical methodological development. Approaches not foreseen by us or by any of the participants
in the Workshop undoubtedly exist. Finally, future developments
in other analytical fields should contribute to improved analytical
methods for vitamin B-6 and to other compounds of nutritional and
biochemical importance. We welcome such developments.

LITERATURE CITED

1. IUPAC-IUB Commission on Biochemical Nomenclature   (1973)
    Nomenclature for vitamin B-6 and related compounds.
    Recommendation (1973) Eur. J. Biochem. 40, 325-327.
2. Nomenclature Policy: Generic descriptors and trivial names
    for vitamins and related compounds (1980) J. Nutr. 110, 8-15.
3. Thanassi, J. W. & Cidlowski, J. A. (1980) A radioimmunoassay
    for phosphorylated forms of vitamin B-6. J. Immuno. Methods
    33, 261-266.

RECOMMENDATIONS FOR STATUS ASSESSMENT OF VITAMIN B-6

James E. Leklem and Robert D. Reynolds

Department of Foods and Nutrition
Oregon State University
Corvallis, OR 97331

and

Beltsville Human Nutrition Research Center
United States Department of Agriculture
Beltsville, MD 20705

Since the discovery of vitamin B-6 and the subsequent eluci-
dation of the various roles that vitamin B-6 plays in the body,
numerous methods for assessing vitamin B-6 status have been developed. The previous paper points out the available methods and
future developments in methodology. A number of direct and indirect
methods have been utilized. Just as there are a variety of methods
available for determining a specific vitamin B-6 metabolite, so
there are an equal variety of approaches to assessing vitamin B-6
status. Both the discussions following each of the papers presented
at this Workshop and the follow-up indepth discussion of the papers
dealing with status assessment pointed out the importance of
recognizing that there is not one "best" method for status assessment.
Also, as stressed in the discussion session of the Workshop, it is
one thing to develop good methodology; it's another matter to put
them into real practical use. The utilization of the methods for
status assessment can be applied to studies of healthy individuals,
evaluation of individuals with specific pathological conditions,
and population studies. However, the choice of the method to be
used must take into account the particular situation being studied.
The use of urinary vitamin B-6 metabolite excretion in a large
population study may be more advantageous than collection of blood
samples. Conversely, in studies of human vitamin B-6 requirements
the assessment of status is probably best done when blood analyses
are included along with other measures. Equally, it is important
to recognize that status assessment in individuals with a particular
disease or pathological condition needs to be evaluated with regard

to the effect that disease may have on tissues which are actively
involved in metabolizing vitamin B-6. For example, patients with
active renal disease may present with abnormal tryptophan metabolism
that is entirely unrelated to an alteration in their vitamin B-6
status. Another aspect of the status assessment problem is the
recognition that tissue levels of the various vitamin B-6 metabolites
would be most desirous. However, present methods and ethical
considerations do not allow this. Therefore, the proper evaluation
of vitamin B-6 status in individuals necessarily must be done with
a knowledge of the dietary intake of vitamin B-6. Often the use
of extensive blood, tissue, and urine analysis is incomplete because
of the failure to determine what foods were consumed prior to
collection of all these samples. Sauberlich aptly points out in
his paper (present proceedings) the lack of vitamin B-6 intake data
in large population studies. Thus, the field of nutrition lacks a
data base that can be used for comparison of other vitamin B-6
intake studies in smaller sub-populations.

The use of intake data by itself does provide a useful understanding of what a person's or population's potential is for
adequate vitamin B-6 status. Additional factors such as bioavailability are important considerations in understanding vitamin B-6
status based on food intake. The question of using only dietary
intake is not recommended and the consensus of those at the
Workshop was that additional biochemical measurements are required.
Intake data as a criterion for status assessment will also improve
as more complete information becomes available on the vitamin B-6
content of foods.

There was expressed at this Workshop the feeling that the
findings reported in the papers of McCoy and Kirksey provide a new
means of evaluating status of the mother. Further studies in this
area will also add needed knowledge of the relationship between
blood levels of vitamin B-6, such as plasma pyridoxal 5'-phosphate,
and milk levels of vitamin B-6.

Plasma pyridoxal 5'-phosphate (PLP), urinary 4-pyridoxic acid
(4PA), and urinary tryptophan metabolite (TM) excretion following
a tryptophan load have been extensively used to evaluate vitamin
B-6 status as well as determine the requirement for vitamin B-6.
For the case of plasma pyridoxal 5'-phosphate, this is a rather
direct measure of the active coenzyme and presumably this is
reflective of tissue levels (1). Urinary 4-pyridoxic acid provides
a measure of the major metabolic end-product of vitamin B-6 (2,3).
Determination of tryptophan metabolites in the urine after a tryptophan load provides an indirect measure of vitamin B-6 status in a
tissue (in this case primarily the liver) because of the numerous
enzyme steps that require PLP (4). This triad of measurements then

gives a rather complete picture of the body's vitamin B-6 status at
that point in time. It is of great importance to recognize that
with these measurements of status one must be aware of any particular pathological or drug-related situation which would either
influence the assay itself or indirectly influence the test. For
example, the use of oral contraceptives influence the metabolism of
tryptophan at several points in the pathway (5,6), but one of these,
tryptophan pyrrolase, does not require PLP. From the discussions
at the Workshop there was a consensus that the use of at least two
of these (i.e. PLP, 4PA, or TM) are necessary to properly assess
vitamin B-6 status. The correlation of PLP and 4PA levels with
dietary intake, as reported by Shultz and Leklem, further strengthens
this consensus. It was pointed out that if one also further takes
into account the protein intake of the individual, there is a better
correlation of each of these with vitamin B-6 intake. Thus, evaluation of status assessment should be done by a combination of dietary
intake (both vitamin B-6 and protein) as well as at least two biochemical measurements. The use of PLP as an indicator of status
is given added strength from animal studies where the tissue levels
correlate quite well with blood levels.

Status assessment as discussed at this Workshop centered around
measurements in younger adults and, to some extent, in infants.
There is relatively little information on status assessment in the
adolescent and pre-adolescent. This at a time when the body is
growing at a relatively rapid rate and there is an increase in
muscle mass. Therefore, status assessment in this group may require
a different approach than in younger adults where their muscle mass
is relatively constant. Likewise, little is available on the vitamin
B-6 status of the elderly, a population in which the muscle mass is
beginning to decrease.

Methionine metabolite excretion has been suggested as another
means of assessing vitamin B-6 status. As discussed at this Workshop, the use of a methionine load test (similar to the tryptophan
load test) has mainly been limited to studies involving vitamin
depletion and repletion. Its use on status assessment remains to
be fully evaluated, but current information (see the paper by
Linkswiler) suggests it may be a sensitive indicator of vitamin B-6
deficiency.

While the methodology of blood aminotransferase activity and
stimulation was evaluated at this Workshop, the use of aminotransferase systems to assess status was not discussed to the same extent.
It was felt that erythrocyte aminotransferase activity and stimulation are probably reflective of relatively long-term dietary
vitamin B-6 intake, but problems of red cell turnover time and

relationship of enzyme activity to other measures of vitamin B-6
status remain to be fully evaluated. Until these problems are
resolved, it cannot be recommended that aminotransferase activity
and stimulation serve as a primary indicator of vitamin B-6 status,
whether in normal individuals or in pathological conditions where
the use of drugs and other therapy need be considered.

As brought out numerous times during the Workshop, perhaps of
primary importance in evaluating vitamin B-6 status is the question
of why one is assessing status. The reason for assessing status
may well dictate the methods to be used. Also as newer methods are
developed and older ones refined, our ability to "fine tune"
vitamin B-6 status assessment will be enhanced. The consensus
concerning status assessment developed at this Workshop does not
imply that we can be comfortable with present approaches. This was
best summed up in the remark of one participant who said, "As a
result of the papers and discussion, this is going to send us back
into the lab to do some work." It is in that spirit that the
Workshop concluded.

LITERATURE CITED

1. Lumeng, L., Ryan, M. P. & Li, T.-K. (1978) Validation of the
    diagnostic value of plasma pyridoxal 5'-phosphate measurements
    in vitamin B-6 nutrition of the rat. J. Nutr. 108, 545-553.
2. Snell, E. E. & Haskell, B. E. (1971) Metabolism of water-
    soluble vitamins. Compr. Biochem. 21, 47-71.
3. Reddy, S. K., Reynolds, M. S. & Price, J. M. (1958) The
    determination of 4-pyridoxic acid in human urine. J. Biol.
    Chem. 233, 691-696.
4. Leklem, J. E., Brown, R. R., Rose, D. P., Linkswiler, H. M. &
    Arend, R. A. (1975) Metabolism of tryptophan and niacin in
    oral contraceptive users receiving controlled intakes of vitamin
    B-6. Am. J. Clin. Nutr. 28, 146-156.
5. Price, J. M., Thorton, M. J. & Mueller, L. M. (1967) Tryptophan
    metabolism in women using steroid hormones for ovulation control.
    Am. J. Clin. Nutr. 20, 452-456.
6. Rose, D. P. & Braidman, I. P. (1971) Excretion of tryptophan
    metabolites as affected by pregnancy, contraceptive steroids,
    and steroid hormones. Am. J. Clin. Nutr. 24, 673-683.

LIST OF PARTICIPANTS

Hemmige Bhagavan
Department of Clinical Nutrition
Hoffman-LaRoche, Inc.
Nutley, New Jersey 07110

George Briggs
Department of Nutritional
    Sciences
University of California
Berkeley, California 94720

Raymond R. Brown
Division of Clinical Oncology
University of Wisconsin
Madison, Wisconsin 53706

Robert A. Campbell
University of Oregon Health
    Science Center
3181 S.W. Sam Jackson Park Road
Portland, Oregon 97201

Stephen P. Coburn
Fort Wayne St. Hospital and
    Training Center
4900 St. Joe Road
Fort Wayne, Indiana 46815

Krishnamurti Dakshinamurti
Department of Biochemistry
University of Manitoba
Winnipeg, Manitoba, Canada R3E OW3

G. Doyle Daves, Jr.
Oregon Graduate Center
19600 N.W. Walker Road
Beaverton, Oregon 97006

Judith A. Driskell
Department of Human Nutrition
Virginia Polytechnic Institute
    & State University
Blacksburg, Virginia 24060

Jesse F. Gregory III
Department of Food Science &
    Human Nutrition
University of Florida
Gainesville, Florida 32611

Betty E. Haskell
Department of Home Economics
University of Texas
Austin, Texas 78712

LaVelle M. Henderson
Department of Biochemistry
University of Minnesota
St. Paul, Minnesota 55108

Avanelle Kirksey
Department of Foods & Nutrition
Purdue University
West Lafayette, Indiana 47907

James E. Leklem
Department of Foods & Nutrition
Oregon State University
Corvallis, Oregon 97331

Ting-Kai Li
Department of Medicine
Indiana University School of
    Medicine
Indianapolis, Indiana 46223

Hellen M. Linkswiler
Department of Nutritional
    Sciences
University of Wisconsin
Madison, Wisconsin 53706

Lawrence Lumeng
Department of Medicine
Indiana University School
    of Medicine
Indianapolis, Indiana 46223

Ernest E. McCoy
Department of Pediatrics
University of Alberta
Edmonton, Alberta, Canada T6G 2G3

Lorraine T. Miller
Department of Foods & Nutrition
Oregon State University
Corvallis, Oregon 97331

George E. Nichoalds
Department of Obstetrics &
    Gynecology
956 Court Street
University of Tennessee
Memphis, Tennessee 38163

Marilyn Polansky
Vitamin & Mineral Nutrition Lab.
USDA Human Nutrition Research
    Center
Beltsville, Maryland 20705

Robert D. Reynolds
Vitamin & Mineral Nutrition Lab.
USDA Human Nutrition Research
    Center
Beltsville, Maryland 20705

Delores Rhody
Raltech Scientific Service
P. O. Box 7545
Madison, Wisconsin 53707

Howerde E. Sauberlich
Letterman Army Institute for
    Research
Presidio of San Francisco
San Francisco, California 94129

Terry D. Shultz
Department of Foods & Nutrition
Oregon State University
Corvallis, Oregon 97331

James H. Skala
Letterman Army Institute for
    Research
Presidio of San Francisco
San Francisco, California 94129

Esmond E. Snell
Department of Microbiology
University of Texas
Austin, Texas 78712

Robert Stokstad
Department of Nutrition Sciences
University of California
Berkeley, California 94720

Ken Strynadka
Department of Pediatrics
University of Alberta
Edmonton, Alberta, Canada T6G 2G3

John A. Sturman
Department of Pathological
    Neurobiology
Institute for Basic Research in
    Mental Retardation
Staton Island, New York 10314

John W. Thanassi
Department of Biochemistry
University of Vermont
Burlington, Vermont 05405

Bert Tolbert
Department of Chemistry
University of Colorado
Boulder, Colorado 80309

Joseph T. Vanderslice
Nutrient Composition Laboratory
USDA Human Nutrition Research
    Center
Beltsville, Maryland   20705

Bob In-Yu Yang
Department of Chemistry
University of Missouri
Kansas City, Missouri   64110